Handbook of Pharmacogenetics

Handbook of Pharmacogenetics

Edited by **Sean Boyd**

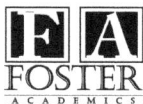

FOSTER
ACADEMICS

New Jersey

Published by Foster Academics,
61 Van Reypen Street,
Jersey City, NJ 07306, USA
www.fosteracademics.com

Handbook of Pharmacogenetics
Edited by Sean Boyd

International Standard Book Number: 978-1-63242-211-8 (Hardback)

Contents

Preface

Over the recent decade, advancements and applications have progressed exponentially. This has led to the increased interest in this field and projects are being conducted to enhance knowledge. The main objective of this book is to present some of the critical challenges and provide insights into possible solutions. This book will answer the varied questions that arise in the field and also provide an increased scope for furthering studies.

This book offers expertly selected information to the readers regarding the field of Pharmacogenetics. The main purpose of the fast developing field of Pharmacogenetics is to identify the genetic factors responsible for the inter-individual variation of drug reaction. These factors make it convenient to classify the patients according to their treatment needs and hence, catalyze drug development and encourage customized, secure and effective treatments. This book provides a wide range of examples discussing various drugs for distinct diseases which reflect different stages of assessment and application. This book is comprehensive and a great source of information to scientists, professionals, practitioners and students alike, since it discusses not just the fundamentals of pharmacogenetics but also focuses on the applications of pharmacogenetics and latest developments in this field along with discussion on its limitations and proposal of ideas to overcome them.

I hope that this book, with its visionary approach, will be a valuable addition and will promote interest among readers. Each of the authors has provided their extraordinary competence in their specific fields by providing different perspectives as they come from diverse nations and regions. I thank them for their contributions.

Editor

Part 1

Pharmacogenetics – Theory and Practice

Pharmacogenetics: Matching the Right Foundation at Personalized Medicine in the Right Genomic Era

Roxana-Georgiana Tauser
University of Medicine and Pharmacy "Gr. T. Popa" Iasi,
Romania

There are more things in heaven and in earth, Horatio,
Than are dreamt of in your philosophy...
W. Shakespeare, Hamlet act I scene 5

1. Introduction

The aim of this chapter is to overview the promises of the pioneering field of pharmacogenetics towards personalized medicine, completely changing the present therapeutic paradigm of "one dose fits all patients" and "trial-and-error" prescriptions to "matching the right dose to the right, specific genetic signature of the patient and at the right time". The review points out the evolution from pharmacogenetics to pharmacogenomics, as well as the impact of genome-wide-associated studies (GWAS) and next generation sequencing technologies on deciphering "missing heritability" and on validation and approval of pharmacogenetic biomarkers as it is reflected both in regulatory authorities recommendations and from consortia perspectives. Pharmacogenetics' translation from bench towards clinical practice in personalized medicine and drug discovery and development underlies the increasing benefits of pipeline pharmacogenetics, especially in the high-priority domains, as well as the emergence of the electronic health records-, biobanking- and bioinformatics-driven pharmacogenetics within extended international networks. More effective and successful integration of pharmacogenetics in clinical practice should address challenges regarding bioethics, insurance and privacy, consensus scientific guidelines, education, pharmacoeconomics and regulatory policy issues. Finally, there are illustrated the promising perspectives opened by: the interrogation of extensive electronic databases comprising clinical phenotype and genotype information; discovery of novel biomarkers by mining epigenoms, "junk DNA", mitochondrial and RNA polymorphisms; and integration of nanotechnologies, in order to achieve the major objective of selecting the right therapeutic strategy endowed with the highest level of efficacy and safety among a predictable segment of the genotyped patients' population.

2. Pharmacogenetics: Conceptual evolution to pharmacogenomics

2.1 Pharmacogenetics: Brief history and definition

The first clinical observations of interpatient variability in clinical response to standard therapeutic doses and the pioneering contributions of Sir Archibald Garrod, Arno Motulsky,

Friedrich Vogel and Werner Kalow led to the concept of pharmacogenetics. In "Inborn Factors of Disease" (1909), Sir Archibald Garrod noticed the implication of the "biochemical individuality" in the interpatient variability of the metabolism and efficacy of the standard regimens. In 1950s there were described sensitivity to primaquin and the risk of hemolytic anemia of the patients with glucose-6-phosphate deficiency (G6PD), slow metabolizers/acetylators of standard doses of isoniasid among tuberculosis patients with increased risk of peripheral neuropathy, prolonged apnea after succynilcholine administration, in relation to hereditary factors. The involvement of genetic factors in the adverse drug reactions was mentioned for the first time by Arno Motulsky – considered the father of the pharmacogenetics – in his paper "Drug Reactions, Enzymes and Biochemical Genetics" (1957). The concept of pharmacogenetics was introduced by Friedrich Vogel in "Moderne problem der humangenetik" (1959) as the study of genetic determinism of the interindividual variability to drugs action. The first monography on pharmacogenetics „Pharmacogenetics: Heredity and the Response to Drugs" (1962) belongs to Werner Kalow, based on his pioneering work on the relation between genetic polymorphisms of butyrilcholinesterase and the risk of prolonged apnea to the standard therapeutic doses of succynilcholine. (Liewei et al., 2011; Grossman & Goldstein, 2009; Tepper & Roubenoff, 2009)

Pharmacogenetics correlates genetic factors to the interindividual variability in drug-response phenotypes and has mainly focused on the association between monogenic polymorphisms and the variation of the drugs' metabolism. (Liewei et al., 2011)

Pharmacogenetics has the potential to increase the clinical benefit and reduce the risk of adverse drug reactions (ADR) in outliers, i.e. people whose drug responses are not "average". (Woodcock & Lesko, 2009)

Pharmacogenetic studies involve the identification of genetic classifiers or markers used to predict interpatient variability concerning drugs' efficacy and/or safety. These genetic markers could be generated through one of the following approaches: candidate gene approach, pathway-based approach or whole genome scan (also cited as Genome Wide Association Studies GWAS) approach.

2.2 Candidate gene, pathway-based and genome-wide studies

In the candidate gene approach, a panel of genes (candidate gene list) is generated based on the hypothesis in question to include drug target and mechanism pathway genes, as well as genes encoding the drug-metabolizing enzymes and membrane transporters involved in absorption, distribution, metabolism and elimination (i.e., drug pharmacokinetics). (Spraggs et al., 2009) The candidate gene approach has been applied by the majority of pharmacogenetics studies to detect associations between known single nucleotide polymorphisms (SNPs) and clinical or pharmacological end points, especially in the cases where there is a major drug metabolism or target gene that has a polymorphism that significantly changes its function. It is a hypothesis-driven approach that enables a study-design adjustment so as to acquire sufficient statistical power. The major drawback resides in its inconsistency in validating genetic markers, especially in cases where allelic variants are not highly penetrant, making the results of these studies difficult to interpret. (Wu et al., 2008 as cited in Sissung et al., 2010; Sissung et al., 2010)

The pathway-based approach uses foreknowledge of both genetic variants and the pathways in which they are involved, therefore this approach has proven particularly useful in identifying and characterizing pharmacogenetics end points within studies aimed to test the interaction between genes. The major obstacles reside in: the necessity of machine learning techniques; complexity of studies requiring larger sample sizes than candidate gene approaches; difficulty to validate gene–gene interactions due to incomplete understanding of the fundamental biology of the pathways' interactions. (Sissung et al., 2010)

The genome-wide approach is useful in determining the most significant SNPs associated with a phenotype amongst a high-density set of polymorphisms. GWAS are most useful to discover SNP associations where prior knowledge (i.e., mechanism, inheritance pattern, protein interactions and so on) is not available. Genome-wide association studies require a careful design of key issues like: a) type of study (case/control or continuous phenotype) according to the key-question and with a well-defined phenotype across all samples; b) sample sizes, dependent on specific effect size and type of study; c) population stratification between cases and controls; d) genotyping technology; e) raw data quality control and processing. (Wu et al., 2008 as cited in Sissung et al., 2010; Shianna, 2009)

GWAS are discovery-driven rather than hypothesis-driven, they evaluate multiple hypotheses and require large sample size, cost and computing power, often resulting in weak statistical signals and false positives (i.e., Type I error). Frequently, GWAS require a two-stage design where discoveries are made using a high-density SNP array and are then validated using additional patient sets and a more hypothesis-driven approach. (Wu et al., 2008 as cited in Sissung et al., 2010) Although recently GWAS application has dramatically increased, few studies have been published partially due to its primarily exploratory nature that requires further replication in large size and independent samples of the initial findings above the genome-wide significance and after correcting for multiple testing. For instance, in the case of antipsychotics drugs (ziprasidone, olanzapine, risperidone, iloperidone) GWAS revealed SNPs located in intergenic regions, but the functions of the variants on the drugs' response are still unknown. (Jian-Ping Zhang, 2011)

The application of GWAS in a population-based cohort allows the study of all possible genetic determinants of a drug response's phenotype in a hypothesis-free (i.e., unbiased) approach and is performed on commercially available, efficient and cost-effective high-throughput, genome-wide genotyping platforms (such as: Illumina's Infinium BeadChips, Affymetrix GeneChips) targeting 100,000 SNPs, or 500,000 SNPs or even 1,000,000 SNPs of the genome. (Spraggs et al., 2009)

Functional SNPs for each selected gene are added based on a literature survey and especially by using a minimum set of "tagging SNPs" (tSNPs) sufficient to capture the common genetic variations (whose minor allele frequency is higher than 2-5%) which allow almost complete genome coverage for the most of genetic diversity in human populations. (Grossman & Goldstein, 2009) Tagging SNPs greatly increase the genomic coverage of genetic variability and they reflect the well-established patterns of linkage disequilibrium, making possible to genotype only the tagging SNPs in order to capture the content of other associated SNPs in the region. The HapMap database with its incorporated software was created by The International HapMap Project (2005) and is an appropriate publicly available resource for selecting globally useful "tagging SNPs" that has been implemented by both commercial companies and academic laboratories. Tagging SNPs are chosen mainly based on r^2 threshold, besides a variety of other criteria (ethnicity, SNP's functional effects etc.). The r^2 threshold is the correlation coefficient between any observed marker and a putative causal allele and is a study-independent measure of SNP utility, being considered a leading standard for evaluating performance of marker sets; the minimum customary pair-wise value for r^2 is 0.7-0.8. (Bakker, 2005 and Pe'er, 2006 as cited in Grossman & Goldstein, 2009) There are currently commercially available arrays (SNP chips) that contain close to 1 million tagging SNPs with excellent genomic coverage for most populations as defined in HapMap Project. For example, Illumina HumanMap 300 has essentially the same statistical genomic coverage as the Affymetrix Mapping 500 K Set, while the Illumina HumanMap 550 array is statistically superior for GWAS. (Hirschhorn & Daly, 2005; Barrett & Cardon, 2006; Pe'er et al., 2006, as cited in Shianna, 2009)

2.3 Pharmacogenomics' scope and goals

The elucidation of the sequence of the human genome in 2001 and the identification and analysis of functional elements in the human genome by the ENCODE (ENCyclopedia Of DNA Elements) Project represented major steps towards a more comprehensive characterization of all functional elements in the human genome. Moreover, the HapMap Project aims to generate a haplotype map of the human genome, describing the common patterns of the human genetic variation which would affect complex, multigenic diseases and responses to drugs and environmental factors. The emergence of the term pharmacogenomics was possible after the availability of the human haplotype map (HapMap) and of high-throughput genotyping platforms that have been facilitating more systematic genetic screens for new and clinically important drug targets. (Passetti et al., 2009) Therefore the concept of pharmacogenomics has progressively evolved from pharmacogenetics and expands beyond monogenic pharmacokinetics traits, making also the transition from associative genetic studies based on candidate gene hypothesis towards genome-wide association/screening studies (GWAS) in order to identify genetic biomarkers with prognostic role for disease progression and predictive capacity for drug responsiveness.

The evolution from pharmacogenetics to pharmacogenomics was due to: a) the integration of –omics technologies and bioinformatics into the genomic medicine and systems pharmacology; b) the acquisition of catalogued genomic and clinical data bases (such as "Pharmacogenetics and Pharmacogenomics Knowledge Base", „Connectivity Map", International HapMap Project); c) identification of SNPs that 'tag' much of the common haplotype variation across any genomic region of a given population; d) positive genetic associations studies between specific genetic signature of patients and variations to standard therapeutic regimens; e) analytical and clinical validation of genetic biomarkers predictive for drug response. (Ayslin et al., 2009)

According to the US Food and Drug Administration (FDA)-approved definitions, pharmacogenetics is 'the study of variations in DNA sequence as related to drug response' (Liewei et al., 2011), and currently is regarded as a subdomain of the much more comprehensive pharmacogenomics that is FDA-defined as 'the study of variations of DNA and RNA characteristics as related to drug response'. (Trent, 2010)

Pharmacogenomics studies the differential expression profiles at the level of the entire human genome in complex interaction to drugs, in a systemic and integrative manner. The identification of all the genetic and epigenetic differences that are the cause of phenotypic variations in patients' responsivity to therapy is a major objective in pharmacogenomics. (Passetti et al., 2009) Each person's phenotype is best determined by the paired combination of the genome and the epigenome. Epigenetics and epigenomics refer to the study of factors that affect gene (or, more globally, genome) function, but without an accompanying change in genes. Typical epigenetic factors might be illustrated by changes in DNA methylation or in chromatin that modify genome structure and hence influence gene expression even in the absence of variations of DNA sequence. (Willard, 2009) Therefore, to achieve the main goal of therapy individualization, pharmacogenomics should also evaluate genetic variation in the context of the individual: gene–gene, gene–drug and gene–environment interactions which might influence the course of a disease and the response to treatment. (Passetti et al., 2009)

Pharmacogenomics is the interface between genomic medicine and systems pharmacology, the two essential pillars supporting the gateway to personalized medicine. (Aislyn et al., 2009) The transdisciplinary field of genomic medicine refers to the use of large-scale genomic information and to the consideration of the full extent of an individual's genome, proteome, transcriptome, metabolome and/or epigenome in the practice of medicine and medical decision-making. Genomic medicine's approaches include gene expression profiling to characterize diseases and define diseases' prognosis, genotyping variants in genes involved in drug metabolism or action in order to select the correct therapeutic dosage for an individual, scanning the entire genome for millions of variants that influence an individual's susceptibility to disease, or analyzing multiple biomarkers to monitor therapy and to provide predictive information in presymptomatic individuals. (Willard, 2009) Genomic medicine brings together knowledge on the relationships between genetics, pathophysiology and pharmacology, thus forming the base for systems pharmacology. Experimental and computational approaches enable systems pharmacology to provide holistic, mechanistic information on disease networks and drug responses, and to identify new drug targets and specific drug combinations. Network analyses of interactions involved in pathophysiology and drug response across multiple scales of organization, from molecular to whole organism, will allow the integration of the systems-level understanding of drug action with genomic medicine, thus generating the personalized medicine. (Aislyn et al., 2009) Personalized medicine refers to a rapidly advancing field of health care that takes into account each person's unique clinical, genomic and environmental information. The goals of personalized medicine are to optimize preventive health care strategies and outcomes of drug therapies for each individual, while people are still healthy or at the earliest stages of disease, by an unprecedented customization or tailoring of medication types and dosages and/or prophylactic measures. (Willard, 2009)

The great promise of pharmacogenomics towards personalized medicine resides mainly in generating an individualized therapeutic guide, highly predictive for much safer and more efficient drug and doses choice for an accurately predicted, homogenously genotype-segment of patients who are responders to the treatment, rather being focused around each individual specifically. (Grossman & Goldstein, 2009)

Pharmacogenomics aims to individualize therapy on the patient's specific genetic profile, by matching the right drug to the right patient at the right time. Pharmacogenomics' translation from bench into clinical practice is broadening the perspective of personalized medicine so as in the near future we might rely on a "DNA chip"/"pharmacogenomic card" specific to each patient and on each genotype preemptively recorded in electronic medical records in order to individualize both the diagnostic procedures and the safest and most efficient medications prior to treatment initiation.

3. Pharmacokinetic pharmacogenetics

Relevant allelic variants to drug treatment's outcome have been discovered in the genes encoding enzymes and transporters involved in drug pharmacokinetics: absorption, distribution, metabolism and excretion (ADME). Enzymes involved in the biotransformation of xenobiotics are classified as phase I or phase II. Phase I enzymes catalyze hydrolysis, reduction and oxidation reactions, while phase II enzymes catalyze conjugation reactions such as sulfation, acetylation and glucuronidation. (Sissung et al. 2010). The majority of phase I reactions are catalyzed by the cytochrome P450 (CYP) enzymes. There are 57 cytochrome P450 (CYP) genes and about the same number of pseudogenes, which are grouped according to their sequence similarity into 18 families and 44 subfamilies. However, only three of those families, CYP1, CYP2 and CYP3, catalyze most phase I reactions of drugs; over 75% of prescribed drugs are metabolized at least in part by three subfamilies: CYP3A, CYP2D6 and CYP2C. (Zanger et al., 2008; van Schaik, 2008, as cited in Sissung et al., 2010) Phase II reactions significantly enable the excretion of drugs by considerably increasing the hydrophilicity of the substrate or deactivate highly reactive species. Key phase II enzymes include N-acetyltransferases 1 and 2 (NAT1 and NAT2), thiopurine S-methyltransferase (TPMT), and the uridine diphosphate glucuronosyltransferase (UGT) family; polymorphisms in these genes have been shown to have clinical implications for a variety of diseases. (Zhou et al., 2008, as cited in Sissung et al., 2010)

3.1 Pharmacogenetics of drug-metabolizing enzymes

Biotransformation of the 200 most often prescribed drugs is catalyzed by members of the CYP3A family (37% of the drugs), followed by CYP2C9 (17%), CYP2D6 (15%), CYP2C19 (10%), CYP1A2 (9%), and CYP2C8 (6%), while CYP2B6 and other CYP isoforms (CYP2A6 and CYP2E1) participate in the metabolism of 4% and 2% of the drugs, respectively. The clinically well-established polymorphisms of CYP2C9, CYP2C19, and CYP2D6 genes are involved in approximately half of these top 200 drugs, since many of the drugs used in high-prevalence diseases in the Western countries are known to be metabolized by these CYPs. (Zanger et al., 2008)

CYP2C9, highly expressed in liver, metabolizes many weakly acidic substances like the anticoagulant warfarin, the anticonvulsants phenytoin and valproic acid, cardiovascular drugs like rosuvastatin and losartan, and several nonsteroidal anti-inflammatory drugs (NSAIDs). Many of these drugs have a narrow therapeutic index, and variations in CYP2C9 activity are among the recognized factors for adverse drug reactions. In vitro and clinical studies have consistently demonstrated that the CYP2C9*2 and *3 alleles are associated with significant, but highly variable, reductions in intrinsic clearance depending on the particular substrate; for instance, CYP2C9*3 allele might be associated to up to 90% reduction in the enzymatic activity of the CYP2C9 protein. The prevalence of CYP2C9*2 and *3 alleles is 35% in Caucasians and much lower in black and Asian populations. Carriers of CYP2C9*2 and CYP2C9*3 alleles are poor metabolizers and have high plasma levels due to low clearance of the substrate-drugs, therefore they experience higher incidences of adverse drug reactions like hypoglycemia from antidiabetic drugs, gastrointestinal bleeding from NSAIDs, and serious bleeding from warfarin treatment. (Pilotto et al., 2007, and Flockhart et al., 2008, as cited in Zanger et al., 2008)

The *CYP2C19* isozyme metabolizes preferentially proton-pump inhibitors (PPI) like omeprazole and pantoprazole indicated in gastroesophageal reflux disease, gastric and duodenal ulcer. The poor metabolizer (PM) phenotype results from two null alleles, leading to the absence of functional CYP2C19 protein, whereas extensive metabolizers carry at least one functional allele. The prevalence of null alleles is about 3–5% to white and black populations, whereas up to 20% of Asians are carriers of two null alleles. The two most common null alleles are *CYP2C19*2* occurring exclusively in Caucasians, and *CYP2C19*3* occurring primarily in Asians. The PPI-efficacy depends on the plasma concentrations achieved over time, which are strongly influenced by *CYP2C19* gene polymorphisms. PM subjects who are carriers of null alleles benefit from their lower metabolism rate because their drug levels are maintained higher for longer periods. On the contrary, subjects with the *CYP2C9 *1/*1* wild-type genotype should receive higher doses of these PPIs in order to achieve stronger acid suppression compared to **1/*2* and **2/*2* subjects. (Kawamura et al., 2007, as cited in Zanger et al., 2008; Zanger et al., 2008; Tomalik-Scharte et al., 2008)

The clinical consequences of pharmacokinetic variability associated to genetic polymorphisms of *CYP2D6* gene for tricyclic and selective serotonin re-uptake inhibitors antidepressants, beta-blockers, anticancer agent tamoxifen, as well as to the *CYP2C9* genetic variants for AT$_1$ (angiotensin II type 1) receptor antagonists (sartans), and anticoagulants (warfarin, acenocoumarol, phenprocoumon), are covered in other chapters of the book.

The *CYP3A4* subfamily contributes to the metabolism of the most diverse group of substrates of all human P450s, as their active sites are flexible enough to bind and metabolize many preferentially lipophilic, structurally large compounds, such as: the immunosuppressants cyclosporin A and tacrolimus, macrolide antibiotics like erythromycin, anticancer drugs like taxol, benzodiazepines, hydroxymethylglutaryl-coenzyme A (HMG-CoA) reductase inhibitors like simvastatin and atorvastatin, and anesthetics. In addition, CYP3A4 is the only human drug-metabolizing P450 that shows a significant sex difference, in that women express approximately 1.5- to 2-fold more CYP3A4 and have higher *in vivo* clearance of several typical CYP3A4 drug substrates than men. Although a number of large-scale sequencing and phenotype–genotype correlation studies have been carried out, the functional effects of *CYP3A4* gene polymorphisms on drugs pharmacokinetic variability remain controversial. (Zanger et al., 2008) However, *CYP3A4* basal and inducible expression phenotype might be influenced by other genes, such as: a) multiple drug resistance gene *MDR1* whose *2677T (Ser893)* allele induced higher basal CYP3A4 expression and activity, whereas the 2677G allele showed a higher rifampicin induction ratio in primary hepatocytes; b) pregnan X receptor *PXR* gene polymorphisms mostly located in promoter or intron 1 regions associated with CYP3A4 basal and inducible expression levels. (Liu, 2007 and Lamba, 2008, as cited in Zanger et al., 2008)

N-acetyltransferase type 2 (NAT2) is a phase II drug metabolizing enzyme responsible for hepatic bioconversion of major antituberculosis agent isoniazid to acetylisoniazid. Isoniazid is a pivotal agent in the treatment of tuberculosis, that remains a global emergency due to the growing prevalence of drug-resistant *Mycobacterium tuberculosis* and of *HIV* infection. *NAT2* gene is affected by a bimodal distribution polymorphism (acetylation polymorphism) described after clinical observation of more frequently and more severely peripheral neuropathy and hepatotoxicity as adverse drug reactions to the slow-acetylators patients. These patients have mean elimination half-lives of 180 min. in comparison with 80 min. for rapid-acetylators. Carriers of at least one wild-type allele (*NAT2*4*) or a high-activity variant allele (*NAT2*12*) have proven high NAT2 enzymatic activity (rapid acetylators), whereas those with two low-activity variants are slow acetylators. Rapid acetylators are more prevalent in East Asia (58-90%) than in Europe (32-43%). Tailoring isoniazid therapy means to increase isoniazid dose to rapid acetylators so as to achieve therapeutic efficacy and to reduce the dose administered to slow-acetylators so as to avoid adverse drug reactions while maintaining the desired antituberculosis effect. (Tomalik-Scharte et al., 2008)

Pharmacogenetics of other phase II drug-metabolizing enzymes is discussed in detail in other chapters for: thiopurine-S-methyl-transferase (*TPMT*) polymorphisms and the necessity to individualize the therapeutic doses of mercaptopurine and azathioprine; dihydropyrimidine dehydrogenase deficiency syndrome noticed during the treatment with standard doses of fluoropyrimidines (5-fluorouracil) to a segment of cancer patients carriers of certain genetic mutations; the pharmacokinetic variability and increased risk of myelotoxicity noticed for the anticancer drug irinotecan as a consequence of genetic polymorphism of UDP-glucuronosyltransferase (*UGT1A1*).

3.2 Pharmacogenetics of transporters

Transporters play a critical role in ADME because they are involved in the efflux and/or influx of drugs via active transport or facilitated diffusion, thus transporters affect drug uptake, bioavailability, targeting, efficacy, toxicity and clearance and they should be considered in combination with metabolic enzymes when discussing drugs' outcomes. Two types of transport superfamilies, ATP-binding cassette (ABC) proteins generally acting as efflux pumps and solute-linked carrier (SLC) proteins as typically influx transporters, are responsible for the majority of drug and endogenous substrates transport. Many transporters have a broad range of substrates; for instance, ABCB1, also known as P-glycoprotein and MRD1, transports several classes of drugs, including anticancer agents, antibiotics, immunosuppressants and statins. (Sissung et al., 2010)

Largely as a result of the Human Genome Project, great advances in molecular biology, sequencing methods and availability of genome-wide technologies, genetic variants across the entire genome, including coding and noncoding regions of multiple transporter genes were identified, functionally characterized and associated with various drug-response phenotypes. Thus, functionally relevant polymorphisms were discovered for the members of ABC and SLC superfamilies of transporters and have been widely studied with positive associations to individual susceptibility to drug-induced adverse events, to variations in drug plasma levels, or renal clearance. (Yee SW et al., 2010) For instance, the organic anion transporting polypeptide polymorphism *SLCO1B1*5* (*Val174Ala, c.521T>C*) is associated with variability in response to statins (atorvastatin, pravastatin, pitavastatin, rosuvastatin, simvastatin), repaglinide, fexofenadine and methotrexate. The *SLCO1B1* genotype affects the transport function and may predict, in a substrate-dependent manner, the attenuated lipid-lowering response to statin therapy. Moreover, stronger evidence has been provided for the role of the *SLCO1B1* genotype in predicting the development of myopathy among patients receiving simvastatin in 40 mg doses. (Yee SW et al., 2010; Romaine et al., 2010) Prescribing relatively low dose of simvastatin to those who are heterozygous for the high risk allele *SLCO1B1* could reduce the incidence of myopathy by nearly 60%, while avoiding simvastatin only to those who are homozygous for the risk allele (nearly 2% of the population analyzed by the SEARCH group) could reduce the incidence of myopathy by 25%. Further investigation is required to identify the optimal therapeutic approach. (Nakamura, 2008)

Furthermore, organic cationic transporter *OCT1* (*R61C, P160L, G401S, 420del* and *G465R*) and *OCT2* (*A270S*) polymorphisms are associated with response's variability to metformin, cisplatin and imatinib. The *ABCG2* genotype (*rs2231142, Gln141Lys, c.421C>A*) is associated with variable pharmacokinetics parameters of atorvastatin, rosuvastatin, gefitinib, sulfasalazine and diflomotecan. *ABCB1* gene polymorphisms (*c.3435C>T, 2677G/T/A*) and/or *ABCC2* (*-24C>T, c.1249G>T, c.3972C>T, c.4544C>T*) are related to therapeutic and adverse effects to anticancer, antiviral and/or antiepileptic drugs. (Yee SW et al., 2010) SNPs of *ABCB1* were found to be associated with moderate-to-severe neutropenia, hand–foot syndrome and diarrhoea in colorectal patients treated with capecitabine or 5-fluorouracil. (Gonzales-Haba et al., 2010)

Nonsynonymous (coding) SNPs generally appear to affect the expression level of the transporter on the plasma membrane and the transporter function in a substrate-dependent manner. In comparison to nonsynonymous variants, noncoding region variants (such as in the proximal promoter region) are more abundant, minor allele frequencies being often higher and the functional consequences are more modest and highly dependent upon the haplotype. The frequency of noncoding polymorphisms are greater in ABC transporters highly expressed in the liver than in SLC predominantly expressed in the kidney. The projected functional map of the 'transporter genome' will characterize gene regions (enhancer regions upstream, downstream and intronic regions of transporter genes) having relevant functional variants and it will be superimposed on the genetic variants resulted from the 1000 Genomes Project in multiple ethnic populations. (Yee SW et al., 2010)

3.3 AmpliChip™ CYP450 test

In 2005, the FDA approved the first pharmacogenetic test AmpliChip™ CYP450 Test (Roche Molecular Systems, Inc., NJ, USA) based on Affymetrix (CA, USA) microarray technology for genotyping 27 alleles in *CYP2D6* and three alleles in *CYP2C19* genes associated with different metabolizing phenotypes. The test is recommended for the assessment of the patient's metabolizing status for each drug that is a substrate for *CYP450* isoenzymes *2D6* and *2C19* and for the dose adjustements in outlier patients who are either ultrarapid- (UM) or poor-metabolizers (PM), in order to achieve the therapeutic efficacy and to avoid the risk of severe adverse reactions. (Squassina et al., 2010) Key genetic mutations associated with clinical relevance on drug plasma concentrations and risk of either lack of efficacy for UM or adverse drug reactions for PM, are used to predict the metabolizer phenotype (ultrarapid, extensive, intermediate and poor metabolizers). FDA has included these biomarkers only as informational pharmacogenetic tests on labels of drugs mainly metabolized by these pathways, such as: *CYP2C19* genotyping for prasugrel, voriconazol, (es)omeprazole, and genotyping *CYP2D6* for tamoxifen, atomoxetine, fluoxetine, paroxetine, amitriptyline, aripiprazole, risperidone, codeine, tramadol, timolol, propranolol, carvedilol. The purpose of these informational pharmacogenetic tests is to improve drug safety by dose optimization based on genotypes predictive for poor- or ultrarapid-metabolizer status, as well as to avoid high plasma concentration when co-administered with other drugs which are *CYP2D6* strong inhibitors. (Squassina et al., 2010)

For instance, patients with poor metabolizer phenotype associated to null alleles *CYP2D6*4, *3, *5, or CYP2D6*6*, will have higher risk of the adverse reaction tardive diskinesia at standard doses of antipsychotics. The individualized doses for these PM patients will be reduced than standard regimens designed for wild-type normally functional allele. On the contrary, to achieve the required level of therapeutic efficacy, ultrarapid metabolizers who are carriers of *CYP2D6*Nxn* multiple functional alleles will be treated with higher doses than those standard recommended for the "average" patients population able to normally metabolize the drugs. However, mothers with phenotype of ultrarapid metabolizers will rapidly convert standard doses of codeine into morphine thus increasing the risk of CNS depression of their breast-fed babies; in such cases of prodrug bioconversion, dose optimization requires to be lower than the standard dose. (Loo et al., 2010)

Although it is widely available in commercial labs, the AmpliChip™ CYP450 Test has still a limited clinical value because it is expensive (over $600/test), time-consuming (i.e. about two weeks), and yet there are no prospective study to demonstrate the cost-effective benefit of genotyping patients and selecting and dosing antipsychotic drugs accordingly. (Jian-Ping Zhang, 2011)

3.4 DMET Plus Panel genotyping platform

While the field of pharmacogenetics is moving towards exploratory, large-scale analyses of the interaction between genetic variation and drug treatment, the Drug Metabolizing Enzymes and Transporters DMET Plus Panel (Affymetrix) genotyping platform has proven a significant research tool. The DMET Plus Panel platform is a low- to mid-scale pathway-based, hypothesis-driven and exploratory pharmacogenetic approach, which interrogates 1936 genetic variations (copy-number variations, insertions/deletions, biallelic and triallelic single nucleotide polymorphisms SNPs) in 225 genes involved in the absorption, distribution, metabolism and elimination (ADME) of a very wide range of therapeutics, as well as a number of genes which regulate intracellular processes that facilitate ADME through indirect relationships, thus comprising biomarkers for all FDA-validated genes and included in the drugs' label. (Sissung et al., 2010; Squassina et al., 2010)

The DMET Plus Panel platform is particularly useful for standardization of exploratory pharmacogenetics and for improvement of the clinical trials' design conducted on smaller patient populations, having more variable end points and polygenetic traits, enabling increased statistical power and reduction of type I error (i.e., false positive) of GWAS. In addition, the application of DMET Plus Panel platform in phase I early clinical trials could identify the polymorphisms consistently associated with drugs' pharmacokinetic variations, determine the recommended dose for later phase II and phase III trials based on genetic profile, thus reducing the attrition rate for new investigational agents. Moreover, besides detection of more common genetic variants, DMET is able to interrogate core biomarkers with an average minor allele frequency below 9%, in comparison with other SNP detection methods for minor alleles with an average frequency of 20%. However, the DMET Plus Panel platform's utility resides mainly in the research setting, since it is not yet FDA approved, not customizable, does not include polymorphisms in many drug targets or in genes that are related to environmental exposures that could influence drug metabolism, and requires prospective clinical validation in order to translate the results in pertinent personalized medicine. (Sissung et al., 2010; Squassina et al., 2010)

Although genetic variation in ADME genes is essential in personalizing therapy, polymorphisms in genes not directly responsible for drug metabolism or transport, but regulating expression of many genes that encode transporters and phase I and phase II enzymes, play critical roles in patients' response to treatment. For example, many SNPs in the nuclear receptors pregnane X receptor (PXR) and constitutive/active androstane receptor genes alter the expression levels of *ABCB1, ABCC2, CYP2C8, CYP3A4, UGTs* and sulfotransferases (*SULTs*) genes and contribute to variability in drug efficacy and safety. (Sissung et al., 2010)

4. Pharmacodynamic pharmacogenetics

Pharmacodynamics can be defined as the study of the biochemical and physiological effects of drugs and their mechanism of action. The effects of drugs result from their interaction with macromolecular components of the organism – receptors, which are grouped in a wide range of structural and functional families. The receptor occupancy by a particular drug class triggers biochemical cascades in target cells and modulates diverse intrinsic signaling pathways and functions, explaining the pharmacodynamic effect. (Ross & Kenakin, 2006)

In addition to genetic polymorphisms of ADME genes, the clinical outcome of standard therapeutic drug regimens is influenced by genetic variations in genes encoding drug targets (receptors, enzymes, ion channels, neurotransmitter's transporter) and pathways affected by drugs.

Since pharmacogenetics of heart diseases therapy, anticoagulants, asthma medication, anticancer agents including thiopurines, antidepressants, osteoporosis and antimalaria drugs, represent other distinct chapters of the book, in order to avoid overlapping information, this chapter will illustrate some functionally relevant polymorphisms of the drug target genes and their role in the interindividual variability of drugs' pharmacodynamics, in a complementary manner to the aforementioned issues.

4.1 Pharmacogenetics of drug hypersensitivity: Human Leukocytes Antigens (HLA) system

In the field of highly active antiretroviral therapy (HAART), abacavir has created a translational roadmap for a pharmacogenetic biomarker from discovery to a test used in real clinical practice. The strong association between abacavir hypersensitivity reaction and *HLA-B*5701* genotype has been demonstrated in both observational and blinded randomized clinical trials in racially diverse populations and represents the best example of the clinical utility of pharmacogenetic screening in HIV medicine. (Mallal et al., 2008)

Hypersensitivity reaction to abacavir was observed during the clinical development program in approximately 5–8% of patients. Hypersensitivity reaction (HSR) symptoms appear early and resolve upon discontinuation of the drug, but worsen (and can be life-threatening) with continued drug administration. Development of an abacavir skin patch assay enabled refinement of the hypersensitivity reaction phenotype. The biomarker *HLA-B*5701,* validated in retrospective and prospective studies, was recommended in the drug label in the EU and USA. The prospective screening for this biomarker in Caucasians as high risk population allows a reduction in HSR frequency from 7.8% to 3.4%. (Trent, 2010) The increased benefit–to–risk ratio and the economic consequences of *HLA-B*5701* pre-screening of HIV-infected patients before abacavir treatment's initiation were demonstrated in a prospective double-blinded clinical trial sponsored by GSK. (Mallal et al., 2008; Roses, 2009; Phillips et al., 2011)

Moreover, consistent data support the association of the HLA class II allele *HLA-DRB*0101* with an increased risk of nevirapine-induced hepatotoxicity, as well as genotype-related peripheral neuropathy, hyperlipidaemia, lipodystrophy to HAART, nucleoside reverse transcriptase inhibitors-related pancreatitis and tenofovir-associated renal proximal tubulopathy. (Tozzi, 2010)

Other recent examples of important HLA associations with drug hypersensitivity include *HLA-B*1502* and Stevens-Johnson syndrome (SJS) and toxic epidermal necrolysis (TEN) that are associated with carbamazepine in Han Chinese; *HLA-B*5801* and SJS/TEN and drug-induced hypersensitivity syndrome/drug reaction with eosinophilia and systemic symptoms associated with allopurinol; *HLA-B*5701* and flucloxacillin-induced liver injury. These pharmacogenetic associations hold the promise to convert the severe and adverse drug reactions into predictable and preventable ones in the future. (Phillips et al., 2011)

4.2 Pharmacodynamic pharmacogenetics of antipsychotics

Pharmacogenetic investigations of schizophrenia susceptibility loci and genes controlling drug target receptors, the blood–brain barrier systems, and epigenetic mechanisms could lead to a molecular classification of treatment response and adverse events of psychotropic drugs. It is estimated that more than 70% of patients with chronic schizophrenia discontinued their antipsychotic drugs, owing to poor effectiveness or tolerability. Most of the pharmacodynamic pharmacogenetic studies in schizophrenia have evaluated treatment response using the candidate gene approach.

The most relevant associations of genetics variants and antipsychotic clinical response were found for −141C *Ins/Del* in dopamine receptor gene *DRD2*, A-1438G in 5-hydroxytriptamine/ serotonin receptor gene *HTR2A*, *His452Tyr* in *HTR2A* gene, *Taq1A* in *DRD2*, *Ser9Gly* in *DRD3*, T102C SNP in *HTR2A*, C759T SNP in *HTR2C* gene. For instance, patients who carry one or two *Del* alleles tend to have less favorable antipsychotic drug responses than patients with the *Ins/Ins* genotype in *DRD2* −141C *Ins/Del* SNPs. Patients with *G/G* genotype for the *HTR2A* A-1438G polymorphism were less likely to respond to clozapine, olanzapine and aripiprazole, especially in negative symptoms, than other polymorphisms at this *HTR2A* locus. For the *His452Tyr HTR2A* genetic variants, the *Tyr/Tyr* genotype predicted poor response to clozapine. Higher risk of the adverse reaction tardive diskinesia was found for carriers of either: A2/A2 genotype at *DRD2 Taq1A* locus, *Gly* allele at *DRD3 Ser9Gly*, or C allele for 5HT2A T102C. (Jian-Ping Zhang, 2011)

Furthermore, single-nucleotide substitutions in the promoter region of serotonin receptor type 2C (*5-HT2C*) could be associated with antipsychotics-induced weight gain and metabolic abnormalities in Han Chinese patients treated over a 10-week period. The *C/C* genotype from *5HT2C SNP C759T* was associated with higher weight gain to clozapine and olanzapine. Comparable results were found in Caucasians treated 9 months with these anti–

psychotics: carriers of the -795T variation gained less weight than study participants without this allele. (Broich & Moeller, 2008)

A repeat length polymorphism of the gene encoding the serotonin transporter, 5-HTTLPR, involves insertion/deletion of a 44-bp segment located upstream of the transcription start site in the promoter region; patients carrying the long allele are about twice as likely to respond to treatment at 4 weeks and reach remission, and less likely to suffer from side effects, than patients with the short/short genotype; short allele is associated with poor response to clozapine and risperidone treatment. (Jian-Ping Zhang, 2011) Moreover, insertion/deletion polymorphism in the promoter region of the serotonin transporter gene is also associated to clinical phenotype response to the antidepressants citalopram, paroxetine and fluoxetine. (Yee SW et al., 2010)

4.3 Pharmacodynamic pharmacogenetics of antidiabetics

Thiazolidinedione drugs (pioglitazone, rosiglitazone) promote the binding of the transcription factor peroxisome proliferator-activated receptor-γ (PPAR-γ) to its DNA response element. Thiazolidinediones promote adipocyte differentiation, increase insulin-stimulated glucose uptake into muscle, insulin suppression of hepatic glucose output, and insulin-stimulated lipolysis. The genetic variation Pro12Ala at the PPARG gene (encoding PPAR-γ) influences the clinical outcome: those carrying the Ala allele have a greater response to rosiglitazone, as well as a lower risk of edema after farglitazar or ragaglitazar therapy, than Pro/Pro homozygotes. (Kang ES et al., 2005 and Hansen et al., 2006, both cited in Pearson, 2009) The hypoglycemic effect of rosiglitazone might also be influenced by adiponectin gene ADIPOQ polymorphisms SNP +45T/G and SNP +276G/T: homozygotes G/G at +45 or +276 have a smaller clinical benefit. (Kang ES et al., 2005 as cited in Pearson, 2009) Sulfonylureas (tolbutamide, glimepiride, glibenclamide) bind to the SUR1 moiety of the pancreatic β-cell K_{ATP} channel causing the channel to close and triggering insulin secretion. The clinical efficacy of sulfonylureas seems to be associated to genetic variations in the KCNJ11 gene (encoding the Kir6.2 subunit of the K_{ATP} channel) and the ABCC8 gene. (Pearson, 2009) The polymorphisms ABCC8 Ser1369Ala and KCNJ11 rs5210 and E23K are in strong linkage disequilibrium and significantly associated with variations in fasting plasma glucose levels induced by sulfonylureas. (Feng Y et al., 2008, Glyon AL et al., 2003 and Sesti G et al., 2006, all cited in Pearson, 2009)

4.4 Pharmacogenetics of hepatitis C virus therapy

Response to pegylated interferon-alfa (PEG-IFN) and ribavirin (RBV) therapy in chronic infection with hepatitis C virus (HCV) is variable and a sustained virological response (SVR) is dependent on genetic factors, hepatitis C viral load, patient age, sex, weight, liver fibrosis stage, and adherence to therapy. Strong predictive, clinically relevant effect of IL28B genotype on SVR shows that C/C genotype at rs12979860 has a greater HCV-genotype 1 RNA decline from days 0-28 than patients with the C/T or T/T genotype. The IL28B genotype may also be considered in conjunction with virological response after 4 weeks: thus, patients with poor viral kinetics and T/T genotype at rs12979860 may decide to stop therapy. In North America, a commercial test for IL28B genotyping is now available and costs approximately $300. (Afdhal et al., 2011)

5. Pharmacogenetics' translation from bench towards clinical practice in personalized medicine and drug design

The great majority of drugs prescribed upon the classical paradigm of "one-drug-fits-all" and "trial-and-error" are effective only in 25-60% of the treated patients. Moreover, 50% from new chemical entities fail in the highly expensive phase III of clinical development. (Spraggs, 2009) Regulatory authorities FDA, European Medicines Agency (EMA) and the Japanese Pharmaceuticals and Medical Devices Agency (PMDA) recognize pharmacogenetics as an essential opportunity to predict drug responsiveness and to personalize therapy, and are increasingly integrating pharmacogenetic information to label updates of approved drugs, as well as incorporating pharmacogenetics into their regulatory review of new medicines. In addition, the regulatory framework that facilitates pharmacogenetics integration into drug development such as the Voluntary Exploratory Data Submissions in the USA and the Pharmacogenomics Briefing Meetings in Europe and Japan, as well as the more recent, formal biomarker qualification by the regulators are developed. (Surh et al., 2010)

5.1 Pharmacogenetic markers validation

Defining clinical guidelines for pharmacogenetic testing has to tackle the following issues: a) establishment of clinical end points; b) validation of pharmacogenetic testing in terms of its sensitivity, specificity, predictive power, cost-efficiency and time to perform; c) interpretation guidelines of the results and their impact on dosing algorithms, population's stratification, clinical trials design, dissemination to clinicians and patients, incorporation into clinical practice without major interference to efficiency and cost of health care system. (Loo et al., 2010)

Pharmacogenetic algorithms should include clinical and genetic factors to guide therapy individualization, should be cost-effective and offer supplementary information over traditional approaches. However, broader dialogue and additional regulatory guidance are needed to reach a consensus regarding: the quantity of pharmacogenetic information in drug labels, indications for physicians (informative *vs.* recommended *vs.* required pharmacogenetic test) and measures to keep this information up to date, relevant sections on the labels (which currently ranges from Warnings to Indications to Clinical Pharmacology), levels of compelling evidence leading to decision-making translation (i.e., type of trial design, sample size, replication, reproducibility, consistency, effect size and other predictor variables). (Surh et al., 2010)

Regulatory recommendations for pharmacogenetic markers concern to: identification of responders and nonresponders; reduction of drug toxicity by minimizing or eliminating ADR; and optimization of the safety and effectiveness of drugs through personalized dosing strategies. This will enhance drug response predictability and safety in preclinical, clinical and postmarket trials. The biomarkers could be classified by their purpose in: improving drug safety, improving drug efficacy and confirming disease status. The FDA has three types of amendments for pharmacogenetic biomarkers, depending on the available evidence and the ability to implement the identified biomarker in clinical practice. These are as follows: information on the biomarker, which is strictly for informational purposes and does not require any action; recommended testing for the biomarker on the label; and mandated testing for the biomarker before drug use. (Squassina et al., 2010; Surh et al., 2010; Burns et al., 2010) Pharmacogenetic tests validated in clinical studies and recommended in the drug labels are detailed in table 1.

Drug Indication	Pharmacogenetic biomarker	Comments
Mandatory, required predictive pharmacogenetic tests in drug label		
Trastuzumab HERCEPTIN® Metastatic BC	*HER2/neu* over-expression	Improve drug efficacy: clinical benefit is limited to the responsive patients, whose tumors overexpress the drug-target *HER2/neu* (IHC or FISH assay)
Lapatinib TYKERB® Metastatic BC	*HER2/neu* over-expression	Improve drug efficacy: clinical benefit limited to tumors overexpressing *HER2/neu* (IHC or FISH assay*)*
Cetuximab ERBITUX® Metastatic CRC	*EGFR expression*	Improve drug efficacy: clinical benefit limited to patients with EGFR-positiv tumors (IHC assay)
Dasatinib SPRYCEL®; Imatinib GLEEVEC® ALL (adults)	*Philadelphia chromosome positive*	Disease confirmation and patients' selection: *BCR-ABL* translocation (Philadelphia chromosome-positiv)
Maraviroc SELZENTRY® HIV (adults)	*CCR-5 C-Cmotif receptor*	Disease confirmation: infection with CCR-5-tropic HIV-1 and resistance to other antiretrovirals
Recommended predictive pharmacogenetic tests in drug label		
Abacavir Ziagen® HIV infection	*HLA-B*5701* allele	Improve drug safety: avoid hypersensitivity reactions to homozygous or heterozygous *HLA-B*5701* genotypes. Screening is also recommended in reinitiation of drug in populations with previous tolerance of abacavir and unknown *HLA-B*5701* status.
Azathioprine, IMURAN®; 6-MP PURINETHOL® ALL, inflammatory bowel disease	*TPMT*	Improve drug safety: avoid myelotoxicity in patients with phenotype or genotype of *TPMT* deficiency or lower activity. Subjects homozygous for *TPMT*3A* are at high risk for life-threatening myelosuppression when treated with standard doses of thiopurines: individualized doses are one tenth to one fifteenth the standard dose, in parallel with careful monitoring to avoid myelotoxicity. Patients with intermediate TPMT levels can safely receive thiopurines at lower doses (30–50% of the standard dose) and safe dose escalation under close monitoring.
Irinotecan CAMPTOSAR® CRC	*UGT1A1*	First FDA approved pharmacogenetic test "Third Wave Technologies, Invader assay" (2005), with dose optimization guidelines dependent on *UGT1A1* genotype: avoid severe (grade III/IV) neutropenia and diarrhoea for those who are at high risk, i.e. homozygous (and possibly heterozygous) for *UGT1A1*28* and *UGT1A1*1* alleles.
Warfarin COUMADIN® Thrombo-embolism	*CYP2C9 and VKORC1 (-1639G>A)*	Improve drug efficacy and safety: avoid increased risk of bleeding to patients homozygous or heterozygous for *CYP2C9*2* or *CYP2C9*3* alleles by prescribing differentiated doses (as compared with those for *CYP2C9*1* homozygous). Pharmacogenetic test: "Nanosphere Verigene Warfarin Metabolism Nucleic Acid Test; therapeutic algorithm based on genotype and clinical factors (http://www.WarfarinDosing.org.)
Clopidogrel (prodrug) PLAVIX® Thrombo-embolism	*CYP2C19*	Improve efficacy and safety: doses adjustment for ultrarapid metabolizers who are carriers of *CYP2C19*17/*17* genotype and for poor metabolizers due to *CYP2C19*2* allele presence.
Carbamazepine TEGRETOL® Epilepsy	*HLA-B*1502* allele	Improve drug safety: avoid serious dermatologic reactions (Stevens–Johnson syndrome and/or toxic epidermal necrolysis).

Drug Indication	Pharmacogenetic biomarker	Comments
Rasburicase ELITEK® Hyperuricemia	G6PD	Improve drug safety: pre-therapy screening to avoid severe hemolytic reactions associated with G6PD deficiency.
Clozapine CLOZARIL® Schizophrenia	HLA-DQB1	Improved safety: pharmacogenetic testing, in parallel with WBC monitoring, avoid prescription to patients with high agranulocytosis risk. Test „PGxPredict: Clozapine"
Tretinoin VESANOID® APL	PML/RARα	Improve drug efficacy and safety. Disease confirmation by t(15;17) cytogenetic marker
Valproic acid DEPAKENE® Seizures	UCD deficiency	Confirm disease: consider evaluation of UCD before therapy with valproate
Only informational pharmacogenetic tests in drug label		
Panitumumab VECTIBIX® Cetuximab ERBITUX® mCRC	K-RAS	Improve efficacy: clinical benefit limited to patients with non-mutated K-RAS.
Imatinib GLEEVEC® GIST	C-KIT	Improve drug efficacy: clinical benefit in patients carriers of the activating C-KIT mutation
Busulfan MYLERAN® CML	Philadelphia chromosome	Improve drug efficacy: responders are positives for Philadelphia chromosome (BCR-ABL)
Capecitabine XELODA® CRC	DPD deficiency	Improve drug safety: decreased DPD and increased level of 5-fluorouracil is associated with severe toxicity (e.g., stomatitis, diarrhoea, neutropenia and neurotoxicity).
Primaquine Malaria	G6PD deficiency	Improve drug safety: avoid acute intravascular hemolytic reactions.
Isoniazid, Pyrazinamide TB	NAT	Improve drug safety: dose adjustements based on NAT-metabolic status, for slow acetylators and fast acetylators to avoid severe adverse reaction of peripheral neuropathy, or lack of efficacy, respectively.
Erlotinib TARCEVA® NSCLC	EGFR mutations	Confirm disease (at least 10% of the cells are EGFR-positive) and response to EGFR tyrosine kinase inhibitors
Lenalidomide REVLIMID® Myelodysplasic syndromes	Deletion of chromosome 5q (del[5q])	Confirm disease: indicated to treat those with transfusion dependent anemia caused by low- or intermediate-risk of myelodysplasic syndromes associated with 5q(del[5q])

IHC: immunohistochemistry; FISH: Flourescence In Situ Hybridization; BC: breast cancer; CRC: colorectal cancer; EGFR: epidermal growth factor receptor; G6PD: glucose-6-phosphate dehydrogenase; ALL: acute lymphoblastic leukemia; 6-MP: 6-mercaptopurine; TPMT: thiopurin-S-methyltransferase; UGT: UDP glucuronyltransferase; CYP: cytochrome P450; VKORC1: vitamin K epoxide-reductase receptor complex 1; HLA: human leukocytes antigens; APL: acute promyelocytic leukemia; PML: progressive multifocal leukoencephalopathy; GIST: gastrointestinal stromal tumor; CML: chronic myelogenous leukemia; DPD: dihydropyrimidine dehydrogenase; NAT: N-acetyltransferase; UCD: urea cycle disorder; WBC: white blood cells; NSCLC: non-small-cell lung cancer.
Data taken from: Burns et al., 2010; Squassina et al., 2010; Loo et al., 2010; Spraggs et al., 2009; Sagreiya et al., 2010; Seip et al., 2010; Pare et al., 2010; Holmes et al., 2010; McDonald et al., 2009; Shuldiner et al., 2009; Mega et al., 2009.

Table 1. Predictive pharmacogenetic tests integrated into drug labels

5.2 Clinical trials with genotype-guided design

Pharmacogenetic cohort studies within randomized controlled clinical trials (RCT) may provide final evidence concerning the impact of specific genetic polymorphisms on the outcome of drug therapy. Patients are randomly assigned to groups receiving either the substance under investigation or the comparison (control) therapy. If pharmacogenetic genotypes are analyzed in all the participants in such studies, genotypes that differentially predict the response to the administered treatments may be identified. (Stingl & Brockmöller, 2011)

Adequate design and well-controlled clinical investigations with randomization elements are defined in the Code of Federal Regulations (CFR) (21CFR 314.126) and they provide the FDA with a legal framework for establishing evidentiary standards for approval of a new molecular entity, that is, they attest to a drug's efficacy and safety when used under label conditions. In a pharmacogenetic context, RCTs can determine whether a genetic test, on average, is beneficial, harmful, or of no clinical value at the population level. When comparing the results of RCTs, there is a potential to find conflicting results due to differences in the null hypothesis, estimated effect size and study power, patient inclusion and exclusion criteria, clinical end points, and methods of data analysis. RCTs also have the potential to underestimate clinical events, for example, adverse reactions, when compared to "real-life" clinical events. (Lesko, 2007)

Although randomized controlled trials (RCT) are considered the gold standard for demonstrating the efficacy of therapeutic interventions, their application for the validation of many biomarkers, especially for multiple SNPs markers derived from GWAS, is limited by large sample sizes, time and financial restraints. Although pharmacogenetic studies as part of RCT allow to distinguish between prognostic markers and "true" predictive pharmacogenetic markers, there might be situations when RCT are unethical to conduct such as: the prescription of azathioprine or 6-mercaptopurine to homozygous carriers of thiopurine methyltransferase deficiency and the prescription of warfarin to combined carriers of low *CYP2C9* activity and low vitamin K epoxide reductase complex subunit 1 *VKORC1* activity. (Lesko, 2007)

Alternatively, carefully designed retrospective and prospective case-control and cohort studies based on large, robust databases and conducted with appropriate power and corrections, will facilitate the discovery and replication of genotype-phenotype associations. Thus, prospective collection and banking of samples with appropriate consent, combined with retrospective DNA testing, is a necessity for exploration and potential validation of pharmacogenetic biomarkers. (Burns et al., 2010; Frueh, 2009; Stingl & Brockmöller, 2011) The case–control study design is the most frequently applied type of observational retrospective study in pharmacogenetics and genotype-related disease susceptibility research. The frequencies of genotypes in persons identified as having specific adverse drug events or poor therapy outcomes ("cases") are compared with those of concurrently sampled controls who have had comparable drug exposure but who do not present the particular outcome. The advantages of case–control studies are: moderate resources, sufficiently high statistical power, performance in the natural settings of populations, focused on one type of well documented drug exposure. However, case–control studies are particularly prone to systematic error, also called "bias" and usually they have a supportive role requiring data replication in differently designed studies. (Stingl & Brockmöller, 2011)

The case–control Study of Hypersensitivity to Abacavir and Pharmacogenetic Evaluation (SHAPE) showed that 100% of both white and black patch test-positive patients carried HLA-B*5701, suggesting a 100% negative predictive value of HLA-B*5701 for abacavir HSR, generalizable across race. (Saag, 2010 as cited in Phillips et al., 2011)

A pharmacogenetic cohort study involves no controls and the group of patients receiving one type of therapeutic intervention is defined at the initiation of therapy and followed over the course of the study. This study design reflects true medical reality, is relatively easy to perform, and produced less biased results. In the time-series modified design, each patient serves as his or her own control because the drug treatment period is interrupted by a placebo period, thus a more precise differentiation between the drug effect and the effects of other factors may be obtained. The major drawbacks of cohort studies are: low statistical power requiring larger samples; a significant risk of confounding if there is heterogeneity in drug treatments, disease stages, and disease severity within the study sample; impossibility to differentiate between predictive and prognostic genotypes; insufficiency to serve as the only basis of therapy recommendations incorporating pharmacogenetics. (Lin & Chen, 2008 as cited in Stingl & Brockmöller, 2011)

Prospective interventional pharmacogenetic trials are based on the sequential pre-post or before-after design and patients receive drug therapies first before genotyping and then again after genotyping; sometimes it is also included a concurrently studied comparison group (parallel-controlled pharmacogenetic study) that implies randomized allocation to either the "therapy-guided by pharmacogenetic" arm or the "therapy as usual" arm. Prospective interventional pharmacogenetic trials allow a comparison between the efficacy of a new mode of treatment and that of the usual therapy and the extent to which the outcome of drug therapy would improve if it is guided by predictive pharmacogenetic testing. Randomized parallel diagnostic trials are more expensive, difficult to blind pharmacogenetic testing and might require larger sample sizes than phase III drug trials. (Haga et al., 2009 as cited in Stingl & Brockmöller, 2011)

Prospective on-going clinical trials with genotype-guided design may be illustrated by: a) IDANAT2 ("Isoniazid Dose Adjustment According to NAT2 Genotype"), initiated in Europe since 2008, aims to comparatively evaluate efficacy and liver toxicity of isoniazid administered in adjusted doses upon slow or fast acetylator status; b) phase II trial in North America on therapeutic strategy choice based on the presence of genotype tymidilate synthase TYMS TSER*3 "increased-risk" allele to the non-responders to fluoropyrimidines; c) phase III trial on rosiglitazone efficacy in Alzheimer's patients stratified by APOE4 allele presence or absence; d) prospective study on Lapatinib (TYKERB) efficacy in metastatic breast cancer overexpressing Her2/ErbB2 to identify biomarkers of acquired chemoresistance to initial anthracyclins, taxans and trastuzumab therapy. (Spraggs et al., 2009)

PREDICT-1 is the first powered, randomized, blinded, prospective trial to evaluate the clinical utility of prospective pharmacogenetic screening for HLA-B*5701 to reduce the incidence of abacavir hypersensitivity in an abacavir-naïve population of HIV-infected subjects. (Hughes et al., 2008)

GENDEP is the largest prospective study to examine the interaction of a moderate effect size between genetic (SLC6A4 variants) and clinical predictors (stressful life event - SLE) on response to antidepressants escitalopram and nortriptyline. The occurrence of antecedent SLEs predicted response to escitalopram and these effects were moderated by two functional polymorphisms *5-HTTLPR* and *STin4* in gene *SLC6A4* encoding the serotonin transporter. (Keers et al., 2011)

The large, randomized controlled clinical trials COAG and EU-PACT (European Pharmacogenetics of Anticoagulant Therapy) will establish the safety and clinical utility of genotype-guided dosing in daily practice for the three main coumarin derivatives (warfarin, acenocoumarol, phenprocoumone) used in Europe, measuring as primary outcome the percentage time in the therapeutic range for international normalized ratio. (van Schie et al., 2009; Squasina et al., 2010) In the meantime, a new rapid and inexpensive Allele-Specific Amplification (ASA)-PCR genotyping assay for vitamin K antagonist pharmacogenetics was validated that may reduce the frequency of over- and undertreatment patients, especially during drug initiation, and thus will improve patient safety. (Spohn et al., 2011)

5.3 Pharmacogenetics in drug design and development

Pharmacogenetics is integrated in all phases of drug discovery and development. A) Preclinically, in high-throughput screening of whole genome expression profile in interaction with drugs and validation of new "druggable" targets; identification the ADME polymorphisms relevant to the investigational substance and evaluate ADME genotyping in all subsequent clinical studies; prediction of the risk of allergy and organ toxicities in carriers of specific genotypes before first application in humans. B) In phase I, identification and validation of pharmacogenetic biomarkers obtained from preclinical data in order to stratify patients into genotypic segments of responders *vs.* non-responders; guide phase II trials design; explain the lack of efficacy or adverse drug reactions, in more cost-effective manner than later, in separate human pharmacogenetic studies. C) In phase II, guide evidenced-based decisions about further development of the investigational substance; potential for further drug/genotype test co-development in phase III. D) Phase III, extensive biomarker research for clear evidence-based data concerning pharmacogenetics for drug labeling (genotype-defined subgroups having particularly high efficacy or high risk for ADR); improving risk–benefit ratio in the case of label extension; identification of innovative treatment principles and drug targets; enrollment in the phase III-IV clinical trials only of the group of patients highly predictable to respond to therapy and excluding those with high risk of adverse drug reactions according to genotype. E) Pharmacovigilance in the post-marketing phase of drugs allows optimization and label changes of approved drugs to include pharmacogenetic genotyping in order to exclude patients who carry genotypes predicting high risk ADR or no response. F) Reconsideration of potentially valuable drugs withdrawn because of adverse drug effects by excluding carriers of risk genotypes and by indicating only to genotypes predictive for high efficacy. (Stingl & Brockmöller, 2011)

Pipeline pharmacogenetics marks the change from the current *lag phase* towards the *log phase*, thus accelerating the rate of marketed new chemical entities, reducing the attrition rate during the expensive late phase clinical development, increasing the benefit to risk ratio through early identification of nonresponders or those individuals with high risk of ADRs, especially if the critical proof of concept for efficacy is prospectively predicted in the protocol for a clinical trial so as to be regarded by regulators as hypothesis testing. Pharmacogenetics has determined a paradigm shift within pharmaceutical industry towards a "mini-blockbuster business model", thus recognizing its significant commercial and success rate contribution. (Lesko, 2007) Among other pipeline pharmacogenetics' benefits for pharmaceutical companies are: the opportunity to reconsider drugs which were initially stopped during development or withdrawn from the market; the ability to avoid investing in unfavorable products at earlier stages of development; the higher quality and more effective clinical trials design; reduction of research and development costs and periods; favorable impact on profit by increasing peak sales correspondent to a higher market share much earlier during the commercial life of the drug. For example, Eli Lilly has applied the tailored therapy strategy for drugs Xigris and Strattera. (Lechleiter, 2009, as cited in Fackler & McGuire, 2009; Roses, 2009)

Stingl and Brockmöller realize a comparative analysis of a variety of pharmacogenetics-related study designs integrated in all phases of drug development and clinical practice, evaluating the following issues: type and quality of evidence gained by each category of study design, their appropriated timeliness, as well as their pros and cons. The authors underline the necessity for new study designs for the clinical application of pharmacogenetics knowledge, as well as for mandatory requirements for the comprehensive characterization of relevant genetic variation in drug development. Future prospective interventional pharmacogenetic-trials in a genotype-preselected or outcomes-preselected population might represent one possible strategy to increase power in pharmacogenetic research at acceptable cost levels, especially to discover and validate the impact of genetic polymorphisms on drug response variability on the difficult-to-treat patients (poor-responders or severe adverse reactions) and in the elderly, on drug–drug interactions, or gene-gene interactions. (Stingl & Brockmöller, 2011)

Successful application of pipeline pharmacogenetics should meet some basic requirements, such as: obtaining the appropriately-documented informed consent; collection and storage of DNA samples for regulatory submission; implementing predictive exploratory pharmacogenetics studies on candidate gene and pathway-associated SNPs (rather than GWAS) during phase I clinical trials to generate hypothesis for early phase IIA, followed by hypothesis testing during phase IIB, in order to increase the statistical significance within a relatively smaller, well-defined group of patients. However, standardized methodologies should be established regarding: specification of sample source, standardization of diagnostic systems and treatments, adequate monitoring, sufficient length of observation, inclusion of possible confounding factors. (Roses, 2009; Spraggs et al., 2009)

The cost of pipeline pharmacogenetics is much lower in comparison with the cost of clinical trials and drug attrition. The advantages of large public-private partnerships at all stages of drug development in order to accelerate new medicines approval and biomarkers qualification and validation for selection of patients for clinical trials, monitoring drug effects and safety risk, regulatory guidelines harmonization and implementation, are illustrated by Eck and Paul. (Eck & Paul, 2010)

6. Pharmacogenetics' perspectives and challenges

High priority directions in the pharmacogenetic research for maximizing its potential benefit for personalized medicine are: 1) Chronic diseases (hypertension, diabetes, asthma, epilepsy, multiple sclerosis etc) which imply: high costs for healthcare system and patients, considerable management care costs; polymedication; low clinical outcomes due to compromised patients' quality of life, continuous suffering and low compliance to medication. 2) Medications with long adjustment periods of therapeutic doses and currently prescribed on "trial-and-error" basis, resulting in reduced compliance rates and increased management care costs. 3) Drugs with narrow therapeutic index (mercaptopurine, warfarin) that require close monitoring and constant dosage adjustment procedures to maintain therapeutic efficacy and minimize adverse reactions. 4) Drugs with severe, life-threatening adverse reactions which require high hospitalization costs (abacavir). 5) Very expensive medications with high clinical efficacy in some segments of population and for which a predictive diagnostic test might be developed (herceptin). (Grossman & Goldstein, 2009)

Pharmacogenetic testing is already implemented in some clinical areas, such as in cardiovascular diseases or in cancer, for selecting and/or dosing a specific medication, while in other fields, such as in psychiatry, the pharmacogenetic approach has been mostly used for the identification, validation and development of new meaningful biomarkers. (Squassina et al., 2010)

Of particular interest is pediatric pharmacogenetics that should consider both variation in gene expression and developmental context in which the genes of interest are functionally active (ontogeny). Apart from the application of pharmacogenetic testing to children for thiopurine-induced myelotoxicity, no other genotype-drug response associations validated in adults have been conclusively validated and no diagnostic or pharmacogenetic dosing algorithms have been so far translated in pediatric patients. (Ross CJ et al., 2011; Becker & Leeder, 2010) In order to achieve this gap, the Canadian Pharmacogenomics Network for Drug Safety (CPNDS) has implemented an active and targeted adverse drug reaction surveillance in pediatric patients with the aim of functional validation of identified gene markers, such as: warfarin-induced bleeding and thrombosis, vincristine-induced peripheral neuropathy, glucocorticoid-induced osteotoxicity, methotrexate-induced mucositis or leukoencephalopathy or nausea and vomiting, anthracycline cardiotoxicity, cisplatine-induced ototoxicity, neurotoxicity and nephrotoxicity. The final objective is to ensure generalizability of clinically significant findings and translation into a pharmacogenetic test of each predictive biomarker evaluated in prospective clinical trials (such as those dedicated to cisplatin ototoxicity and codeine-induced mortality in breastfed infants by mothers who are *CYP2D6* ultrarapid metabolizers and *UGT2B7*2* homozygous carriers), as well as to provide a cost–benefit analysis for validated predictive biomarker. (Loo et al., 2010)

6.1 Translational challenges

Successful integration of pharmacogenetics into future clinical practice and personalized medicine should overcome further translation barriers related to: a) global problems of scarcity of data demonstrating pharmacogenetic testing's clinical validity and utility; b) standardized and powerful statistical correlations between genotype and drug-response phenotype across different populations; c) education of health professionals and public; d) pharmacoeconomics issues; e) bioethical and social aspects; f) more favorable regulatory policy for clinical uptake of pharmacogenetics via sustaining large-scale industry-academia collaborations; g) the adoption of harmonized and standardized guidelines for biorepository and data sharing across multi-national networks; h) lack of incentives for the private sector to invest in the development and licensing of pharmacogenetics diagnostic tests for improving the safety and efficacy of out-of-patent drugs. (Spraggs et al., 2009; Gurwitz et al., 2009)

Scientific community and International Society of Pharmacogenomics Education Forum have called for the enhanced implementation of pharmacogenomics and personalized medicine into core medical teaching curricula and practice, in order to fill in the gap between intensive research on validated pharmacogenetic testing and its appropriate, effective clinical integration and interpretation in routine individualized therapy. (Squassina et al., 2010) For instance, Pharmacogenomics Education Program (PharmGenEd™) is an educational platform for dissemination of evidence-based clinically relevant pharmacogenomics, fostering educational and scientific collaboration among educators, researchers and clinicians (http://pharmacogenomics.ucsd.edu). PharmGenEd also participates along with Pharmacogenomics Knowledge Base (PharmGKB) and National Institute of Health Pharmacogenomic Research Network (NIH PGRN), in the Clinical Pharmacogenetics Implementation Consortium (CPIC) to create a curated resource for storing, annotating and updating specific data relevant for clinical implementation of pharmacogenetic testing. (Kuo et al., 2011)

The adoption of the pharmacogenetics tests for personalized medicine depends on clinical- and cost-effectiveness analyses on which the reimbursement for their routine use will be based. (Liewei et al., 2011) In the context of pharmacoeconomic models, pharmacogenetic testing might be regarded more cost-effective than cost-saving, or at least cost-effective for particular combinations of treatment, genetic polymorphisms and disease, depending greatly on the differences among healthcare systems and reimbursement policies. (Squassina et al., 2010; Trent, 2010)

Appropriate protection for privacy and confidentiality of databases with large amount of genotypic, phenotypic and demographic data regarding individuals is crucial in order to avoid the possible risk of psychosocial harm, genetic and social discrimination, privacy and possible implications for employment and access to life and health insurance. (Squassina et al., 2010) Moreover, pharmaceutical companies could voluntarily ignore, for economic reasons, patients with rare or complex genetic conditions or those who are not responding to any known treatment, leading to consequent deprivation of effective treatments. These concerns are attenuated by USA specific regulations, such as the Genetic Information Nondiscrimination Act (GINA), the Health Insurance Portability and Accountability Act Privacy Rule, and the Genomics and Personalized Medicine Act (GPMA), as well as by founded nonprofit organizations of major key stakeholders (pharmaceutical companies, healthcare providers and payers, patient advocacy groups, industry policy organizations, academic institutions and government agencies), like the Personalized Medicine Coalition and Pharmacogenetics for Every Nation Initiative (PGENI). (Squassina et al., 2010)

Taking into account the ethical, legal and social issues of pharmacogenetics research, as well as the multi-disciplinary opinions of the key stakeholders, Howard and colleagues have identified six outstanding ethical issues raised by the informed consent process in pharmacogenetics research and proposed valuable recommendations for the development of future practical pharmacogenetics consent guidelines, such as: 1) scope of consent; 2) consent to pharmacogenetics 'add-on' studies; (3) confidentiality, privacy protection and coding of personal information in long-term databases, especially in those controlled by private pharmaceutical companies; (4) intellectual property and commercialization policy of pharmacogenetics research projects with financial benefit-sharing plan; (5) disclosure of the possibility of deposition and sharing in public repository of the samples and data, at the onset of the pharmacogenetics study; (6) potential risks stemming from population-based research so as to avoid overgeneralizations and undermining the moral, cultural and religious standards. (Howard et al., 2011)

6.2 Pharmacogenetics' perspectives by next generation sequencing

GWAS are particularly useful to determine the most significant SNPs associated with a phenotype amongst a high-density set of polymorphisms, in cases where there are large cohorts to evaluate, clinical end points are simple to define without variability, and the genetic factors associated with the end points are highly penetrant. However, GWAS are discovery- rather than hypothesis-driven, result in weak statistical power and false positives, need large sample size, cost and computing power requirements. Therefore, GWAS imply a two-stage design where discoveries made using a high-density SNP array are then validated using a hypothesis design on replicative populations. (Sissung et al., 2010) Nonetheless, for ADR with a significant genetic component that confers a large effect (carbamazepine-induced Stevens–Johnson syndrome, abacavir-induced hypersensitivity, statin-induced myopathy and gefitinib-induced diarrhoea), associations can be identified with a relatively small number of samples (10–100 cases). (Loo et al., 2010; Davis & Johnson, 2011)

Rare variants in complex mixtures of DNA might be quantitatively measured by mass spectrometry-based genotyping. Fluidigm's microfluidic device ("lab-on-chip"), able to mix 96 samples and 96 primer sets in nano-scale assay chambers that support over 9000 parallel qRT-PCR reactions, could be also used for genotyping and targeted sequence capture; thus filling the gap between biomarker evaluation of a few candidate genes and the hundreds of markers GWAS-discovered. (Gibson, 2011)

The development of next-generation sequencing (NGS) or massively parallel sequencing, as well as nanopore sequencing technologies, through whole-genome, whole-exome and whole-transcriptome analysis, allows fast, inexpensive, reliable production of large volumes of DNA or RNA sequence data. (Metzker, 2011; Tucker et al., 2009) NGS comprises a number of methods that are grouped broadly as template preparation, sequencing and imaging, genome alignment and assembly, and data analysis. The unique combination of specific protocols distinguishes one technology from another and determines the type of data produced from commercial platforms such as: Roche/454, Illumina/Solexa, Life/APG and Helicos BioSciences, the Polonator instrument and the Pacific Biosciences. The NGS technologies, their broad applications and guidelines for platform selection to address biological questions of interest are reviewed by Metzker (Metzker, 2011). Having aligned the digested fragments of individuals' targeted regions of genome to a reference genome, 'SNP calling' identifies variable sites, whereas 'genotype calling' determines the genotype for each individual at each site, thus revealing principal types of genome alterations (like nucleotide substitutions, small insertions and deletions, copy number alterations, chromosomal rearrangements). (Rasmus et al., 2011) Computational, biological and clinical analyses of the resulting genome data will assess reproducibility and statistical significance; links to pathways and the functional relevance of mutated genes to disease; and the relationships of genome alterations with cancer prognosis and response to therapy, respectively. (Meyerson et al., 2010)

Over a relatively short time frame, DNA sequencing has become cheaper and faster (US$ 1,000 price tag for a whole human genome sequence now seems feasible) and even more with the foreseeable third-generation DNA sequencers utilizing single molecules and avoiding initial cloning or amplification steps. (Trent, 2010; Pushkarev et al., 2009)

In addition to NGS rapid technological developments, the promotion of alternative strategies for delivery of healthcare through nontraditional pathology laboratories, such as direct-to-consumer (DTC) DNA tests and point-of-care DNA testing, will expand the integration of pharmacogenetics into clinical practice by assisting health practitioner to make on-the-spot decisions about the individualisation of drug and dose directly at the bedside in the intensive care unit or consulting room. (Trent, 2010)

6.3 New players in pharmacogenetics: Alternative splicing, miRNAs and structural RNA polymorphisms

In addition to polymorphisms in protein-coding genes (nonsynonymous SNPs) associated to complex diseases, alternative splicing in protein-coding genes and variations in microRNAs and other noncoding RNAs have emerged as new players in pharmacogenetics and they should be considered in an integrative approach in deciphering the genotype-induced inter-individual variability of drugs' tolerance, efficacy and metabolism.

Alternative splicing of pre-mRNAs was proposed 30 years ago by the Nobel Prize winner Walter Gilbert as a way of generating different mRNAs from a single gene and it is regarded as one of the most elegant and important mechanisms for proteome diversity generation. Alternative splicing in protein-coding genes can affect the biological activity of proteins, having major consequences on drug metabolism and drug response phenotype. Generation of wrong alternative splicing variants is a common feature of complex diseases and also an important player in drug resistance and ADME. For example, alternative splicing variants in the BCR–ABL fused gene were correlated with Imatinib mesylate resistance in chronic myelogenous leukemia patients (Gruber et al., 2006, as cited in Passetti et al., 2009); whereas splicing isoforms of nuclear pregnane and constitutive androstane receptors can affect the pharmacokinetics and pharmacodynamics of docetaxel and doxorubicin in Asian patients. (Horr et al., 2008, as cited in Passetti et al., 2009) The functional relevance of alternative splicing of pre-mRNAs and generated splice variants in the context of whole genome studies instead of a single gene would reveal how they will affect cellular networks and pathways. (Passetti et al., 2009)

The noncoding RNAs (ncRNAs) are a large group of transcripts lacking protein-coding potential, having variable size range from approx. 18 to 25 nucleotides for the families of microRNAs (miRNAs) and small interfering RNAs (siRNAs), approx. 20 to 300 nucleotides for small RNAs commonly found as transcriptional and translational regulators, or up to and beyond 10 000 nucleotides in length for RNAs involved in various other processes. (Costa FF, 2008, as cited in Passetti et al., 2009) miRNAs are noncoding RNAs that can regulate gene expression by Watson–Crick base pairing to target several mRNAs in a gene regulatory network. The binding of miRNAs to their target mRNAs is critical for regulating mRNA levels and therefore protein expression. miRNAs are master regulators of important gene and transcriptome networks in eukaryotic cells, they can block mRNA translation and affect both the expression of at least 30% of all protein-coding genes by targeting their 3'-UTR sequences and long ncRNAs. A growing number of reports have been showing the associations of deregulated expression of miRNAs in complex diseases (cancer, obesity, diabetes, schizophrenia) by altering the regulation of expression of many important genes. One miRNA can downregulate multiple target proteins by interacting with different target mRNAs ('one hit multiple targets' concept), thus pointing out the particular therapeutic relevance of miRNAs as an attractive drug target. (Wurdinger & Costa, 2007, as cited in Passetti et al., 2009) Moreover, polymorphisms in miRNAs represent a newly identified type of genetic variability that can influence the risk of diseases and also variability in pharmacokinetics and pharmacodynamics of drugs. For instance, polymorphisms in miRNA target sites of protein-coding genes are associated to cancer, hypertension, asthma, cardiovascular disease, and polymorphisms in microRNAs are associated with schizophrenia, Parkinson. (Passetti et al., 2009) In addition, long ncRNAs, increasingly seen as functional genes, have been involved in disease progression, such as: *ZNFX1-NA1* in breast cancer, *SPRY4-IN* in melanoma; *NEAT1* long ncRNA in Alzheimer. (Gibson, 2011)

Alternative splicing might affect microRNA regulation and subsequently microRNAs are able to regulate hundreds of effector genes in a multilevel regulatory mechanism that allow individual miRNAs to profoundly affect the gene expression program in the cells. Both microRNA regulation and alternative splicing will induce changes in proteome diversity that can affect the way drugs are metabolized by patients, and this will have major implications for both drug design and personalized medicine in the future. Furthermore, genetic variations in the sequence of miRNAs, target sites of miRNAs and alternative splicing will affect gene regulatory networks and pathways responsible for drug metabolism and resistance, thus emerging as a new paradigm clearly redefining the pharmacogenomics field and personalized medicine. (Passetti et al., 2009)

Structural RNA SNPs (srSNPs) designate genetic polymorphisms in the transcribed regions of genes that affect RNA functions and represent ~49% (synonymous SNPs, 2%; those in 5'- and 3'-untranslated regions, 2%; intronic, 45%) from disease-associated SNPs derived from GWAS, whereas nonsynonymous (coding cSNPs) account for only ~9% and regulatory SNPs (rSNPs; SNPs in intergenic regions that alter transcription of protein-coding genes) for ~43%. (Hindorff et al., 2009, as cited in Sadee et al., 2011) Structural RNA SNPs affect RNA functions such as splicing, turnover and translation, having tissue-specific effects, while regulatory single-nucleotide polymorphisms (rSNPs) affect transcription. (Sadee et al., 2011)

Recent GWAS and next-generation sequencing of the transcriptome have opened path for large-scale exploration of mRNA expression quantitative trait loci (eQTLs) which are commonly categorized as rSNPs affecting transcription and altering mRNA expression levels in target tissues. (Sadee, 2009, as cited in Sadee et al., 2011) Furthermore, the evaluation of allelic ratios of transcripts would enable the detection of rSNPs and srSNPs, by revealing any deviation from unity expected in an autosomal gene - termed "allelic expression imbalance" (AEI) – that indicates the presence of cis-regulatory factors and represents a more precise relative measure of transcript activity as compared with total mRNA levels. (Johnson, 2008, as cited in Sadee et al., 2011) Structural RNA polymorphisms will likely prove essential to fill gaps in the "missing heritability", substantially contributing to discover pharmacogenetic biomarkers of increased predictive power. The clinical relevance of rSNPs and srSNPs has greatly contributed the available validated predictive genetic variants. For example, there are validated srSNPs and rSNPs in DME (*CYP2C19, CYP2D6, CYP3A5, UGT1A1, NAT1, ABCB1, ABCC2*) associated with variability in the bioactivation, pharmacokinetics and clinical outcome of clopidogrel, tamoxifen, statins, efavirenz, tacrolimus, paclitaxel, antiretrovirals. Moreover, validated srSNPs and rSNPs in genes that encode drug targets (D2 dopamine receptor gene *DRD2*) are associated with poor response to antipsychotics or with risk for metabolic syndrome (rSNPs in gene *TPH2* encoding tryptophan hydroxylase). (Sadee et al., 2011)

6.4 Pharmacogenetics' perspectives by biobanking and electronic health records

Global surveys conducted by the Industry Pharmacogenomics Working Group (I-PWG) in order to determine current industry and institutional review boards/ ethical committee (IRB/EC) practices, policies and standards, for prospective biospecimens' collection and storage for pharmacogenomics research, emphasize the significant value of pharmacogenetics research and biobanking for personalized medicine, as well as the necessity for harmonization and standardization across the industry and the key stakeholders in regulations concerning: sample acquisition and data privacy protection, pharmacogenetics-related language in informed consent, outsourcing of DNA sample storage, "clinical relevance" of the genetic information to be returned to the patients, benefits and foreseeable risks. (Franc et al., 2011a, 2011b; Warner et al., 2011; Ricci et al., 2011)

The creation of a biorepository that are closely link with electronic medical records (EMR) may be an economically efficient approach to genomic medicine and especially to GWAS that require DNA sample from large populations with robust phenotypic data. The Geisinger MyCode Biorepository is perhaps the first large-scale biobanking project around EMR. In addition, a data warehouse project – the Clinical Decision Information System – initiated in 2006 aims to assembly in a single point of reference 40 different data sources regarding patients' clinical phenotype, biobanks, clinical trials databases, as well as financial, administrative, operational and patient survey databases. Such data warehouses allow optimizing performance, maintaining control and privacy aspects, reliability, robustness and fast-response. (Gerhard et al., 2009)

Large multi-national consortia have been already established, such as NIH-funded PGRN, and NIH-funded Electronic Medical Records and Genomics Network (eMERGE), which are catalogued in Pharmacogenomics Knowledge Base. (McCarty & Wilke, 2010)

The convergence of the rapidly expanding biomedical informatics, high-throughput genotyping, DNA biobanks and EMR across large health-care networks, plays a pivotal role in pharmacogenomics' translation to the bedside. Through real-time monitoring of multiple de-identified EMR databases integrated in sophisticated cross-institutional networks (e.g., the PGRN, the eMERGE network, and the HMO Research Network, Harvard University/Partners Healthcare system i2b2, the Vanderbilt BioVu), highly accurate quantifying disease phenotypes and treatment outcomes could be efficiently extracted by the application of natural language processing (NLP), semantic interoperability, data normalization strategies and novel bioinformatics platforms. The following translational mechanisms are envisaged: (i) retrospective assessment of previously known findings in a clinical practice-setting; (ii) discovery of new associations in huge observational cohorts; (iii) prospective application in a setting capable of providing real-time decision support; iv) enhance pharmacovigilance, especially during the postmarketing phase; vi) validation of previous conventional cohort-driven GWAS, in a cost-effective, earlier and more accurately manner. (Wilke et al., 2011; Kohane, 2011) In addition, electronic health records-driven genomic research (EDGR) will provide a rich set of comprehensive clinical phenotypes, in close to real time, at a low cost and a high degree of timeliness, matched to the corresponding DNA samples from biorepositories. The cost-efficiency advantage of EDGR comes from maximizing the research utility of that clinical-care investment such that it is only a fraction of a *de novo* research cohort pipeline. Other advantages of EDGR include: ability to assess in-depth the clinical significance of genomic associations; great representation of a clinical population; data on environmental exposures; broad and accurate reflection of clinical phenotypes and controls; identification of confounders. (Kohane, 2011) In the future, as standardization across national biobanks-linked EMR, consent procedures and ownership of the derived intellectual property will be adopted, genetic data will be recorded preemptively into each patient's EMR, and robust biomedical informatics platforms will interrogate this information during the process of clinical decision making, providing efficient real-time decision support at the point of care. (Wilke et al., 2011; Kohane, 2011)

Development of simple, up-to-date, easily accessible, reliable clinical algorithms and guidelines must guide physicians in the interpretation of genetic data, decision making about diagnostic testing and follow-up clinical care. These point-of-care tools will be embedded in electronic health records system and it will be crucial to accelerate the individualized medicine. (Fackler & McGuire, 2009; Liewei et al., 2011)

In addition, the implementation of robust health information technology able to electronically manage all different types of -*omics* biomarker data and phenotypic characterization of research study participants, might be illustrated by software platforms like: Hewlett-Packard's Gateway for Integrated Genomics - Proteomics Applications and Data (GIGPAD) or Microsoft's Amalga. (Fackler & McGuire, 2009)

The National Institute of Health's Pharmacogenomics Research Network (PGRN) is a collaborative partnership of research groups funded "to lead discovery and advance translation in genomics in order to enable safer and more effective drug therapies", with the ultimate goal to predict and personalize medicine in routine clinical practice. (Long & Berg, 2011) PGRN's accomplishments and future projects to provide peer-reviewed, updated, evidence-based, freely accessible guidelines for gene/drug pairs, so as to facilitate the translation and interpretation of preemptive pharmacogenomic tests for the most relevant pharmacogenes from laboratory, through electronic medical records system, into decision-making prescription recommendations, have been extensively discussed. (Long & Berg, 2011; Roden & Tyndale, 2011; Relling & Klein, 2011)

6.5 Further perspectives in pharmacogenomics

Further perspectives for pharmacogenomics to emerge as an important piece in the puzzle of personalized medicine will concern: a) the integration of pharmacogenomics with additional, non-drug-related patient characteristics, individual disease factors, and environmental aspects (Kroemer, 2010); b) tissue-specific epigenetic changes, microRNAs or "junk DNA" (Trent, 2010); c) discovery of useful pharmacogenetic markers in the mitochondrial DNA (mtDNA) within transmitochondrial cell lines or cybrids in order to optimize antibiotherapy (Squassina et al., 2010); d) biomarkers validation for drug therapy in organ transplantation and for complex diseases characterized by a great phenotypic and genetic variability; e) coordinated implementation into certified laboratories of the pharmacogenes' next-generation-sequencing, according to GCP guidelines; f) the adaptation of the regulatory and reimbursement environment. (Fackler & McGuire, 2009)

Moreover, nanotechnology is projected to play a critical role in personalized medicine, greatly dependent on the evolutionary development of a systems biology approach to clinical medicine based upon "-omic" technology analysis and integration. In a comprehensive review, Sakamoto and colleagues analyse: the current state of nano-based products over a vast array of clinical indications and patient specificity; rational design of nanotechnologies for individualized therapy; nano-based injectable therapeutics, implantable drug-delivery devices; nanotechnology and tissue engineering; nanowires and cantilevers arrays that are used to detect minute amount of protein biomarkers. (Sakamoto et al., 2010)

7. Conclusions

Pharmacogenomics is the interface between genomic medicine and systems pharmacology and its translation from bench into clinical practice is broadening the perspective of personalized medicine so as in the near future we might rely on a "DNA chip"/"pharmacogenomic card" specific to each patient and on each genotype preemptively recorded in EMR, in order to individualize both the diagnostic procedures and the safest and most efficient medications prior to treatment initiation. Although it is still regarded as an elusive dream due to limited marketed drug–test companion products and actually implemented clinical practices, pharmacogenomics translation into personalized medicine has become a more imminent reality. Advances in next-generation sequencing technology to uncover the contribution of "missing heritability" to biomarker-guided therapeutic individualization, the convergence of biorepositories- and electronic health records-pharmacogenomics research, the encouraging initiatives for policy and guidelines harmonization, as well as extensive collaborations across large pharmacogenomic networks, will hopefully overcome the current challenges ahead on the road to personalized medicine and will play a pivotal role in pharmacogenomics' translation to the bedside.

8. References

Afdhal NH, McHutchison JG, Zeuzem S, Mangia A, Pawlotsky JM, Murray JS, Shianna KV, Tanaka Y, Thomas DL, Booth DR, Goldstein DB. (2011) Hepatitis C pharmacogenetics: state of the art in 2010. *Hepatology*. Vol.53, No.1, pp.336-45

Aislyn DW, Seth IB, Ravi I. (2009) Systems pharmacology and genome medicine: a future perspective. *Genome Medicine*, No. 1, pp. 11-20

Becker ML, Leeder JS. (2010) Identifying genomic and developmental causes of adverse drug reactions in children. *Pharmacogenomics*. 11(11), pp.1591-602

Broich K., Moeller H.J. (2008) Pharmacogenetics, pharmacogenomics and personalized psychiatry: Are we there yet? *Eur Arch Psychiatry Clin Neurosci,* 258[Suppl 1]:1–2.

Burns DK, Hughes AR, Power A, Wang SJ, Patterson SD. (2010) Designing pharmacogenomic studies to be fit for purpose. *Pharmacogenomics.* 11(12), pp.1657-67

Davis HM, Johnson JA. (2011) Heart failure pharmacogenetics: past, present, and future. *Curr Cardiol Rep. Jun;* 13(3), pp.175-84

Eck SL, Paul SM. (2010) Biomarker qualification via public-private partnerships. *Clin Pharmacol Ther.* 87(1), pp. 21-3

Fackler JL, McGuire AL. (2009) Paving the Way to Personalized Genomic Medicine: Steps to Successful Implementation. *Curr Pharmacogenomics Person Med.* 1;7(2), pp.125-132

Franc MA, Cohen N, Warner AW, Shaw PM, Groenen P, Snapir A. (2011a) Industry Pharmacogenomics Working Group. Coding of DNA samples and data in the pharmaceutical industry: current practices and future directions--perspective of the I-PWG. *Clin Pharmacol Ther.* 89(4), pp. 537-45

Franc MA, Warner AW, Cohen N, Shaw PM, Groenen P, Snapir A. (2011b) Current practices for DNA sample collection and storage in the pharmaceutical industry, and potential areas for harmonization: perspective of the I-PWG. *Clin Pharmacol Ther.* 89(4), pp.546-53

Frueh FW. (2009) Back to the future: why randomized controlled trials cannot be the answer to pharmacogenomics and personalized medicine. *Pharmacogenomics.* 10(7), pp. 1077-81

Gerhard GS, Langer DR, Carey JD & Stewart FW. (2009) Electronic Medical Records in Genomic Medicine Practice and Research. In *Genomic and Personalized Medicine,* Edited by Huntington F. Willard & Geoffrey S. Ginsburg, Academic Press, pp. 233-241

Gibson G. (2011) Biomarkers in the next decade. Conference Scene - The Inaugural Australian Biomarker Discovery Conference. *Pharmacogenomics* 12(2), pp. 155–157

Gonzalez-Haba E, García MI, Cortejoso L, et al. (2010) ABCB1 gene polymorphisms are associated with adverse reactions in fluoropyrimidine-treated colorectal cancer patients. *Pharmacogenomics.* 11(12), pp. 1715-23

Grossman I., Goldstein DB. (2009) Pharmacogenetics and Pharmacogenomics. In *Genomic and Personalized Medicine,* Edited by Huntington F. Willard & Geoffrey S. Ginsburg, Academic Press, pp. 321-334

Gurwitz D, Zika E, Hopkins MM, Gaisser S, Ibarreta D. (2009) Pharmacogenetics in Europe: barriers and opportunities. *Public Health Genomics.* 12(3), pp.134-41

Holmes DR Jr, Dehmer GJ, Kaul S, Leifer D, O'Gara PT, Stein CM. (2010) ACCF/AHA clopidogrel clinical alert: approaches to the FDA "boxed warning": a report of the American College of Cardiology Foundation *J Am Coll Cardiol.* 56, pp.321-341

Howard HC, Joly Y, Avard D, Laplante N, Phillips M, Tardif JC. (2011) Informed consent in the context of pharmacogenomic research: ethical considerations. *Pharmacogenomics J.* 11(3), pp. 155-61

Hughes S, Hughes A, Brothers C, Spreen W, Thorborn D. (2008) CNA106030 Study Team. PREDICT-1 (CNA106030): the first powered, prospective trial of pharmacogenetic screening to reduce drug adverse events. *Pharm Stat.* 7(2), pp.121-9

Jian-Ping Zhang, Anil KM. (2011) Pharmacogenetics and Antipsychotics: Therapeutic Efficacy and Side Effects Prediction. *Expert Opin Drug Metab Toxicol.* 7(1), pp. 9–37

Keers R, Uher R, Huezo-Diaz P, Smith R, et al. (2011) Interaction between serotonin transporter gene variants and life events predicts response to antidepressants in the GENDEP project. *Pharmacogenomics J.* 11(2), pp.138-45

Kohane IS. (2011) Using electronic health records to drive discovery in disease genomics. *Nat Rev Genet.* 12(6), pp.417-28

Kroemer HK, Meyer zu Schwabedissen HE. (2010) A piece in the puzzle of personalized medicine. *Clin Pharmacol Ther.* 87(1), pp.19-20

Kuo MG, Ma DJ, Lee KC, Halpert RJ, Bourne EP, Ganiats GT, Taylor P. (2011) Pharmacogenomics Education Program (PharmGenEd™): bridging the gap between science and practice. *Pharmacogenomics* 12(2), pp. 149–153

Lesko LJ. (2007) Personalized medicine: elusive dream or imminent reality? *Clin Pharmacol Ther.* 81(6), pp. 807-16

Liewei W., McLeod HL, Weinshilboum RM. (2011) Genomics and Drug Response, *N Engl J Med*, 364, pp.1144-1153

Long RM, Berg JM. (2011) What to expect from the Pharmacogenomics Research Network. *Clin Pharmacol Ther.* 89(3), pp. 339-41

Loo TT, Ross CJ, Sistonen J, Visscher H, Madadi P, Koren G, Hayden MR, Carleton BC. (2010) Pharmacogenomics and active surveillance for serious adverse drug reactions in children. *Pharmacogenomics.* 11(9), pp.1269-85

Mallal S, Phillips E, Carosi G, et al. (2008) HLA-B*5701 screening for hypersensitivity to abacavir. *N Engl J Med* 358, pp.568-579

McCarty CA, Wilke RA. (2010) Biobanking and pharmacogenomics. *Pharmacogenomics.* 11(5), pp. 637-41

McDonald MG, Rieder MJ, Nakano M, Hsia CK, Rettie AE. (2009) CYP4F2 is a vitamin K1 oxidase: an explanation for altered warfarin dose in carriers of the V433M variant. *Mol Pharmacol.* 75, pp.1337-1346

Mega JL, Close SL, Wiviott SD, et al. (2009) Cytochrome P-450 polymorphisms and response to clopidogrel. *N Engl J Med* 360, pp.354-362

Metzker ML. (2011) Sequencing technologies - the next generation. *Nature Reviews Genetics,* 12, pp. 31-46

Meyerson M, Stacey G, Gad G. (2010) Advances in understanding cancer genomes through second-generation sequencing. *Nature Reviews Genetics,* 11, pp. 685-696

Nakamura Y. (2008) Pharmacogenomics and Drug Toxicity. *N Engl J Med.* 359, pp. 856-858

Pare G, Mehta SR, Yusuf S, et al. (2010) Effects of CYP2C19 genotype on outcomes of clopidogrel treatment. *N Engl J Med* 363, pp.1704-1714

Passetti F, Ferreira CG, Costa FF. (2009) The impact of microRNAs and alternative splicing in pharmacogenomics. *The Pharmacogenomics Journal* 9, pp. 1–13.

Pearson ER. (2009) Pharmacogenetics of Diabetes. *Current Diabetes Reports,* 9, pp. 172–181.

Phillips EJ, Chung WH, Mockenhaupt M, Roujeau JC, Mallal SA. (2011) Drug hypersensitivity: pharmacogenetics and clinical syndromes. *Allergy Clin Immunol.* 127(3 Suppl):S60-6

Pushkarev D, Neff NF, Quake SR. (2009) Single-molecule sequencing of an individual human genome. *Nature Biotech.* 27, pp. 847–852

Rasmus Nielsen, Joshua S. Paul, Anders Albrechtsen, Yun S. Song. (2011) Genotype and SNP calling from next-generation sequencing data. *Nature Reviews Genetics,* 12, pp.443-451

Relling MV, Klein TE. (2011) CPIC: Clinical Pharmacogenetics Implementation Consortium of the Pharmacogenomics Research Network. *Clin Pharmacol Ther.* 89(3), pp.464-7

Ricci DS, Broderick ED, Tchelet A, Hong F, Mayevsky S, Mohr DM, Schaffer ME, Warner AW, Hakkulinen P, Snapir A. (2011) Global requirements for DNA sample collections: results of a survey of 204 ethics committees in 40 countries. *Clin Pharmacol Ther.* 89(4), pp.554-61

Roden DM, Tyndale RF. (2011) Pharmacogenomics at the tipping point: challenges and opportunities. *Clin Pharmacol Ther.* 89(3), pp.323-7

Romaine SP, Bailey KM, Hall AS, Balmforth AJ. (2010) The influence of SLCO1B1 (OATP1B1) gene polymorphisms on response to statin therapy. *Pharmacogenomics J.* 10(1), pp.1-11

Roses AD. (2009) The medical and economic roles of pipeline pharmacogenetics: Alzheimer's disease as a model of efficacy and HLA-B*5701 as a model of safety. *Neuropsychopharmacology.* 34(1), pp.6-17.

Ross EM, Kenakin TP. (2006) Pharmacodynamics. Mechanisms of Drug Action and the Relationship Between Drug Concentration and Effect. In *Goodman & Gilman's The Pharmacological Basis of Therapeutics.* 11th edition, McGraw-Hill New York, pp. 31-44.

Ross CJ, Visscher H, Rassekh SR, Castro-Pastrana LI, Shereck E, Carleton B, Hayden MR (2011) Pharmacogenomics of serious adverse drug reactions in pediatric oncology. *J Popul Ther Clin Pharmacol,* Vol 18, No 1, e134-151

Sadee W, Wang D, Papp AC, Pinsonneault JK, Smith RM, Moyer RA, Johnson AD. (2011) Pharmacogenomics of the RNA world: structural RNA polymorphisms in drug therapy. *Clin Pharmacol Ther.* 89(3), pp.355-65

Sagreiya H, Berube C, Wen A, et al. (2010) Extending and evaluating a warfarin dosing algorithm that includes CYP4F2 and pooled rare variants of CYP2C9. *Pharmacogenet Genomics* 20, pp.407-413

Sakamoto JH, van de Ven AL, Godin B, Blanco E, et al. (2010) Enabling individualized therapy through nanotechnology. *Pharmacol Res.* 62(2), pp. 57-89

Seip RL, Duconge J, Ruaño G. (2010) Implementing genotype-guided antithrombotic therapy. *Future Cardiol.* 6(3), pp.409-24

Shianna KV. (2009) Genome-Wide Association Studies and Genotyping Technologies. In *Genomic and Personalized Medicine,* Edited by Huntington F. Willard & Geoffrey S. Ginsburg, Academic Press, pp. 101-107

Shuldiner AR, O'Connell JR, Bliden KP, et al. (2009) Association of cytochrome P450 2C19 genotype with the antiplatelet effect and clinical efficacy of clopidogrel therapy. *JAMA* 302, pp. 849-857

Sissung TM, English BC, Venzon D, Figg WD, Deeken JF. (2010) Clinical pharmacology and pharmacogenetics in a genomics era: the DMET platform. *Pharmacogenomics.* Vol. 11, No 1, Jan. 2010, pp 89-103

Spohn G, Geisen C, Luxembourg B, Sittinger K, Seifried E, Bönig H. (2011) Validation of a Rapid and Inexpensive Allele-Specific Amplification (ASA)-PCR Genotyping Assay for Vitamin K Antagonist Pharmacogenomics. *Mol Diagn Ther.* 1;15(1), pp.13-9

Spraggs FC, Koshy TB, Edbrooke RM, Roses DA. (2009) Role of Pharmacogenomics in Drug Development. In *Genomic and Personalized Medicine,* Edited by Huntington F. Willard & Geoffrey S. Ginsburg, Academic Press, pp. 343-356

Squassina A, Manchia M, Manolopoulos VG, Artac M, et al. (2010) Realities and expectations of pharmacogenomics and personalized medicine: impact of translating genetic knowledge into clinical practice. *Pharmacogenomics.* 11(8), pp. 1149-67

Stingl Kirchheiner JC, Brockmöller J. (2011) Why, when, and how should pharmacogenetics be applied in clinical studies?: current and future approaches to study designs. *Clin Pharmacol Ther.* 89(2), pp.198-209

Surh LC, Pacanowski MA, Haga SB, Hobbs S, Lesko LJ, Gottlieb S, et al. (2010) Learning from product labels and label changes: how to build pharmacogenomics into drug-development programs. *Pharmacogenomics.* 11(12), pp.1637-47

Teichert M, Eijgelsheim M, Rivadeneira F, et al. (2009) A genome-wide association study of acenocoumarol maintenance dosage. *Hum Mol Genet* 18, pp.3758-3768

Tepper IR., Roubenoff R. (2009) The Role of Genomics and Genetics in Drug Discovery and Development. In *Genomic and Personalized Medicine,* Edited by Huntington F. Willard & Geoffrey S. Ginsburg, Academic Press, pp.335-342

The International Warfarin Pharmacogenetics Consortium. (2009) Estimation of the warfarin dose with clinical and pharmacogenetic data. *N Engl J Med* 360: 753-764

Tomalik-Scharte A, Lazar A, Fuhr U, Kirchheiner J. (2008) The clinical role of genetic polymorphisms in drug-metabolizing enzymes. *The Pharmacogenomics Journal,* 8, pp. 4-14.

Tozzi V. (2010) Pharmacogenetics of antiretrovirals. *Antiviral Res.* 85(1), pp.190-200

Trent RJ. (2010) Pathology practice and pharmacogenomics. *Pharmacogenomics.* 11(1), pp.105-11

Tucker T, Marra M, Friedman JM. (2009) Massively parallel sequencing: the next big thing in genetic medicine. *Am. J. Hum. Genet.* 85, pp.142–154

van Schie RM, Wadelius MI, Kamali F, Daly AK, Manolopoulos VG, de Boer A, Barallon R, Verhoef TI, Kirchheiner J, Haschke-Becher E, Briz M, Rosendaal FR, Redekop WK, Pirmohamed M, Maitland van der Zee AH. (2009) Genotype-guided dosing of coumarin derivatives: the European pharmacogenetics of anticoagulant therapy (EU-PACT) trial design. *Pharmacogenomics.* 10(10), pp.1687-95

Warner AW, Bhathena A, Gilardi S, Mohr D, Leong D, Bienfait KL, Sarang J, Duprey S, Franc MA, Nelsen A, Snapir A. (2011) Challenges in obtaining adequate genetic sample sets in clinical trials: the perspective of the industry pharmacogenomics working group. *Clin Pharmacol Ther.* 89(4), pp. 529-36

Wilke RA, Xu H, Denny JC, Roden DM, Krauss RM, McCarty CA, Davis RL, Skaar T, Lamba J, Savova G. (2011) The emerging role of electronic medical records in pharmacogenomics. *Clin Pharmacol Ther.* 89(3), pp.379-86

Willard F.H. (2009). Organization, Variation and Expression of the Human Genome as a Foundation of Genomic and Personalized Medicine. In *Genomic and Personalized Medicine,* Edited by Huntington F. Willard & Geoffrey S. Ginsburg, Academic Press, pp. 4-21

Woodcock J, Lesko LJ. (2009) Pharmacogenetics – Tailoring Treatment for the Outliers, *N Engl J Med* 360(8), pp. 811-813

Yee SW, Chen L, Giacomini KM. (2010) Pharmacogenomics of membrane transporters: past, present and future. *Pharmacogenomics.* 11(4), pp.475-9

Zanger UM, Turpeinen Miia, Klein Kathrin, Schwab M. (2008) Functional pharmacogenetics/genomics of human cytochromes P450 involved in drug biotransformation. *Anal Bioanal Chem.* 392, pp.1093–1108

Multiplexed Pharmacogenetic Assays for SNP Genotyping: Tools and Techniques for Individualizing Patient Therapy

Susan J. Hsiao[1] and Alex J. Rai[1,2,*]
[1]Department of Pathology, Columbia University Medical Center, New York, NY,
[2]Special Chemistry Laboratory, New York Presbyterian Hospital,
Columbia University Medical Center, New York, NY,
USA

1. Introduction

In this article, we provide an overview of the cytochrome P450 drug metabolism system, a major target for pharmacogenetics assays. We discuss briefly the major enzyme subfamilies and highlight some of the important members of each. We then delve into the currently available methodologies that are used for genotyping including single base (primer) extension, hybridization, ligation, and sequencing. The various methods have distinct requirements but all can be used for the interrogation of single nucleotide polymorphisms. These genetic differences may confer altered properties in the encoded enzymes including differences in the ability to metabolize drugs. Methods to identify such differences can help select subsets of patients who may or may not be able to effectively utilize particular medications. In such a manner, these techniques allow for the appropriate triage of patients to therapies that are targeted for their genotype, allowing for a tailored, individualized treatment regimen. Pharmacogenetic testing of this nature can help to usher in the era of personalized medicine.

2. Genotypic variation in cytochrome P450s and effects on drug metabolism

Adverse drug reactions are important causes of morbidity and mortality, and have been reported to result in significantly increased healthcare costs and longer hospital lengths of stay. Adverse drug reactions can result from comorbid diseases that affect drug metabolism such as renal or hepatic insufficiency, from drug-drug interactions, and from genetic factors affecting drug pharmacokinetics. Reduction of adverse drug reactions associated with comorbid conditions and drug-drug interactions is potentially achievable through increased awareness and reporting; however prevention of adverse drug reactions due to individual genetic differences requires a different approach – efficient and cost-effective determination of individual genotypic profiles of the enzymes involved in drug metabolism.

---

* Corresponding Author

Drugs are metabolized through a series of reactions, the majority of which are carried out by cytochrome P450 (CYP), a monooxygenase superfamily of enzymes with over 60 members. The CYP genes are highly polymorphic in humans, with hundreds of single nucleotide polymorphisms (SNPs), insertions and deletions, and copy number variations described to date. These genetic polymorphisms give rise to different metabolic phenotypes: ultrarapid metabolizers (UM), extensive metabolizers (EM), intermediate metabolizers (IM) and poor metabolizers (PM). Individuals with the EM phenotype have two normal alleles and have normal metabolism; those with the IM phenotype have one defective allele and may have reduced drug metabolism; and those with the UM phenotype have gene duplications and have increased drug metabolism. The PM phenotype is characterized by two defective alleles, resulting in markedly decreased drug metabolism and in particular situations, higher levels of drugs and increased risk for adverse drug reactions.

Of the many isoforms of CYP, CYP1A2, CYP2B6, CYP2C9, CYP2C19, CYP2D6, CYP2E1, and CYP3A4, are responsible for the metabolism of the majority of clinically important drugs. (Table 1)

	#SNPs	Clinically significant alleles or %poor metabolizers	Examples of substrates
CYP1A2	>30	N.D.	Caffeine, estradiol, clozapine, olanzapine, theophylline
CYP2B6	>70	CYP2B6*6: 15-40% Asians, >50% African-Americans	Bupropion, methadone, ifosphamide, efavirenz, selegiline
CYP2C9	>50	CYP2C9*2: 8-19% Caucasians, 3.2% African-Americans CYP2C9*3: 8.3% Caucasians, 3.3% Asians	NSAIDs, angiotensin receptor blockers, sulfonylureas, warfarin
CYP2C19	>30	PM: 3-5% Caucasians, 15-20% Asians	Proton pump inhibitors, anti-epileptics, clopidogrel
CYP2D6	>100	PM: <1% Asians, 2-5% African-Americans, 6-10% Caucasians	Tricyclic antidepressants, SSRIs, opiods, anti-psychotics, tamoxifen, beta blockers, anti-arrhythmics
CYP2E1	10	N.D.	Anesthetics
CYP3A4	>30	N.D.	Macrolide antibiotics, benzodiazepines, anti-retrovirals, anti-histamines, calcium channel blockers, HMG CoA reductase inhibitors

Table 1. Common CYP polymorphisms affect the metabolism of clinically important drugs. N.D.= not determined.

CYP1A2 metabolizes several drugs including clozapine (used in the treatment of schizophrenia), theophylline (used to treat respiratory disorders such as COPD and asthma), and caffeine. Greater than 30 SNPs have been identified to date , but a genotype-phenotype relationship has not yet been established. Similarly, a genotype-phenotype relationship has not yet been established for CYP2E1, a CYP protein responsible for the metabolism of most anesthetics.

CYP2B6 is highly polymorphic (>70 SNPs) and metabolizes approximately 8% of clinically important drugs including the anti-retroviral drugs efavirenz and nevirapine, which are used in the treatment of HIV infection. The CYP2B6*6 allele, which is found commonly in Asians and African-Americans, results in decreased metabolism and response to efavirenz.

Greater than 50 SNPs have been identified for CYP2C9, which metabolizes approximately 10% of all clinically prescribed medications. One of the most important drugs metabolized by CYP2C9 is warfarin, a widely used anticoagulant. CYP2C9*2 and CYP2C9*3 alleles which are relatively common in Caucasians (approximately 8%) have been implicated as playing a large role in the interindividual variation in the metabolism of this drug. These alleles have been demonstrated to reduce enzymatic activity *in vitro*, *2 by 70% and *3 by 30%, respectively.

CYP2C19 plays a role in the metabolism of several drugs, but perhaps has been best studied for its role in the metabolism of proton pump inhibitors which are used to treat gastroesophageal reflux disorders. 3-5% of Caucasians and 15-20% of Asians are CYP2C19 poor metabolizers. PMs have reduced metabolism of proton pump inhibitors, leading to increased plasma levels of drug and increased response to treatment. Recently, 2C19 has become popular because of its involvement in the metabolism of Plavix, an antiplatelet drug used to prevent strokes and heart attacks. Important alleles include *2 and *3 which reduce enzymatic activity, and *17 which produces an ultrarapid metabolizer phenotype. Of great interest, 2C19 shares homology with 2C9. In fact, >90% of the amino acid sequence is identical between these two isoforms. Despite their near identity at the amino acid level, the active site of the two enzymes differs, and thus accounts for the differences in substrate specificity.

CYP2D6 is highly polymorphic with greater than 100 SNPs thus far characterized. These genetic polymorphisms play a significant role in affecting the metabolism of ~20% of clinically important drugs including anti-depressants, anti-psychotics, anti-arrhythmics, and beta blockers. These features make CYP2D6 an attractive target for pharmacogenetic assays. The PM phenotype is found in < 1% of Asians, 2-5% of African-Americans, and 6-10% of Caucasians. Interestingly, only six alleles of CYP2D6 account for >99% of the poor metabolizers in the Caucasian population (Roberts et al. 2006). Hence, a targeted approach to interrogate these six SNPs could provide a useful assay to identify such individuals in this limited cohort.

The CYP3A family of isoforms are crucial drivers of drug metabolism in the liver. In fact, CYPs 3A4 and 3A5 are responsible for 40-50% of all such activity. CYP3A4 metabolizes a large range of clinically important drugs, and over 30 SNPs have been described. However, no significant interindividual variability has yet been reported , suggesting that genetic variation may not play a large role in regulating CYP3A4 activity. Interestingly however, the *3 allele which results in a variant with a reduced metabolism phenotype is found in ~30% of Caucasians. The 3A5 isoform is less well characterized but shares overlapping substrate specificity with 3A4.

In summary, hundreds of SNPs have been identified within the multiple members of the SNP superfamily and other genes involved in drug metabolism, making these genes an important target for SNP genotyping in pharmacogenetics and personalized medicine. Various techniques for SNP genotyping are described in the following section.

3. SNP genotyping methods

Many SNP genotyping strategies have been developed, ranging from small scale, low-throughput approaches to interrogate one of few SNPs, to large scale, high-throughput approaches that can genotype hundreds of SNPs. Both small and large scale approaches have been applied for pharmacogenetics studies. These approaches generally detect SNP alleles using one of the following strategies: primer extension, hybridization, ligation, or sequencing.

3.1 Single base (primer) extension

Single base (primer) extension is a process that involves the use of a SNP probe with the 3′ end a single base upstream of the SNP of interest. The SNP probe is then extended by a single base, and the incorporated base is detected. Detection can be either through fluorescence, if a fluorophore is incorporated into the dideoxynucleotides and an appropriate detector is used, or can be done based on sizing of fragments if a size separation technique, such as mass spectrometry, is used.

As an example, we have developed an assay using this technology to determine the genotype profile of genes affecting the metabolism of warfarin. Warfarin is a widely used anticoagulant. However, the combination of variable, genetically-based, individual responses to warfarin and a narrow therapeutic window with potentially serious complications, make this an ideal situation in which pharmacogenetics testing could be beneficial. As described above, the CYP2C9*2 and CYP2C9*3 alleles have been shown to be important in the metabolism of warfarin. In addition, warfarin inhibits Vitamin K epoxide reductase complex subunit 1 (VKORC1), an enzyme complex that reduces vitamin K 2,3 epoxide to its active form. Multiple SNPs have been identified in VKORC1, leading to either low-dose or high-dose phenotypes. VKORC1 polymorphisms, which are found commonly in many populations, have been estimated to account for approximately 25% of the variability in warfarin dose requirement. Finally, gamma-glutamyl carboxylase (GGCX) is an enzyme that catalyzes the post-translational modification of vitamin K-dependent proteins and has been reported to have a modest effect on warfarin metabolism.

Four SNPs for these genes were examined simultaneously in a multiplexed assay. Genomic DNA was isolated from whole blood and the region of interest was amplified by PCR. SNP primers (each of different length) were designed with the sequence ending one nucleotide upstream of the SNP of interest. The primer was then extended a single base with a fluorescently labelled dideoxynucleotide terminator (ddNTP). The reaction product was then separated by capillary electrophoresis and analyzed. (Fig 1)

This method has several advantages. It is an accurate procedure that can be performed with minimal hands-on effort. It lends itself to custom design and is flexible in that oligonucleotide probes used to detect SNPs of interest can be added or removed quickly from an existing panel. In our hands, this method gave results that were 100% concordant with traditional sequencing results. This method has the additional benefit of a short turnaround time- the entire analysis may be performed in less than 24 hours, the majority of which is needed for incubation steps and for the automated electrophoretic separation.

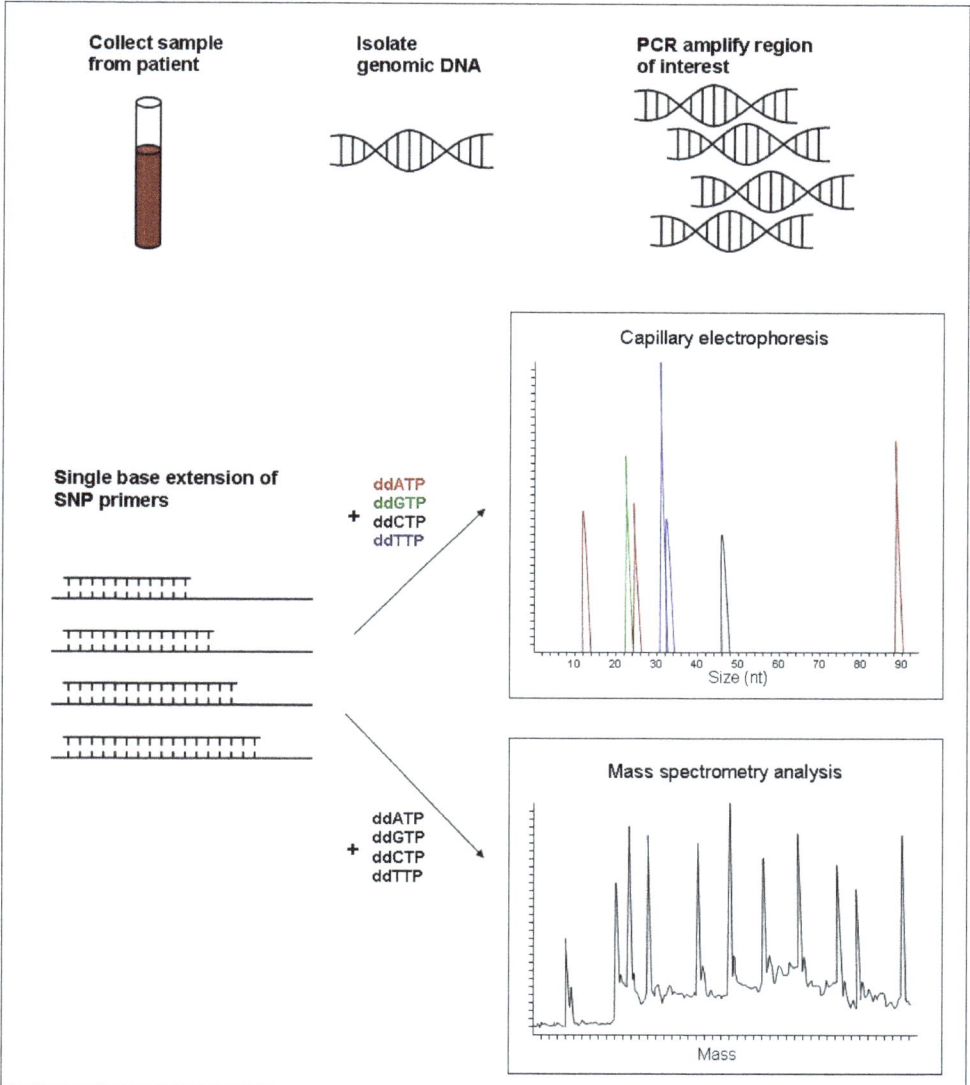

Fig. 1. Detection of SNPs by single base primer extension. Blood is collected from a patient and genomic DNA is isolated from lymphocytes. A multiplex PCR reaction is performed to amplify DNA fragments containing the SNP of interest. This is followed by a multiplex SNP reaction whereby oligonucleotides ending one base pair upstream of the SNP of interest are added and then extended with nucleotide terminators. In the case of capillary electrophoresis, detection is based on fluorescence whereby the ddNTPs are tagged with various fluorophores. In contrast, for mass spectrometry detection is based on accurate sizing of modified nucleotide terminators.

In addition to the assay described above for assessing warfarin metabolism, we have successfully used the same approach to interrogate 8 SNPs of CYP2D6. As described in the previous section, CYP2D6 is highly polymorphic and plays a role in the metabolism of approximately one-fourth of clinically important drugs. We sought to interrogate these SNPs to characterize the PM phenotype. One limitation of this approach (and capillary electrophoresis in general) is in the resolving capacity of this technique, which under our conditions is ~2 nt. In our procedure, we are resolving and visualizing oligonucleotides for SNP interrogation in a window from 10-95 nt, the maximum number of fragments that can be resolved is ~12. This resolving capacity is inherent to the capillary electrophoresis methodology and commercial analyzers of which several are available, all share this limitation.

A similar approach can be used to multiplex a larger number of SNPs, and can thus overcome the limitations described above. Such a genotyping approach needs to exploit methods that are of higher resolution (relative to capillary electrophoresis), such as mass spectrometry. Using this technique, genomic DNA is isolated, the region of interest is amplified by PCR, and SNP primers are hybridized, as described above. These SNP primers are extended by a single base with unlabelled dideoxynucleotide terminators.

The SNP allele is then detected by the mass of the extension product, as a function of the time required to traverse the time-of-flight tube. (Fig 1) We have recently used this technique to interrogate 11 SNPs simultaneously from a single sample. This technique is (theoretically) capable of resolving up to 35-40 SNPs in one well, and thus a greater number of SNPs can be interrogated (relative to capillary electrophoresis), whether they reside in one gene or many genes. Such a methodology is ideal when the number of SNPs of interest is within these parameters.

Several commercial platforms offer larger scale SNP genotyping using single base extension as an approach. The MassARRAY system (Sequenom), an example of a mass spectrometric based platform as described above, can interrogate ~35-40 SNPs simultaneously. The SNPstream assay (Beckman Coulter) is able to interrogate either 12 or 48 SNPs simultaneously in a 384-well plate. A fluorescently labelled nucleotide is added to a tagged SNP probe by single base extension. Each well of the 384-well plate contains tagged oligonucleotides at specific positions within the well. These tagged oligonucleotides are complementary to one of the 12 or 48 tagged SNP probes. The genotype of the SNP is identified by determination of the position of fluorescence in the well.

3.2 Hybridization-based approaches

Hybridization-based approaches for SNP genotyping depend on stringent hybridization conditions (conducive to the ability or inability to form Watson-Crick base pairs) as a means to distinguish one or more alleles. As compared to single base primer extension, hybridization assays are sensitive to variations on length and sequence of both probe and target oligonucleotides. Similar to primer extension, hybridization assays can also interrogate many SNPs simultaneously within the same sample. For example, the Affymetrix GeneChip is an array of oligonucleotides that allows genome-wide interrogation of SNPs.

In hybridization-based approaches, genomic DNA is isolated, regions of interest are amplified, cleaved, and then tagged, for example with biotin. The tagged products are subsequently hybridized under stringent conditions to allele-specific oligonucleotides on a solid matrix, such as a bead or array. These allele-specific oligonucleotides differ by only one or few bases, and correspond to the various alleles of the DNA fragment of interest. The reaction is performed under conditions whereby mismatched targets, i.e. those that do not hybridize perfectly, can be washed away. This leaves only the stably hybridized DNA fragments, i.e. those that have a perfect match to their corresponding target, that are fluorescently labelled. Subsequent detection of the fluorescent signal allows for the determination of the SNP genotype. The specificity of the assay can be increased by using multiple probes for each SNP allele (Figure 2).

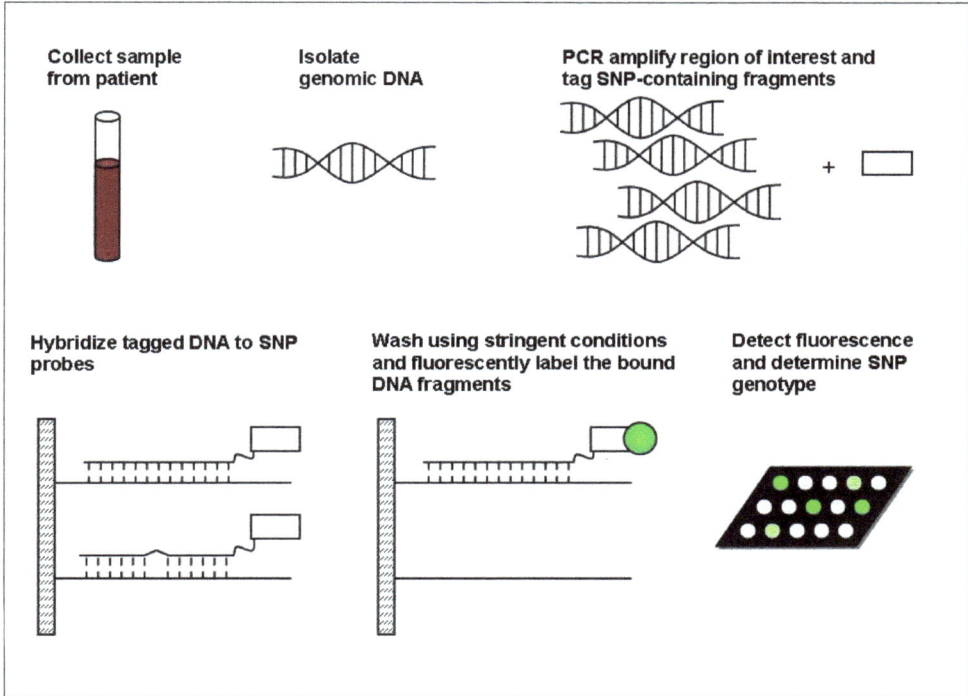

Fig. 2. Detection of SNPs by hybridization. Blood is collected from a patient and genomic DNA is isolated from lymphocytes. A PCR reaction is performed to amplify and tag DNA fragments containing the SNP of interest. Tagged DNA fragments are hybridized to SNP probes bound to a solid matrix, and mismatched fragments are washed away. Hybridized fragments are fluorescently labelled and detected to determine the SNP genotype.

Dynamic allele-specific hybridization (DASH) is another assay that utilizes differential hybridization for SNP genotyping. In DASH, genomic DNA is isolated, and the region of interest is amplified using a biotinylated primer. The biotin tag allows for the attachment of a single stranded DNA fragment to a bead. This is then hybridized with a SNP-specific oligonucleotide. Now, a fluorescent molecule that intercalates into the double-stranded DNA is added, and the fluorescence signal is measured over an increasing temperature gradient. A melting curve can thus be established. (Fig 3) A complete match between the genomic DNA and the SNP-specific oligonucleotide results in the expected melting temperature curve, whereas mismatches result in a curve showing lowered melting temperatures. This technique was used in a study of 13 SNPs in the adiponectin gene which has been linked to type 2 diabetes.

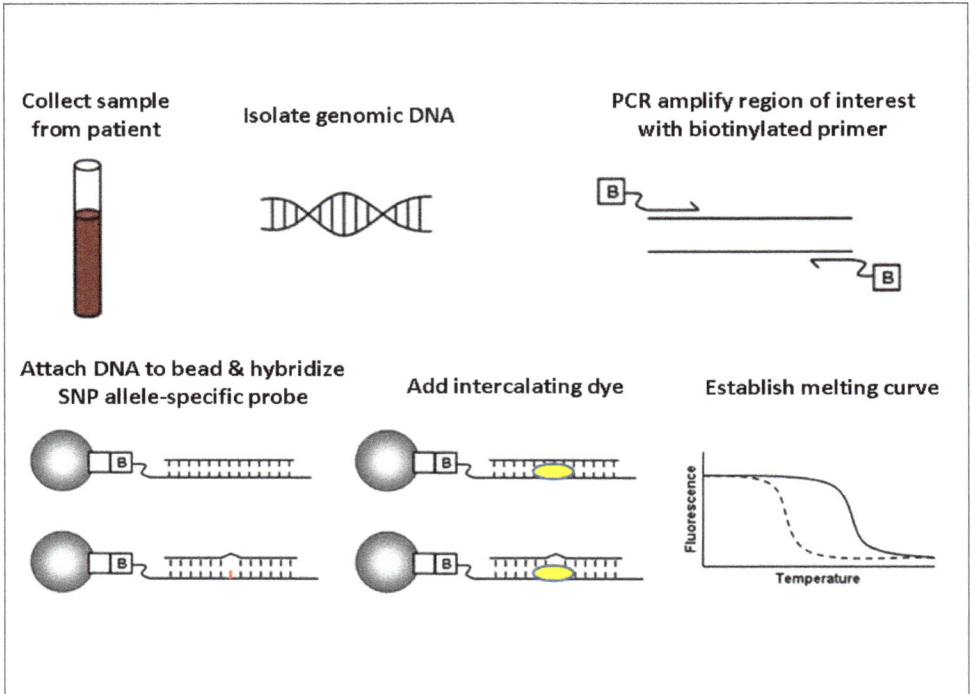

Fig. 3. Dynamic allele-specific hybridization (DASH). Blood is collected from a patient and genomic DNA is isolated from lymphocytes. A PCR reaction is performed to amplify and tag DNA fragments containing the SNP of interest. The DNA fragment is attached to a streptavidin bead, and is hybridized to a SNP probe. A fluorescent intercalating DNA dye is added, and a melting curve is determined. A mismatch (dashed line) will result in a lower melting temperature.

A unique take on the use of hybridization for SNP genotyping involves the use of molecular beacons. A molecular beacon is an oligonucleotide hairpin with a fluorophore at one end and a fluorescence quencher at the other end with a sequence complementary to the SNP allele nested in the middle. In the unbound state, no fluorescent signal will be emitted as the fluorophore and the fluorescence quencher are in close proximity at the stem of the hairpin structure. When the molecular beacon hybridizes with a perfect match to a genomic DNA fragment, the hairpin structure of the molecular beacon is linearized, separating the fluorophore and the fluorescence quencher, allowing fluorescence signal to be emitted (Figure 4).

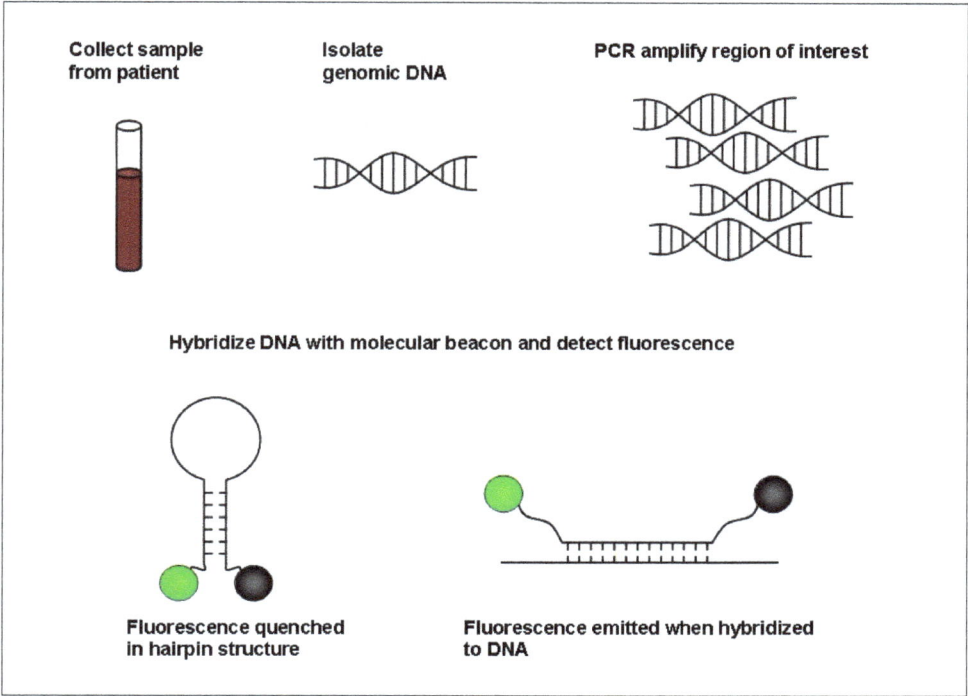

Fig. 4. Interrogation of SNPs using molecular beacons. Blood is collected from a patient and genomic DNA is isolated from lymphocytes. A PCR reaction is performed to amplify DNA fragments containing the SNP of interest. The DNA fragment is hybridized to a molecular beacon. When the molecular beacon is not bound to the DNA fragment, the fluorophore and fluorescence quencher are held in close proximity to each other and no fluorescence signal is emitted. When the molecular beacon hybridizes with the DNA fragment, the flurophore and fluorescence quencher are separated and fluorescence is emitted.

The TaqMan (Applied Biosystems) assay is a widely used assay that utilizes hybridization to determine SNP genotypes. This assay takes advantage of the 5′ nuclease activity of Taq polymerase to detect SNP alleles. In this assay, the region of interest is amplified by PCR. In addition to the forward and reverse primers, an allele-specific probe is also hybridized under stringent conditions to the template DNA. The allele-specific probe has a fluorophore at the 5′ end and a fluorescence quencher at the 3′ end. When the allele-specific probe perfectly complements the template DNA, it is stably bound, whereas when there is a mismatch, the probe will not hybridize stably with the template DNA and will not be a substrate for the 5′ nuclease activity of Taq polymerase. When Taq polymerase reaches the allele-specific probe as it extends DNA from the primer, the 5′ fluorophore is released by the 5′ nuclease activity of Taq polymerase, and the probe is displaced. Release of the 5′ fluorophore separates the fluorophore from the 3′ fluorescence quencher, allowing fluorescence to be emitted and subsequently measured (Figure 5). The Taqman assay was recently used to interrogate 121 SNPs to analyze Y-chromosome variation in 264 samples.

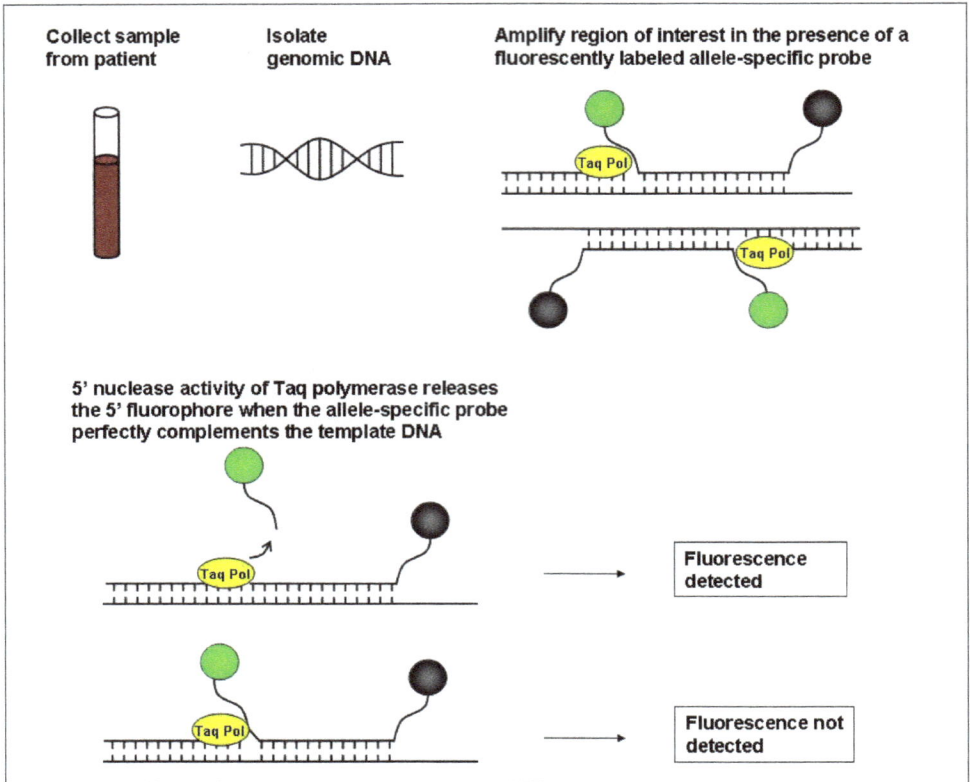

Fig. 5. SNP interrogation utilizing the 5′ nuclease activity of Taq polymerase. Blood is collected from a patient and genomic DNA is isolated from lymphocytes. A DNA fragment containing the SNP of interest is amplified by PCR in the presence of an allele-specific probe labelled with a fluorophore at one end, and with a fluorescence quencher at the other end. When the allele-specific probe complements the DNA, the 5′ nuclease activity of Taq polymerase will release the fluorophore, and fluorescence signal will be detected.

3.3 Ligation-based approaches

The ligation-based approach to interrogate SNPs exploits the ability of DNA ligase to ligate two adjacent oligonucleotides bound to a template DNA. In this assay, two oligonucleotides are required; an allele-specific oligonucleotide which has its 3′ end complementary to the SNP nucleotide to be interrogated, and a second oligonucleotide with its 5′ end designed to anneal immediately adjacent to the 3′ end of the first oligonucleotide. Both oligonucleotides are hybridized to the target DNA. DNA ligase is then added to the reaction. Only if the 3′ end of the first oligonucleotide is indeed complementary to the SNP allele, will ligation occur, as DNA ligase is sensitive to 3′ mismatches. The ligated and unligated products are of different sizes and can thus be detected using a separation technique, for example capillary electrophoresis or mass spectrometry analysis. This approach can also be scaled up for high throughput analysis. (Fig 6)

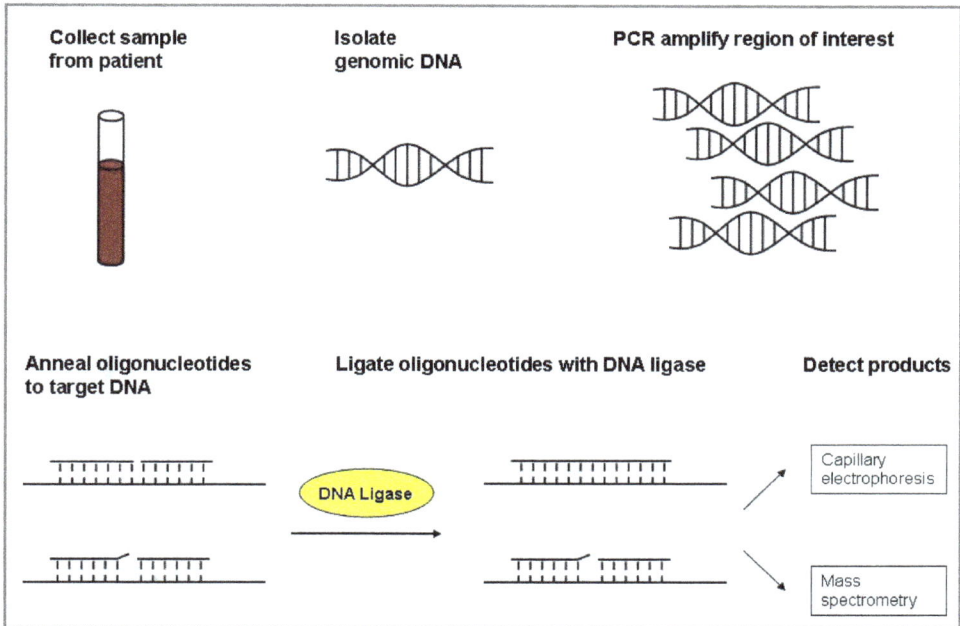

Fig. 6. SNP allele detection by ligation. Blood is collected from a patient and genomic DNA is isolated from lymphocytes. A DNA fragment containing the SNP of interest is amplified by PCR. Two oligonucleotides are annealed to the DNA fragment, flanking the SNP site to be interrogated. If the allele-specific oligonucleotide is complementary to the SNP allele, DNA ligase will be able to ligate the oligonucleotides, and the ligated product can be detected by capillary electrophoresis or mass spectrometry.

The oligonucleotide ligation and capillary electrophoresis method is used in the SNPlex assay (Applied Biosystems), a platform which allows multiplexing for the detection of multiple SNPs simultaneously. The SNPlex assay has been used in multiple studies; in a recent study it was used to detect SNPs in 528 members of families with sarcoidosis.

3.4 Sequencing based strategies: Pyrosequencing and other next generation sequencing methods

Conventional capillary electrophoresis based Sanger sequencing was developed in the (late) 1970s and became widely adopted thereafter. It revolutionized life science research in the subsequent years by providing a critical tool that was fundamental in the elucidation of genetic sequence information. Despite this, the technology suffers from limitations in speed, resolution, throughput and scalability

Next-generation sequencing technologies have recently been developed and have made possible cost-efficient, high-throughput sequencing, that can overcome these drawbacks. An example of next-generation sequencing is pyrosequencing, a sequencing-by-synthesis technique. The pyrosequencing technique sequences approximately 250 bases per read. In pyrosequencing, each added base is detected in real-time by fluorescence. Specifically, genomic DNA is isolated, and the region of interest is amplified by PCR. A sequencing primer is then annealed to the template DNA, and the reaction components are added: DNA polymerase, ATP sulfurylase, luciferase, apyrase, adenosine 5′ phosphosulfate (APS), and luciferin. One of four deoxynucleotide triphosphates (dTTP, dCTP, dGTP, or dATPαS) is then added (dATPαS is used in place of dATP as it can be incorporated by DNA polymerase, but is not a substrate for luciferase). If the added dNTP is complementary to the template DNA, the dNTP is incorporated by DNA polymerase, releasing pyrophosphate (PPi). The released PPi is converted to ATP by ATP sulfurylase with adenosine 5′ phosphosulfate as a substrate. The ATP serves to drive the conversion of luciferin to oxyluciferin by the luciferase enzyme. Oxyluciferin generates visible light proportional to the amount of ATP. This visible light is measured and used to determine if a dNTP was incorporated, and if so, the number of dNTPs added. The unincorporated dNTPs and ATP is degraded by apyrase. This cycle of reactions is repeated with the next dNTP. By this process of sequential addition of dNTPs, the sequence can be determined. (Fig 7)

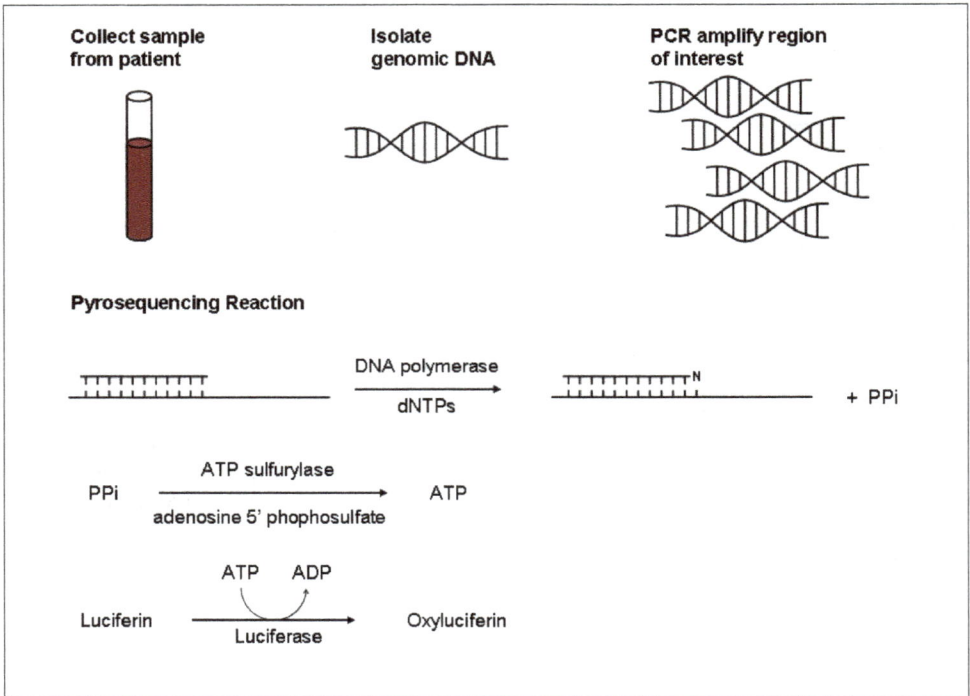

Fig. 7. Pyrosequencing. Blood is collected from a patient and genomic DNA is isolated from lymphocytes. A DNA fragment containing the SNP of interest is amplified by PCR. A sequencing primer is added, as are the sequencing reaction components: DNA polymerase, one of four dNTPs (dTTP, dCTP, dGTP, or dATPαS). If the nucleotide is incorporated, PPi is released, which is then converted by ATP sulfurylase to ATP. The ATP drives the conversion of luciferin to oxyluciferin by luciferase. Oxyluciferin generates visible light proportional to the amount of ATP.

A high-throughput application of pyrosequencing, termed 454 pyrosequencing, was developed in 2005 by 454 Life Sciences. In this technique, the target DNA is attached to a bead and placed in a picoliter-sized well of a fiberoptic slide (containing 1.6 million wells). The substrates for the pyrosequencing reaction are added to the wells in waves via a flow-chamber, the light signal is detected, and the sequence is determined. This parallelized pyrosequencing technology allows the determination of mega- to gigabase amounts of DNA in a fast and cost-efficient manner.

Illumina (Solexa) sequencing is another next-generation sequencing technology that has recently been developed for high-throughput sequencing. DNA is sequenced by repeated cycles of single base extension. As in standard single base extension, DNA is extended a single base with a fluorescently labelled nucleotide terminator. The nucleotide terminator in this case is not a dideoxynucleotide; instead it is a modified, reversible terminator. The identity of the incorporated base is determined by detection of fluorescence. Next, the flurophore is removed and the terminator is reversed, and the cycle of single base extension is repeated. In this manner, approximately 75 bases can be read at a time.

A third important next-generation sequencing technology is SOLiD sequencing (Sequencing by Oligonucleotide Ligation and Detection), a technology developed by Applied Biosystems. Rather than utilizing a polymerase, this technology utilizes an elegant system of hybridization and ligation steps to determine the sequence of target DNA. In brief, DNA is attached to a flow cell and is hybridized and ligated to one of a set of fluorescently labelled probes. The fluorescence is detected, then cleaved and the process is repeated to extend the sequence. A combination of repeated hybridization and ligation steps and use of primers with different offsets allows not only the sequence to be determined, but also provides a "two-base" read to improve accuracy. This technology can provide sequence data of approximately 50 bases with each individual read. This individual sequencing reaction is performed across millions of templates in a massively parallel fashion. Thus, in a rapid manner, large stretches of DNA can be sequenced spanning entire genomes. In fact, the amount of DNA sequence data that is generated is staggering, exceeding hundreds of gigabytes of information from a single run. A single instrument today can generate more information in a 24 hour period than was possible using multiple instruments with standard technology operating over a decade, in the 1980s, 1990s, and even in the 2000s.

3.5 Other SNP genotyping methods

The Invader assay (Third Wave Technologies) utilizes the ability of Flap endonuclease (FEN) to cleave specific DNA structures to determine SNP alleles. Flap endonuclease is a 5' nuclease that recognizes DNA structures with a single stranded 5' overhang, or flap. Flap endonuclease will cleave DNA at the junction of the single and double stranded DNA. In this assay, genomic DNA is isolated and the region of interest is amplified by PCR. Two probes are hybridized to the target DNA: an Invader oligonucleotide and an allele-specific oligonucleotide. The Invader oligonucleotide is designed to anneal with its 3' end immediately upstream to the SNP site. The allele-specific oligonucleotide, which has a 5' fluorophore and a 3' fluorescence quencher, anneals to the SNP site and to the downstream sequence. In addition, the allele-specific oligonucleotide has additional 5' sequence not complementary to upstream sequence that extends from the bound DNA, forming a structure recognized by FEN. Cleavage of the allele-specific oligonucleotide by FEN separates the 5' fluorophore from the 3' fluorescence quencher, and allows fluorescence to be emitted. If the allele-specific oligonucleotide does not complement the SNP site exactly, the resulting structure is not recognized by Flap endonuclease and no fluorescence signal will be detected. (Fig 8)

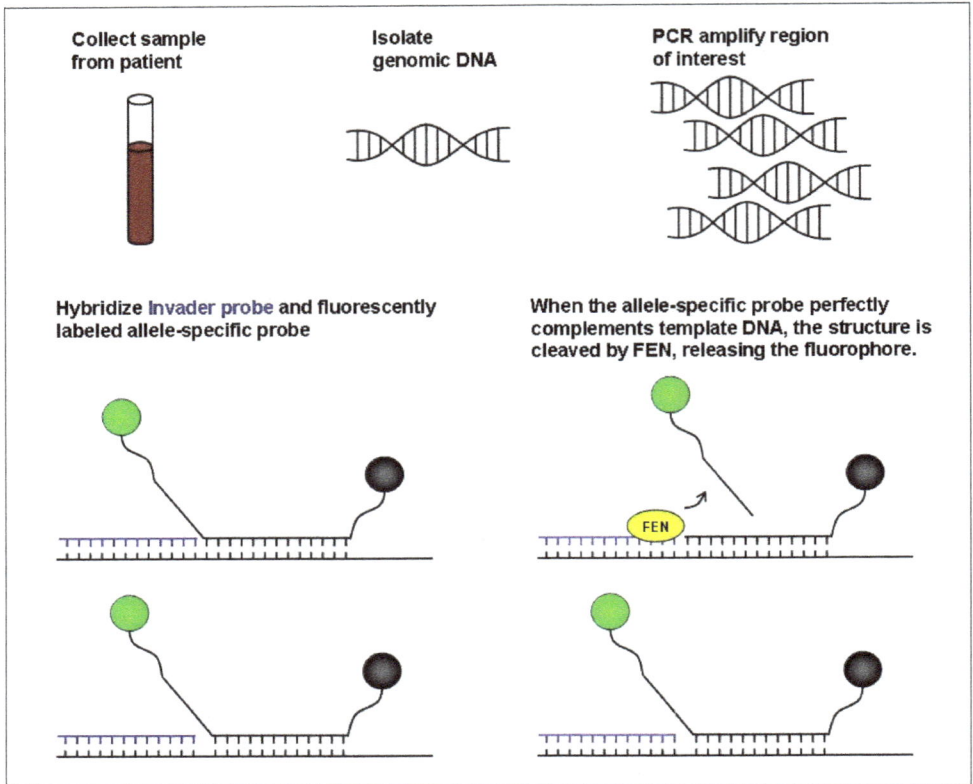

Fig. 8. Invader assay for SNP interrogation. Blood is collected from a patient and genomic DNA is isolated from lymphocytes. A DNA fragment containing the SNP of interest is amplified by PCR. An Invader probe (blue) and an allele-specific probe labelled with a flurophore and a fluorescence quencher are hybridized to the DNA fragment. FEN recognizes the resulting structure and cleaves it, releasing the fluorophore.

The Invader assay was successfully used (in conjunction with other SNP genotyping methods) to genotype 122 SNPs in 9 candidate genes associated with diabetes. In a study by Ozaki et al., a multiplexed Invader assay was used to interrogate 92,788 SNPs from 94 individuals in a genome-wide association study.

4. Considerations in the selection of the appropriate SNP genotyping tool

Several factors merit consideration and are important for the judicious selection of an appropriate SNP genotyping assay. Accuracy, reliability, and establishment of quality control are intermingled and readily apparent as important factors. These elements are critical to the development of a robust assay and the validation of such. The accuracy and reliability of results is paramount since these data are used to inform clinical decision making by allowing for optimized selection of therapy for the patient. The inclusion and establishment of an appropriate quality control paradigm ensures the integrity of reagents, test conditions, and experimental and technical workflow. These features form the basis of, and are a prerequisite to, generating an accurate and reliable result.

There are additional factors that will affect more widespread adoption of these assays and make individualized patient therapy available and accessible to most patients. Such considerations include: speed, automation, customizability, and the requirement for specialized equipment and /or technical training. These set of factors deal with the logistics in operationalizing the implementation of such assays.

The speed at which results are obtained and the test's ease of use can directly affect the clinical utility of the assay and further dictate where the assay is performed and who can conduct testing (regulatory requirements differ by country, and within the United States they may also differ by state, e.g. New York). For example, under certain conditions it may be favourable for testing to be conducted by a healthcare provider in an outpatient setting where results are immediately used to make treatment decisions. If an assay is fairly straightforward & easy to use and the chances of obtaining an accurate result are high, it may be advantageous to perform outside the clinical laboratory. On the contrary, it may be beneficial for testing to be sent to a centralized laboratory and performed by a trained, licensed technologist. This is the ideal situation for a higher complexity test. However, in this situation, results may not be immediately available and thus there will be a delay in using the information to change clinical management of the patient.

Assays in which little hands-on effort is required and can be automated will increase speed, throughput, and will help to reduce errors. In cases where numerous SNPs are interrogated, a single, multiplexed reaction allows for the simultaneous investigation of several SNPs, reducing time and cost. The number of SNPs identified and characterized as playing a role in drug metabolism to date has been a relatively manageable size; however, as more SNPs are identified, both multiplexed and high-throughput assays could further reduce costs

Customized assays are advantageous in that they are designed to answer focused questions, and can be tailored to specific patient populations. In addition, they are flexible and can be rapidly changed as new clinically significant SNPs are identified and need to be incorporated. A requirement for specialized training and/or equipment may slow widespread adoption of a SNP genotyping assay but is necessary for conducting high complexity testing of this nature. Finally, cost also can play an important role, particularly in an environment of increasing healthcare expenditures. In recent years, pharmacogenetic testing (and other molecular diagnostics assays) have come under greater scrutiny and the debate over appropriate reimbursement scales by insurance payers continues.

The methodologies described in the previous section have all been used successfully to genotype SNPs, however they have different advantages and limitations that factor into their usefulness in individualized SNP genotyping assays. (Table 2) The ideal assay would combine the advantages of each methodology, and eliminate the common requirement for either large amounts of DNA or for an initial PCR step. New technologies that would increase sensitivity or reduce the need for multiplexed PCR would be necessary to make the simultaneous interrogation of hundreds or thousands of SNPs faster and more cost-effective.

Methodology	Multiplexed assays?	High-throughput assays?	Advantages	Limitations
Single base (primer) extension	Yes	Yes	High accuracy of incorporation by DNA polymerase	Multiple steps for detection/ separation
Hybridization	More difficult	Yes	Widely available; not dependent on enzymatic reaction	Requirement for optimization of probes and hybridization conditions
Ligation	Yes	Yes	High specificity of DNA ligase	Multiple steps for detection/ separation
Sequencing	More difficult	Yes	Sequencing of 50-250 bases; speed	Specialized equipment required

Table 2. Comparison of SNP genotyping methodologies.

5. Conclusions

Multiple genetic differences between individuals have been described in the Cytochrome P450 family of drug metabolizing enzymes. These genetic differences may confer altered properties including differences in the ability to metabolize drugs. Methods to identify such differences can help select subsets of patients who may or may not be able to effectively utilize particular medications. Several widely used methods with differing approaches and advantages have been highlighted above. Further technological advances will help these technologies become more widely adopted. These techniques allow for the appropriate triage of patients to therapies that are targeted for their genotype, allowing for a tailored, individualized treatment regimen. Pharmacogenetic testing of this nature will help to usher in this new era of personalized medicine.

6. References

Ahmadian, A., B. Gharizadeh, A. C. Gustafsson, F. Sterky, P. Nyren, M. Uhlen & J. Lundeberg (2000) Single-nucleotide polymorphism analysis by pyrosequencing. *Anal Biochem*, 280, 103-10.

Alderborn, A., A. Kristofferson & U. Hammerling (2000) Determination of single-nucleotide polymorphisms by real-time pyrophosphate DNA sequencing. *Genome Res*, 10, 1249-58.

Bentley, D. R., S. Balasubramanian, H. P. Swerdlow, G. P. Smith, J. Milton, C. G. Brown, K. P. Hall, D. J. Evers, C. L. Barnes, H. R. Bignell, J. M. Boutell, J. Bryant, R. J. Carter, R. Keira Cheetham, A. J. Cox, D. J. Ellis, M. R. Flatbush, N. A. Gormley, S. J. Humphray, L. J. Irving, M. S. Karbelashvili, S. M. Kirk, H. Li, X. Liu, K. S. Maisinger, L. J. Murray, B. Obradovic, T. Ost, M. L. Parkinson, M. R. Pratt, I. M. Rasolonjatovo, M. T. Reed, R. Rigatti, C. Rodighiero, M. T. Ross, A. Sabot, S. V. Sankar, A. Scally, G. P. Schroth, M. E. Smith, V. P. Smith, A. Spiridou, P. E. Torrance, S. S. Tzonev, E. H. Vermaas, K. Walter, X. Wu, L. Zhang, M. D. Alam, C. Anastasi, I. C. Aniebo, D. M. Bailey, I. R. Bancarz, S. Banerjee, S. G. Barbour, P. A. Baybayan, V. A. Benoit, K. F. Benson, C. Bevis, P. J. Black, A. Boodhun, J. S. Brennan, J. A. Bridgham, R. C. Brown, A. A. Brown, D. H. Buermann, A. A. Bundu, J. C. Burrows, N. P. Carter, N. Castillo, E. C. M. Chiara, S. Chang, R. Neil Cooley, N. R. Crake, O. O. Dada, K. D. Diakoumakos, B. Dominguez-Fernandez, D. J. Earnshaw, U. C. Egbujor, D. W. Elmore, S. S. Etchin, M. R. Ewan, M. Fedurco, L. J. Fraser, K. V. Fuentes Fajardo, W. Scott Furey, D. George, K. J. Gietzen, C. P. Goddard, G. S. Golda, P. A. Granieri, D. E. Green, D. L. Gustafson, N. F. Hansen, K. Harnish, C. D. Haudenschild, N. I. Heyer, M. M. Hims, J. T. Ho, A. M. Horgan, et al. (2008) Accurate whole human genome sequencing using reversible terminator chemistry. *Nature*, 456, 53-9.

Bertilsson, L. (1995) Geographical/interracial differences in polymorphic drug oxidation. Current state of knowledge of cytochromes P450 (CYP) 2D6 and 2C19. *Clin Pharmacokinet*, 29, 192-209.

Butler, M. A., M. Iwasaki, F. P. Guengerich & F. F. Kadlubar (1989) Human cytochrome P-450PA (P-450IA2), the phenacetin O-deethylase, is primarily responsible for the hepatic 3-demethylation of caffeine and N-oxidation of carcinogenic arylamines. *Proc Natl Acad Sci U S A*, 86, 7696-700.

Classen, D. C., S. L. Pestotnik, R. S. Evans, J. F. Lloyd & J. P. Burke (1997) Adverse drug events in hospitalized patients. Excess length of stay, extra costs, and attributable mortality. *JAMA*, 277, 301-6.

Desta, Z., X. Zhao, J. G. Shin & D. A. Flockhart (2002) Clinical significance of the cytochrome P450 2C19 genetic polymorphism. *Clin Pharmacokinet*, 41, 913-58.

Eichelbaum, M., M. Ingelman-Sundberg & W. E. Evans (2006) Pharmacogenomics and individualized drug therapy. *Annu Rev Med*, 57, 119-37.

Eiermann, B., G. Engel, I. Johansson, U. M. Zanger & L. Bertilsson (1997) The involvement of CYP1A2 and CYP3A4 in the metabolism of clozapine. *Br J Clin Pharmacol*, 44, 439-46.

Field, T. S., B. H. Gilman, S. Subramanian, J. C. Fuller, D. W. Bates & J. H. Gurwitz (2005) The costs associated with adverse drug events among older adults in the ambulatory setting. *Med Care*, 43, 1171-6.

Flockhart, D. A. (2007) Drug Interactions: Cytochrome P450 Drug Interaction Table. Indiana University School of Medicine. *http://medicine.iupui.edu/clinpharm/ddis/table.asp*, Accessed April 25, 2011.

Floyd, M. D., G. Gervasini, A. L. Masica, G. Mayo, A. L. George, Jr., K. Bhat, R. B. Kim & G. R. Wilkinson (2003) Genotype-phenotype associations for common CYP3A4 and

CYP3A5 variants in the basal and induced metabolism of midazolam in European- and African-American men and women. *Pharmacogenetics,* 13, 595-606.

Grossman, P. D., W. Bloch, E. Brinson, C. C. Chang, F. A. Eggerding, S. Fung, D. M. Iovannisci, S. Woo & E. S. Winn-Deen (1994) High-density multiplex detection of nucleic acid sequences: oligonucleotide ligation assay and sequence-coded separation. *Nucleic Acids Res,* 22, 4527-34.

Guan, S., M. Huang, X. Li, X. Chen, E. Chan & S. F. Zhou (2006) Intra- and inter-ethnic differences in the allele frequencies of cytochrome P450 2B6 gene in Chinese. *Pharm Res,* 23, 1983-90.

Gurwitz, J. H., T. S. Field, J. Judge, P. Rochon, L. R. Harrold, C. Cadoret, M. Lee, K. White, J. LaPrino, J. Erramuspe-Mainard, M. DeFlorio, L. Gavendo, J. Auger & D. W. Bates (2005) The incidence of adverse drug events in two large academic long-term care facilities. *Am J Med,* 118, 251-8.

Ha, H. R., J. Chen, A. U. Freiburghaus & F. Follath (1995) Metabolism of theophylline by cDNA-expressed human cytochromes P-450. *Br J Clin Pharmacol,* 39, 321-6.

Hall, J. G., P. S. Eis, S. M. Law, L. P. Reynaldo, J. R. Prudent, D. J. Marshall, H. T. Allawi, A. L. Mast, J. E. Dahlberg, R. W. Kwiatkowski, M. de Arruda, B. P. Neri & V. I. Lyamichev (2000) Sensitive detection of DNA polymorphisms by the serial invasive signal amplification reaction. *Proc Natl Acad Sci U S A,* 97, 8272-7.

Howell, W. M., M. Jobs, U. Gyllensten & A. J. Brookes (1999) Dynamic allele-specific hybridization. A new method for scoring single nucleotide polymorphisms. *Nat Biotechnol,* 17, 87-8.

Ingelman-Sundberg, M., Daly, A.K., Nebert, D.W., eds. (2008) Human Cytochrome P450 (CYP) Allele Nomenclature Committee *http://www.cypalleles.ki.se/,* Last updated Sept 4, 2008, Accessed April 23, 2011.

Kalow, W., S. V. Otton, D. Kadar, L. Endrenyi & T. Inaba (1980) Ethnic difference in drug metabolism: debrisoquine 4-hydroxylation in Caucasians and Orientals. *Can J Physiol Pharmacol,* 58, 1142-4.

Kawamura, M., S. Ohara, T. Koike, K. Iijima, H. Suzuki, S. Kayaba, K. Noguchi, S. Abe, M. Noguchi & T. Shimosegawa (2007) Cytochrome P450 2C19 polymorphism influences the preventive effect of lansoprazole on the recurrence of erosive reflux esophagitis. *J Gastroenterol Hepatol,* 22, 222-6.

King, C. R., E. Deych, P. Milligan, C. Eby, P. Lenzini, G. Grice, R. M. Porche-Sorbet, P. M. Ridker & B. F. Gage (2010) Gamma-glutamyl carboxylase and its influence on warfarin dose. *Thromb Haemost,* 104, 750-4.

Landegren, U., R. Kaiser, J. Sanders & L. Hood (1988) A ligase-mediated gene detection technique. *Science,* 241, 1077-80.

Lang, T., K. Klein, J. Fischer, A. K. Nussler, P. Neuhaus, U. Hofmann, M. Eichelbaum, M. Schwab & U. M. Zanger (2001) Extensive genetic polymorphism in the human CYP2B6 gene with impact on expression and function in human liver. *Pharmacogenetics,* 11, 399-415.

Lazarou, J., B. H. Pomeranz & P. N. Corey (1998) Incidence of adverse drug reactions in hospitalized patients: a meta-analysis of prospective studies. *JAMA,* 279, 1200-5.

Lin, Y. S., A. L. Dowling, S. D. Quigley, F. M. Farin, J. Zhang, J. Lamba, E. G. Schuetz & K. E. Thummel (2002) Co-regulation of CYP3A4 and CYP3A5 and contribution to hepatic and intestinal midazolam metabolism. *Mol Pharmacol*, 62, 162-72.

Livak, K. J. (1999) Allelic discrimination using fluorogenic probes and the 5' nuclease assay. *Genet Anal*, 14, 143-9.

Livak, K. J., S. J. Flood, J. Marmaro, W. Giusti & K. Deetz (1995) Oligonucleotides with fluorescent dyes at opposite ends provide a quenched probe system useful for detecting PCR product and nucleic acid hybridization. *PCR Methods Appl*, 4, 357-62.

Lyamichev, V., A. L. Mast, J. G. Hall, J. R. Prudent, M. W. Kaiser, T. Takova, R. W. Kwiatkowski, T. J. Sander, M. de Arruda, D. A. Arco, B. P. Neri & M. A. Brow (1999) Polymorphism identification and quantitative detection of genomic DNA by invasive cleavage of oligonucleotide probes. *Nat Biotechnol*, 17, 292-6.

Margulies, M., M. Egholm, W. E. Altman, S. Attiya, J. S. Bader, L. A. Bemben, J. Berka, M. S. Braverman, Y. J. Chen, Z. Chen, S. B. Dewell, L. Du, J. M. Fierro, X. V. Gomes, B. C. Godwin, W. He, S. Helgesen, C. H. Ho, G. P. Irzyk, S. C. Jando, M. L. Alenquer, T. P. Jarvie, K. B. Jirage, J. B. Kim, J. R. Knight, J. R. Lanza, J. H. Leamon, S. M. Lefkowitz, M. Lei, J. Li, K. L. Lohman, H. Lu, V. B. Makhijani, K. E. McDade, M. P. McKenna, E. W. Myers, E. Nickerson, J. R. Nobile, R. Plant, B. P. Puc, M. T. Ronan, G. T. Roth, G. J. Sarkis, J. F. Simons, J. W. Simpson, M. Srinivasan, K. R. Tartaro, A. Tomasz, K. A. Vogt, G. A. Volkmer, S. H. Wang, Y. Wang, M. P. Weiner, P. Yu, R. F. Begley & J. M. Rothberg (2005) Genome sequencing in microfabricated high-density picolitre reactors. *Nature*, 437, 376-80.

Mehlotra, R. K., M. J. Bockarie & P. A. Zimmerman (2007) CYP2B6 983T>C polymorphism is prevalent in West Africa but absent in Papua New Guinea: implications for HIV/AIDS treatment. *Br J Clin Pharmacol*, 64, 391-5.

Nuckols, T. K., S. M. Paddock, A. G. Bower, J. M. Rothschild, R. J. Fairbanks, B. Carlson, R. J. Panzer & L. H. Hilborne (2008) Costs of intravenous adverse drug events in academic and nonacademic intensive care units. *Med Care*, 46, 17-24.

Rai, A. J., N. Udar, R. Saad & M. Fleisher (2009) A multiplex assay for detecting genetic variations in CYP2C9, VKORC1, and GGCX involved in warfarin metabolism. *Clin Chem*, 55, 823-6.

Rai, A. J., J. Yee & M. Fleisher (2010) Biomarkers in the era of personalized medicine - a multiplexed SNP assay using capillary electrophoresis for assessing drug metabolism capacity. *Scand J Clin Lab Invest Suppl*, 242, 15-8.

Roberts, R.L., M.A. Kennedy (2006) Rapid detection of common cytochrome P450 2D6 alleles in Caucasians. Clin Chim Acta, 366(1-2):348-351.

Sconce, E. A., T. I. Khan, H. A. Wynne, P. Avery, L. Monkhouse, B. P. King, P. Wood, P. Kesteven, A. K. Daly & F. Kamali (2005) The impact of CYP2C9 and VKORC1 genetic polymorphism and patient characteristics upon warfarin dose requirements: proposal for a new dosing regimen. *Blood*, 106, 2329-33.

Tyagi, S., D. P. Bratu & F. R. Kramer (1998) Multicolor molecular beacons for allele discrimination. *Nat Biotechnol*, 16, 49-53.

Tyagi, S. & F. R. Kramer (1996) Molecular beacons: probes that fluoresce upon hybridization. *Nat Biotechnol*, 14, 303-8.

Vargas, E., A. Terleira, F. Hernando, E. Perez, C. Cordon, A. Moreno & A. Portoles (2003) Effect of adverse drug reactions on length of stay in surgical intensive care units. *Crit Care Med*, 31, 694-8.

Xie, H. G., H. C. Prasad, R. B. Kim & C. M. Stein (2002) CYP2C9 allelic variants: ethnic distribution and functional significance. *Adv Drug Deliv Rev*, 54, 1257-70.

Part 2

Pharmacogenetics in Oncology

3

Pharmacogenomics of Thiopurine S-Methyltransferase: Clinical Applicability of Genetic Variants

Sonja Pavlovic, Branka Zukic and Gordana Nikcevic
Institute of Molecular Genetics and Genetic Engineering,
University of Belgrade, Belgrade,
Serbia

1. Introduction

Sequence variability among individual human genomes has become a key resource for modern medicine in the search for genetic markers affecting disease susceptibility, disease manifestation and response to treatment. Genetic markers have been used for years as an indispensable tool for the diagnosis and follow-up of a number of diseases. They are also used as prognostic and predictive markers. Their application as pharmacogenetic markers is especially important.

Pharmacogenetics is referred to as the study of the variations in a DNA sequence as related to drug efficacy and toxicity. It began with studying differences among individuals. However, as it developed, it became clear that genetic differences between populations should also be taken into account. Following great progress in understanding the molecular basis of health and disease, pharmacogenetics has evolved into pharmacogenomics, a much newer discipline which can be described as the whole-genome application of pharmacogenetics. More precisely, pharmacogenomics is the study of variations of DNA and RNA characteristics as related to drug response.

Genetic variability can affect various aspects of drug therapy: disposition of the drug (pharmacokinetics), efficacy of the drug (pharmacodynamics) and adverse drug reactions (ADRs). Genetic factors are estimated to account for 15-30% of inter-individual differences in drug metabolism and response.

The ultimate goal of pharmacogenetic testing is to aid physicians in the prescription of the appropriate medication at the correct dose prior to the initiation of the therapy. This would lead to minimizing adverse events and toxicity and maximizing efficacy by excluding those who are unlikely to benefit (non-responders) or who may be harmed (adverse responders).

Here, we provide an overview of the genetic variants of thiopurine S-methyltransferase (*TPMT*) gene that influence inter-individual dosing of thiopurine drugs, to highlight a tangible benefit of translating genomic knowledge into clinical practice. Particular single nucleotide polymorphisms (SNPs) in *TPMT* gene have proven to be applicable for optimising the dosage in pursuit of maximum efficacy and minimum adverse effects. Thus, they set an important paradigm of the implementation of pharmacogenomics in mainstream clinical practice.

2. Pharmacogenetics

The role of genetics in response to drugs was first predicted by Sir Archibald Garrod in the early 1930s (Garrod 1931). Pharmacogenetics, as it is known today, originated as a new scientific discipline in the late 1950s by the merging of two older ones: pharmacology and genetics. Pharmacogenetics examines the role of inherited individual differences in response to drugs. It is a branch of science that explains variability in response to drugs and genetic basis as the cause of this variability. Initially, the focus was on individual human differences, but over time the area of interest of this science extended to genetic differences between populations. Many professionals from this field deal exclusively with humans, but this science has applied its principles to all living organisms that are able to respond to a drug or other chemicals.

Research in the field of pharmacogenetics is being developed into two main directions: first, the identification of specific genes and their products that are associated with various diseases and that could represent targets for new therapeutics; and second, the identification of genes and allelic variants of genes that might influence the response to already existing drugs (Wolf et al., 2000).

3. Human genetic variations

In 2003, after more than a decade, the Human Genome Project was completed. It was clear that the information obtained from the Project had the potential to forever transform healthcare and that genome-based medicine, frequently called personalized medicine, is the future of healthcare. Ever since, the main goal was achieving faster and cheaper sequencing of the whole human genome. The key advantage is the possibility to identify very rare or new, "private" genetic variants. Among a patient's personal genome data, the most important data is about inter-individual genetic differences.

More than ninety-nine percent of the DNA sequence is identical among individuals. The remaining DNA is responsible for genetic diversity (Kidd et al., 2004). Polymorphisms are common genetic variations in the human genome. They represent sequence variations that occur with a frequency >1% in the general population. The most studied polymorphisms are SNPs (single nucleotide polymorphisms). They are distributed over the whole genome. The number of SNPs is estimated to range from 0.3 to 1 SNP per 100 base pairs (bp). Besides SNPs, there are other important classes of polymorphisms, such as VNTRs (variable number of tandem repeats, polymorphic sequence containing 20-50 copies of 6-100 bp repeats), STRs (short tandem repeats, a subclass of VNTR in which repeat unit consists of only 2-7 nucleotides) and CNPs (copy number polymorphisms, variation in the number of copies (CNV) of a DNA sequence in the > 1 kb size range, which are common and widely distributed in the human genome).

The totality of these genetic variations found in an individual, a variome, should carry an answer about inborn diseases, compliance with drug therapies and other processes - all specific to that individual. However, in order to be fully understood and finally translated into the everyday clinical practice, variome data needs to be adequately interpreted. The most important approach of interpretation is to correlate genetic variation with clinical data.

4. Thiopurine S-methyltransferase (TPMT)

One of the best examples of the application of pharmacogenetics in clinical practice is the discovery that different individual responses to purine antagonists as therapeutics are caused by individual variations in thiopurine S-methyltransferase (TPMT) enzyme activity (Weinshilboum *et al.*, 1980). Patients who have reduced TPMT enzyme activity can develop toxic effects after the application of standard doses of these drugs (Weinshilboum *et al.*, 1980). On the other hand, there are patients in whom the activity of this enzyme is extremely high and they do not respond to standard doses of drugs (Weinshilboum *et al.*, 1980). The characterization of mutations within the *TPMT* gene enabled the explanation of these inter-individual differences in enzyme activity. Consequently, the goal of pharmacogenetics, the individualization of therapy, becomes a step closer. The characterization of mutations in *TPMT* gene is also a model system that illustrates how knowledge in the field of pharmacogenetics is successfully used in clinical practice.

5. Thiopurine drugs

Antimetabolites or structural analogs are compounds analogous to natural cell compounds such as folic acid, purines and pyrimidines. The mechanism of their action is based on the fact that they replace natural metabolites in the biochemical processes of cells. Antimetabolites have the greatest impact on the biochemical pathways that are involved in the metabolism of nucleotides and nucleic acids. Purine antagonists as thiopurine drugs have been widely used in medical practice for over 50 years. The structural analogues of purines are 6-mercaptopurine (6-MP), 6-thioguanine (6-TG) and azathioprine (AZA) (Coulthrad *et al.*, 2005).

Thiopurine drugs are indicated for the treatment of various diseases. 6-MP and 6-TG are mainly used in the treatment of hematologic malignancies, such as acute leukemia and lymphoma in children and adults. In childhood acute lymphoblastic leukemia (ALL), 6-TG is primarily used in the induction phase, and 6-MP in the consolidation phase of ALL therapy. The immunosuppressive drug AZA is the drug of choice in the treatment of inflammatory bowel diseases, rheumatoid arthritis, autoimmune hemolytic anemia, systemic lupus erythematosus, as well as in transplantation medicine.

Thiopurine drugs were synthesized in 1951 (Elion 1986). It was shown that newly synthesized drugs inhibit the use of natural purines and act upon the reduction of some tumors in rats (Elion 1967). Soon the activity of these drugs was confirmed in childhood ALL. At that time, the prognosis of this disease was extremely poor. The discovery that 6-MP can lead to the complete remission of childhood ALL, resulted in the approval of the use of these drugs in medical practice by the U.S. Food and Drug Administration in 1953 (Burchenal *et al.*, 1953). AZA was introduced in therapy later, in 1963, after its successful use in kidney transplantation (Murray *et al.*, 1963).

The basic principle of how thiopurine drugs act is the inhibition of many pathways in nucleic acid biosynthesis. Consequently they prevent proliferation of cells involved in determination and amplification of the immune response, causing suppression of the immune system. Thiopurine drugs are also used in cancer treatment (Katzung 2004). An important biochemical feature of cancer cells is excessive synthesis of nucleic acids. Thiopurine drugs are able to stop this synthesis, and thus prevent the division of neoplastic cells (Katzung 2004). Anticancer and immunosuppressive activity is accomplished through the incorporation of thioguanine nucleotides, metabolic products of thiopurine drugs, into DNA.

Thiopurine drugs are inactive in their original form. They are precursors of the active drug, so-called pro-drugs, and they have to be metabolized first in order to exhibit cytotoxic, therapeutic effect (Lennard 1992). The first step is the non-enzymatic degradation of AZA to 6-MP and imidazole group. 6-MP and 6-TG go through metabolic changes prior to the expression of their cytotoxic effects. After metabolic conversion, 6-MP and 6-TG are incorporated into the DNA and RNA molecules as thioguanine nucleotides (6-TGN) (Bertino 1991). 6-MP can also inhibit *de novo* synthesis of purine nucleotides (Dervieux *et al.,* 2001; Coulthard *et al.,* 2002). 6-TGN are incorporated into DNA as "false" bases, causing DNA damage by single strand breaking, inter-strand cross-linking and DNA-protein cross-linking (Maybaum *et al.,* 1981; Maybaum *et al.,* 1983; Christie *et al.,* 1984; Tay *et al.,* 1969; Pan *et al.,* 1990; Bodell 1991). Also, the inhibition of normal DNA replication may occur, through the partial inhibition of DNA polymerase and DNA ligase (Ling *et al.,* 1992) as well as through the significant inhibition of RNase H (Krynetskaia *et al.,* 1999).

6. Metabolism of thiopurine drugs

As already mentioned, 6-MP and 6-TG are metabolically converted to 6-TGN before expressing their cytotoxic effect (Fig 1). Metabolic conversion begins with the enzyme hypoxanthine-guanine phosphoribosyltransferase (HPRT, EC: 2.4.2.8). After a series of metabolic steps, 6-TGN are formed and incorporated into DNA and RNA molecules.

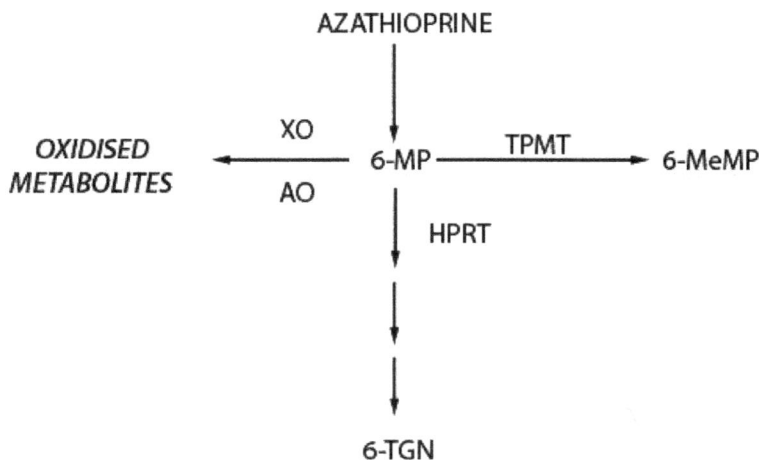

Fig. 1. Thiopurine drug metabolism. The figure shows a simplified representation of thiopurine drug biotransformation, with azathioprine being converted *in vivo* to 6-mercaptopurine (6-MP), followed by the metabolic activation of 6-MP mediated by hypoxanthine-guanine phosphoribosyltransferase (HPRT), to form 6-thioguanine nucleotides (6-TGN). 6-MP is inactivated by xanthine oxidase (XO), aldehyde oxidase (AO) or thiopurine S-methyltransferase (TPMT). TPMT enzyme uses S-adenosyl-L-methionine as a methyl group donor. One of the reaction products is methyl-6-mercaptopurine (6-MeMP).

Thiopurine drugs are inactivated in the organism by oxidation (mediated by aldehyde oxidase (AO, EC 1.1.3.13) and xanthine oxidase (XO, EC 1.1. 3.22)) and methylation (mediated by thiopurine S-methyltransferase (TPMT, EC 2.1.1.67)), reactions which are needed to prevent high drug concentrations and adverse drug-related events. XO and AO produce metabolites that have little or no cytotoxic effect. XO activity in hematopoietic tissue is very low, almost insignificant. This is the reason why the main pathway of thiopurine drug inactivation goes through the TPMT enzyme (Remy 1963).

The influence of TPMT enzyme activity on cytotoxicity induced by thiopurine drugs was first documented in 1987 (Van Loon *et al.*, 1987).

7. TPMT allozymes

Thiopurine S-methyltransferase is a cytosolic monomeric enzyme that catalyzes S-methylation of heterocyclic aromatic sulfhydryl compounds, and consequently, partial inactivation of immunosuppressive thiopurine medications. The molecular weight of TPMT protein is 28.18 kDa and it consists of 245 amino acids. The natural substrate for TPMT is unknown, although this enzyme is expressed in nearly all human tissues (Weinshilboum *et al.*, 1978). Structural and biochemical analyses of TPMT protein revealed the existence of certain protein variants with altered activity. In some individuals, TPMT enzyme activity is significantly decreased or increased compared to the normal TPMT activity level.

One of the first studies of TPMT activity in red blood cells determined the distribution of TPMT activity to be trimodal. Namely, it was found that approximately 90% of individuals express high TPMT activity. These individuals are referred to as high methylators. Intermediate methylators represent approximately 10% of the population. Low or undetectable TPMT activity is reported in 0.3% individuals (Weinshilboum *et al.*, 1980). This study initially identified the hereditary nature of the TPMT deficiency in humans. Trimodal frequency distribution of TPMT activity corresponds to monogenic co-dominant inheritance. Additionally, ultra-high methylators have been observed (Spire-Vayron de la Moureyre *et al.*, 1999; Roberts *et al.*, 2008). It has been shown that these different TPMT allozymes are defined by certain *TPMT* gene polymorphisms.

8. Genetic variants in *TPMT* gene

Human *TPMT* gene (NG_012137, NM_000367, GeneBank: 7172 or MIM: 187680) was discovered using a "classical" molecular biology strategy. Firstly, TPMT enzyme from kidneys was purified and a partial amino acid sequence was obtained (Van Loon *et al.*, 1982). This information served for the successful cloning of human *TPMT* cDNA (Honchel *et al.*, 1993).

Initially, on chromosome 18q.21.1 the pseudogene for *TPMT* has been discovered, containing a similar sequence to the *TPMT* gene (Lee *et al.*, 1995). The human gene for *TPMT* was cloned and mapped on the short arm of chromosome 6, at the position 6p22.3 (Szumlanski *et al.*, 1996). *TPMT* gene comprises a region of 34 kb and 10 exons, 8 of which encode *TPMT* protein. Krynetski et al. thoroughly characterized the *TPMT* gene and its adjacent sequences (Krynetski *et al.*, 1997).

TPMT gene exhibits significant genetic heterogeneity. It has been shown that certain polymorphisms in *TPMT* gene define different TPMT allozymes with different enzyme activity. At present, the *TPMT* allele nomenclature comprises at least 27 *TPMT* alleles (Feng *et al.*, 2010), with wild type allele designated as *TPMT*1*. There are several *TPMT* variant alleles comprising one or more SNPs (Table 1).

TPMT variant allele	Genetic variant	Molecular alteration	Position in the TPMT gene	Reference
*TPMT*1*	Wt			
*TPMT*1A*	-178C>T		Exon 1	Spire-Vayron de la Moureyre *et al.*, 1998b
*TPMT*1S*	c.474T>C	p.Ile158Ile	Exon 7	Alves *et al.*, 1999
*TPMT*2*	c.238G>C	p.Ala80Pro	Exon 5	Krynetski *et al.*, 1995
*TPMT*3A*	c.460G>A and c.719A>G	p.Ala154Thr and p.Tyr240Cys	Exon 7, Exon 10	Tai *et al.*, 1997
*TPMT*3B*	c.460G>A	p.Ala154Thr	Exon 7	Szulmanski *et al.*, 1996; Tai *et al.*, 1996
*TPMT*3C*	c.719A>G	p.Tyr240Cys	Exon 10	Szulmanski *et al.*, 1996; Tai *et al.*, 1996
*TPMT*3D*	c.460G>A, c.719A>G and c.292G>T	p.Ala154Thr, p.Tyr240Cys and p.Glu98STOP	Exon 7, exon 10 and exon 5	Otterness *et al.*, 1997
*TPMT*4*	IVS9–1G>A	exon 10 is shortened as a result of use of the cryptic splice site created by G>A substitution	intron 9/exon 10	Otterness *et al.*, 1998
*TPMT*5*	c.146T>C	p.Leu49Ser	Exon 4	Otterness *et al.*, 1997
*TPMT*6*	c.539A>T	p.Tyr180Phe	Exon 8	Otterness *et al.*, 1997
*TPMT*7*	c.681T>G	p.His227Glu	Exon 10	Spire-Vayron de la Moureyre *et al.*, 1998b
*TPMT*8*	c.644G>A	p.Arg215His	Exon 10	Hon *et al.*, 1999
*TPMT*9*	c.356A>C	p.Lys119Thr	Exon 5	Schaeffeler *et al.*, 2004
*TPMT*10*	c.430G>C	p.Gly144Arg	Exon 7	Colombel *et al.*, 2000
*TPMT*11*	c.395G>A	p.Cys132Tyr	Exon 6	Schaeffeler *et al.*, 2003
*TPMT*12*	c.374C>T	p.Ser125Leu	Exon 6	Hamdan-Khalil *et al.*, 2003
*TPMT*13*	c.83A>T	p.Glu28Val	Exon 3	Hamdan-Khalil *et al.*, 2003
*TPMT*14*	c.1A>G	p.Met1Val	Exon 3	Lindqvist *et al.*, 2004
*TPMT*15*	IVS7–1G>A	p.Arg140_Cys165del (deletion of the entire exon 8 in the final protein, resulting in a frame shift and a premature stop codon in exon 9)	intron 7/ exon 8	Lindqvist *et al.*, 2004

TPMT variant allele	Genetic variant	Molecular alteration	Position in the TPMT gene	Reference
TPMT*16	c.488G>A	p.Arg163His	Exon 7	Schaeffeler et al., 2004
TPMT*17	c.124C>G	p.Gln42Glu	Exon 3	Schaeffeler et al., 2004
TPMT*18	c.211C>A	p.Gly71Arg	Exon 4	Schaeffeler et al., 2004
TPMT*19	c.365A>C	p.Lys122Thr	Exon 5	Hamdan-Khalil et al., 2005
TPMT*20	c.712A>G	p.Lys238Glu	Exon 10	Schaeffeler et al., 2006
TPMT*21	c.205C>G	p.Leu69Val	Exon 4	Schaeffeler et al., 2006
TPMT*22	c.488G>C	p.Arg163Pro	Exon 7	Schaeffeler et al., 2006
TPMT*23	c.500C>G	p.Ala167Gly	Exon 8	Lindqvist et al., 2007
TPMT*24	c.537G>T	p.Gln179His	Exon 8	Garat et al., 2008
TPMT*25	c.634T>C	p.Cys212Arg	Exon 10	Garat et al., 2008
TPMT*26	c.622T>C	p.Phe208Leu	Exon 9	Kham et al., 2009
TPMT*27	c.319T>G	p.Tyr107Asp	Exon 5	Feng et al., 2010
TPMT*28	c.611T>C	p.Ile204Thr	Exon 9	Appell et al., 2010

HGVS nomenclature has been applied. IVS-intron

Table 1. Summary of the currently known SNPs in the TPMT gene.

The common nonfunctional alleles include TPMT*2 (containing a single c.238 G>C polymorphism), TPMT*3A (containing both c.460 G>A and c.719 A>G polymorphisms), TPMT*3B (containing a single c.460 G>A polymorphism), TPMT*3C (containing a single c.719 A>G polymorphism) and TPMT*4 (containing a single nucleotide G>A substitution at the 3'end of intron 9) (Krynetski et al., 1995; Tai et al., 1996; Loennechen et al., 1998; Otterness et al., 1998). Most of these SNPs are located in the coding region of the TPMT gene and lead to non-synonymous amino acid substitutions (p.Ala80Pro, p.Ala154Thr and p.Tyr240Cys for c.238 G>C, c.460 G>A and c.719 A>G polymorphisms, respectively), which cause a decrease in activity of TPMT enzyme in comparison to the wild type. On the contrary, TPMT*4 allele contains a frameshift within exon 10, leading to low-enzyme activity.

The majority of genetic variants detected in the TPMT gene represent sequence variations that alter the encoded amino acid (Weinshilboum et al., 2006). Besides these, there are genetic variants that influence transcription and mRNA splicing, resulting in variable TPMT gene expression.

Recently, a great deal of evidence has confirmed the existence of such modifiers of TPMT activity within non-coding regions of the TPMT gene. In particular, it has been demonstrated that the presence of variable number of tandem repeats, VNTRs, ranging from three to nine, in the TPMT gene promoter, directly alters TPMT activity, most likely due to the alteration of promoter cis-regulatory elements (Zukic et al., 2010; Pavlovic 2009; Pavlovic et al., 2010; Georgitsi et al., 2011).

TPMT promoter VNTRs include GC-rich blocks that are putative binding sites of various transcriptional factors (Krynetski *et al.*, 1997, Fessing *et al.*, 1998). The VNTR region architecture is defined by three types of repeats (A, B and C) that vary amongst each other by length and nucleotide sequence. Repeats are always arranged in the same order: A is followed by B and then C, with no intervening sequences. The number of A and B repeats varies, while the C repeat is always present in only one copy (Spire-Vayron de la Moureyre *et al.*, 1999). An inverse correlation between the total number of repeats and the enzymatic activity was observed (Spire-Vayron de la Moureyre *et al.*, 1998a), while findings from Zukic and co-workers suggest that on top of the total number of VNTRs, the type/architecture of the repeat has crucial impact on *TPMT* gene transcriptional regulation as well (Zukic *et al.*, 2010).

Recently, trinucleotide repeat variants in the *TPMT* promoter region have been described which may explain the 1-2% of Caucasians who demonstrate ultra-metabolizer phenotype (Roberts *et al.*, 2008).

9. Functional characterization of TPMT allozymes

The functional characterization and expression analysis in human cells and yeast system (Tai *et al.*, 1997; Otterness *et al.*, 1997; Hamdan-Khalil *et al.*, 2003; Lindqvist *et al.*, 2004; Schaeffeler *et al.*, 2006; Ujiie *et al.*, 2008), revealed that alleles *TPMT*2*, *TPMT*3A*, *TPMT*5*, *TPMT*12*, *TPMT*14*, and *TPMT*22* encode for TPMT enzymes that have a very reduced activity in comparison to wild type allele designated as *TPMT*1*. In addition, it has been shown that *TPMT*18* allele encodes for an enzyme that has a slightly reduced activity compared to wild-type allele. Alleles *TPMT*9*, *TPMT*19* and *TPMT*24* express TPMT proteins whose activity is not statistically different from the activity of wild-type enzyme (Garat *et al.*, 2008; Hamdan-Khalil *et al.*, 2005). Polymorphisms in the alleles *TPMT*4* and *TPMT*15* cause alternative processing of *TPMT* mRNA and consequently, the expression level of the TPMT enzyme is reduced. They belong to the so-called quantitative polymorphisms (Otterness *et al.*, 1998; Lindqvist *et al.*, 2004). The molecular mechanism that leads to the reduction of TPMT activity was studied in the most common *TPMT* genetic variants. Expression studies of *TPMT*2* and *TPMT*3A* alleles showed that both alleles are about 100 times less expressed than wild type, *TPMT*1* allele (Tai *et al.*, 1997). Also, the expression of *TPMT*2* and *TPMT*3A* allelic variants was not in correlation with the activities of TPMT*2 and TPMT*3A proteins. The mechanism of accelerated degradation of TPMT*2 and TPMT*3A proteins is responsible for the reduced level of TPMT proteins and thereby for the reduced catalytic ability of enzymes (Tai *et al.*, 1997). More detailed studies have confirmed that in the accelerated degradation of TPMT*3A protein, through a ubiquitin-mediated system, the molecular chaperones from the family of heat shock proteins are involved (Wang *et al.*, 2003).

10. Population-specific distribution of *TPMT* variant alleles

Pharmacogenetics is generally focused on inter-individual differences in drug metabolism and on variations in response to drugs. The frequency of pharmacogenetic markers studied so far, is different between certain racial and ethnic groups. Historically, the practical application of pharmacogenetic achievements, i.e., the individualization of therapy, has been based on studies conducted on Caucasians. With time, other ethnic groups have been included in clinical trials, and it became clear that responses to drug therapy may depend on ethnic background (Relling *et al.*, 2011a). Thus, if the metabolism of drugs varies among different ethnic groups, then the pharmacogenetic data of one population cannot be extrapolated to another one without prior assessment. Knowledge of the pharmacogenetic differences between populations can be of great importance for the pharmaceutical industry.

The distribution of clinically relevant *TPMT* alleles is population specific (Spire-Vayron de la Moureyre *et al.*, 1998a; Hon *et al.*, 1999; Collie-Duguid *et al.*, 1999; Schaffeler *et al.*, 2004). The *TPMT*3A* allele is the most common variant allele in Caucasians (frequency approximately 3.5%) (Relling *et al.*, 2011a), while *TPMT*3C* is predominant in subjects with Asian or African ancestry (frequencies of 0.3–5.3% and 2.4–10.9 % respectively) (Kubota *et al.*, 2001; Hongeng *et al.*, 2000; Hon *et al.*, 1999; McLeod *et al.*, 1999). Additionally, *TPMT*8* has been reported to be common in the African population (Hon *et al.*, 1999; Oliveira *et al.*,2007; Alves *et al.*, 2004).

The common *TPMT* variant alleles in Caucasian include *TPMT*2*, *TPMT*3A*, *TPMT*3B* and *TPMT*3C* (Krynetski *et al.*, 1995; Tai *et al.*, 1996; Loennechen *et al.*, 1998). These variant alleles are detected in over 80-95% of Caucasians characterized to have low or intermediate TPMT activity (Yates *et al.*, 1997).

11. Methodology for TPMT phenotype and genotype testing

The TPMT phenotype and genotype can be defined in several ways. Phenotypic analysis of TPMT enzyme activity could be performed by radiochemical activity assays (McLeod *et al.*, 1995; Weinshilboum *et al.*, 1978), or an assay based on high performance liquid chromatography (HPLC) method (Kroplin *et al.*, 1998). Genotyping is performed using PCR-based methods (Yates *et al.*, 1997; Coulthard *et al.*, 1998), denaturing high performance liquid chromatography (DHPLC) (Hall *et al.*, 2001; Schaeffeler *et al.*, 2001), Real Time-PCR (Lindqvist *et al.*, 2003), a combination of microchip and sequencing (arrayed primer extension - APEX) (Yi *et al.*, 2002), molecular haplotype analysis (McDonald *et al.*, 2002) and pirosequencing (Haglund *et al.*, 2004).

Methods based on PCR are used to detect the most common *TPMT* variant alleles that lead to reduced TPMT activity. These analyses are helpful in identifying individuals with a high risk of developing potentially fatal hematologic toxicity caused by thiopurine drugs. Measurement of TPMT enzyme activity was, until recently, very expensive and relatively inaccessible to patients. A concordance of more than 95% exists between actual TPMT enzyme activity and the prediction of its activity based on detection of *TPMT* variant alleles (McLeod *et al.*, 2000; Schwab *et al.*, 2001). Therefore, molecular genetic analysis represents a quick and efficient method to identify patients at risk for toxicity and adverse effects-free guidance of the therapy.

Commercially available genetic tests change over time. Many of them include only the *2, *3A, *3B and *3C alleles. There is no doubt that sequencing of the *TPMT* gene remains the most accurate, although expensive method.

12. Clinical applicability of *TPMT* genetic variants: Individualization of thiopurine therapy

All patients with decreased TPMT activity are at risk of hematologic toxicity owing to the accumulation of high levels of 6-thioguanine nucleotides (Weinshilboum 2003). Thiopurine-induced myelosuppression can result in increased morbidity, hospitalization and/or treatment discontinuation (Leung *et al.*, 2009; Ugajin *et al.*, 2009). Myelosuppression increases an individual's risk of developing an infection and sepsis (Campbell *et al.*, 2001; Posthuma *et al.*, 1995; Connell *et al.*, 1993; Schütz *et al.*, 1993). The incidence of mild leukopenia is approximately 5-25% (Gurwitz *et al.*, 2009). Rare, but severe leukopenia can develop suddenly and unpredictably in approximately 3% of patients (Carter *et al.*, 2004). A 27-year analysis showed that AZA contributed to the incidences of myelosuppression in 5% of patients (Connell *et al.*, 1993). Over an 18-year period, 2% of patients with IBD experienced 6-MP-induced leukopenia that resulted in hospitalization (Present *et al.*, 1989). The incidence of myelosuppression occurred more frequently during the first eight weeks after treatment initiation, and was more likely to occur with a higher drug dose (Present *et al.*, 1989; Lewis *et al.*, 2009).

Consequently, thiopurine drug dose reduction is necessary to avoid toxicity (Weinshilboum *et al.*, 1980). Therefore, it is of great importance to determine TPMT status before initiating thiopurine therapy (Relling *et al.*, 2011a; Gurwitz *et al.*, 2009; Schmiegelow, K. *et al.*, 2009; Relling *et al.*, 2010). TPMT genotyping is commonly used for determination of TPMT status.

Patients who are homozygotes or compound heterozygotes for nonfunctional genetic variants, treated with standard drug doses, develop severe, eventually fatal, myelosuppression and require AZA, 6-MP or TG reduced doses by at least 10-fold (Schwab *et al.*, 2001; Evans *et al.*, 2001; Schwab *et al.*, 2002; Slanar *et al.*, 2008; Relling *et al.*, 2011a).

Patients with intermediate TPMT activity, heterozygous carriers of nonfunctional genetic variants in the *TPMT* gene, also require dose reduction (Weinshilboum *et al.*, 1980; Dokmanovic *et al.*, 2006). The initial dose of AZA or 6-MP should be reduced by 30-70%. The AZA dose can be titrated as tolerated. The 6-MP dose should be adjusted based on the severity of myelosuppression and disease-specific guidelines. The initial dose of 6-TG should be reduced by 30-50%, and adjusted based on the severity of myelosuppression and disease-specific guidelines (Weinshilboum 2001; Krynetski *et al.*, 2003; Weinshilboum 2003; Dokmanović *et al.*, 2008; Relling *et al.*, 2011b).

In addition, 1 - 2% of patients are ultra-high methylators, who experience thiopurine treatment resistance and hepatotoxicity as a result of treatment with elevated 6-MP concentrations (Spire-Vayron de la Moureyre *et al.*, 1999; Roberts *et al.*, 2008). These patients often do not respond to therapy, although doses of drugs up to 50% higher than the standard doses are given. (Schaeffeler *et al*, 2004; Spire-Vayron de la Moureyre *et al.*, 1998a; Dokmanovic *et al.*, 2006).

13. Guidelines for thiopurine dosing based on *TPMT* genotype

The Clinical Pharmacogenetics Implementation Consortium (CPIC), as a part of the National Institutes of Health's Pharmacogenomics Research Network, developed the first guideline for the dosing of thiopurines based on *TPMT* genotype (updates at http://www.pharmgkb.org) (Relling *et al.*, 2011b).

Dose adjustments based on *TPMT* genotype have reduced thiopurine induced adverse effects without compromising the desired antitumor and immunosuppressive therapeutic effects in several clinical settings (Relling *et al.*, 2011a).

Although the information on *TPMT* genotype is recommended rather than required as part of thiopurine drug treatment, some groups (Relling *et al.*, 2011a; Gurwitz *et al.*, 2009; Relling *et al.*, 2010) advocate testing for *TPMT* status prior to initiating thiopurine therapy, so that starting dosages can be adjusted accordingly. This is very important, since, if one starts with low doses in all patients in order to avoid severe toxicity, in the minority with a *TPMT* defect, one risks disease progression during the period of upward dosage titration (Sandborn 2001). Therefore, the use of this genetic test in routine clinical practice is recommended, while clinicians should continue to evaluate markers of disease progression and/or myelosuppression to adjust thiopurine doses upward or downward from the genotype-directed starting doses (Relling *et al.*, 2011a).

Besides CPIC guideline, there are recommendations and guidelines offered by other groups (Nguyen *et al.*, 2011). Namely, the Royal Dutch Association for the Advancement of Pharmacy Pharmacogenomic Working Group recommends for patients who are intermediate metabolizers that the dose of AZA or 6-MP should be reduced by 50% and titrated based on hematologic monitoring and efficacy. For patients who are poor metabolizers, the dose of AZA or 6-MP should be reduced by 90% and titrated based on hematologic monitoring and efficacy. Moreover, patients who are intermediate or poor metabolizers should not be treated with 6-TG as there are "insufficient data to allow calculation of dose adjustment" (Swen *et al.*, 2011).

The US Food and Drug Administration (FDA) and prescribing information for AZA and 6-MP recommend either TPMT genotyping or phenotyping prior to initiating therapy to help identify patients who are at an increased risk of developing toxicity (http://www.fda.gov/Drugs/ScienceResearch/ResearchAreas/Pharmacogenetics/ucm083378. htm). The prescribing information for 6-TG indicates that patients with TPMT deficiency "may be unusually sensitive to the myelosuppressive effects of 6-TG. Substantial dosage reductions may be required to avoid the development of life-threatening bone marrow suppression". In addition, the American College of Gastroenterology treatment guidelines prefer TPMT phenotyping over genotyping in patients who are being treated with thiopurines for ulcerative colitis (Korbluth *et al.*, 2010).

On the other hand, there are research groups that do not advocate for TPMT genotyping before treatment with thiopurines (Booth *et al.*, 2011). The Agency for Healthcare Research and Quality (AHRQ) concluded that "there is currently insufficient evidence regarding the effectiveness of determining TPMT status prior to thiopurine treatment in terms of improvement in clinical outcomes and incident myelotoxicity in comparison with routine monitoring of full blood counts and adverse events" (http://www.ahrq.gov/clinic/tp/tpmttp.htm#Report).

Also, the British Society of Gastroenterology does not require either TPMT genotyping or phenotyping as a prerequisite to initiating thiopurine therapy because the use of AZA has been shown to be safe in patients with Crohn's disease or ulcerative colitis (Carter *et al.*, 2004).

14. From TPMT pharmacogenetics to TPMT pharmacogenomics

It is worth noting that there is no clear boundary between the low and intermediate, or intermediate and high methylators. Even individuals within the same "methylation" group show different enzymatic activity, and these differences are genetically determined (Vuchetich *et al.*, 1995). Also, there are many patients with wild type *TPMT* who develop toxicity. All this leads to the conclusion that the association of a particular genetic variation with adverse drug effects could be softened or enhanced by the other genetic variations present in the same individual that influence other processes (drug absorption, transportation, metabolism, *TPMT* gene transcription and consequently the abundance of TPMT protein). Moreover, the effects and clinical relevance of genetic variants in another gene, encoding an enzyme involved in mercaptopurine metabolism (inosine-triphospate-pyrophosphatase, *ITPA*), on mercaptopurine pharmacogenetics has been demonstrated (Stocco *et al.*, 2010).

Finally, a myriad of other genetic factors, which influence interactions between thiopurines and other drugs, could play an important role in the final TPMT activity phenotype.

Therefore, more comprehensive study of the modifying role of different genetic factors in TPMT pharmacogenetics, will in time lead to our understanding of controversial results published in our era. The new era of pharmacogenomics will bring more consistent and reliable guidelines for thiopurine dosing based on patient's genotype.

In recent years, the term pharmacogenomics is more and more present alongside the term pharmacogenetics. Due to rapid technological development and the great success of the human genome sequencing project, the variations and interactions of multiple genes, rather than variations in individual genes, have been recognized as the cause of diverse responses to drugs (O'Brien *et al.*, 1999; Kennedy *et al.*, 2003). Genotyping methods, the application of microarrays and GWAS analyses (Genome Wide Association Studies) that are used in pharmacogenomics, provide an insight into a number of individual genes at one time, their possible interactions and changes in their expression. The final goal of pharmacogenomics is the individualization of therapy in accordance with a patient's genotype and gene expression profile. Thus, by using the appropriate therapeutics and adequate doses without side effects, the cheapest, fastest and the most efficient treatment for patients would be achieved. Under these conditions, patients would not be faced with complications, time and money for additional drugs and hospital days would not be wasted for treatment of complications, while the primary disease progresses. Unfortunately, widely available pharmacogenomic tests for particular diseases still do not exist. The individualization of therapy in medical practice, if at all implemented, is conducted based on pharmacogenetic achievements, by testing polymorphisms in a single gene.

15. Conclusions

Although pharmacogenetics is one of the most promising fields of biomedicine, only a few pharmacogenetic markers have been introduced in routine clinical practice. Among them are genetic variants in the *TPMT* gene which can be used for determination of the cause of unusual therapeutic response in patients treated with thiopurine drugs.

TPMT genotyping is recommended prior to initiating thiopurine therapy by several groups and consortia, so that starting dosages can be adjusted accordingly. Doses customized on the basis of *TPMT* status reduce the likelihood of acute myelosuppression without compromising disease control.

Nowadays, *TPMT* genetic testing comprise the analysis of DNA sequence at each of the important single-nucleotide polymorphism in the *TPMT* gene associated with altered level of enzyme activity.

However, the understanding of a single genetic variation is far more complex when it is put in the context of other genetic variations. In that sense, the future of personalized medicine is heading towards variomics - the study of the overall genetic variations found in an individual.

Although the knowledge of pharmacogenomics is incomplete and still in expansion, evidence presented in this chapter show that up to date knowledge can already be used for more successful, personalized patient treatment. There is no doubt that pharmacogenomics together with gene therapy will change the future of medicine and will steadily pave the path to personalized medicine.

16. Acknowledgment

This work has been funded by a grant No. III 41004, Ministry of Education and Science, Republic of Serbia.

17. References

[1] Alves S, Prata MJ, Ferreira F, Amorim A. Thiopurine methyltransferase pharmacogenetics: alternative molecular diagnosis and preliminary data from northern Portugal. Pharmacogenetics 1999; 9:257-261.

[2] Alves S, Rocha J, Amorim A, Prata MJ. Tracing the origin of the most common thiopurine methyltransferase (TPMT) variants: preliminary data from the patterns of haplotypic association with two CA repeats. Ann Hum Genet 2004; 68:313-323.

[3] Appell ML, Wennerstrand P, Peterson C, Hertervig E, Martensson LG. Characterization of a novel sequence variant, TPMT*28, in the human thiopurine methyltransferase gene. Pharmacogenet Genomics 2010; 20:700-707.

[4] Bertino JR. Improving the curability of acute leukemia: Pharmacologic approaches. Seminars in Hematology 28:9–11, 1991.

[5] Bodell WJ. Molecular dosimetry of sister chromatid exchange induction in 9L cells treated with 6-thioguanine. Mutagenesis 1991; 6:175–177.

[6] Booth RA, Ansari MT, Loit E, Tricco AC, Weeks L, Doucette S, Skidmore B, Sears M, Sy R, Karsh J. Assessment of Thiopurine S-Methyltransferase Activity in Patients Prescribed Thiopurines: A Systematic Review. Ann Intern Med 2011; 154:814-823.

[7] Burchenal JH, Murphy ML, Ellison RR. Clinical evaluation of a new antimetabolite, 6-mercaptopurine, in the tratement of acute leukaemia and allied diseases. Blood 1953; 8:965–999.

[8] Campbell S, Ghosh S. Is neutropenia required for effective maintenance of remission during azathioprine therapy in inflammatory bowel disease? Eur J Gastroenterol Hepatol. 2001; 13:1073-1076.

[9] Carter MJ, Lobo AJ, Travis SP, IBD Section, British Society of Gastroenterology. Guidelines for the management of inflammatory bowel disease in adults. Guts 2004; 53 (Suppl 5):v1-16.

[10] Christie NT, Drake S, Meyn RE, Nelson JA. 6-Thioguanineinduced DNA damage as a determinant of cytotoxicity in cultured chinese hamster ovary cells. Cancer Res 1984; 44:3665–3671.

[11] Collie-Duguid ES, Pritchard SC, Powrie RH, Sludden J, Collier DA, Li T, McLeod HL. The frequency and distribution of thiopurine methyltransferase alleles in Caucasian and Asian populations. Pharmacogenetics 1999; 9:37–42.

[12] Colombel JF, Ferrari N, Debuysere H, Marteau P, Gendre JP, Bonaz B, Soulé JC, Modigliani R, Touze Y, Catala P, Libersa C, Broly F. Genotypic analysis of thiopurine S-methyltransferase in patients with Crohn's disease and severe myelosuppression during azathioprine therapy. Gastroenterology 2000; 118:1025-1030.

[13] Connell WR, Kamm MA, Ritchie JK, Lennard-Jones JE. Bone marrow toxicity caused by azathioprine inflammatory bowel disease: 27 years of experience. Gut 1993; 34:1081-1085.

[14] Coulthard SA, Howell C, Robson J, Hall AG. The relationship between thiopurine methyltransferase activity and genotype in blasts from patients with acute leukemia. Blood 1998; 92:2856-2862.

[15] Coulthard SA, Hogarth LA, Little M, Matheson EC, Redfern CP, Minto L, Hall AG. The effect of thiopurine methyltransferase expression on sensitivity to thiopurine drugs. Mol Pharmacol 2002; 62:102–109.

[16] Coulthard S, Hogarth L. The thiopurines: an update. Invest New Drugs 2005; 23:523-532.

[17] Dervieux T, Blanco JG, Krynetski EY, Vanin EF, Roussel MF, Relling MV. Differing contribution of thiopurine methyltransferase to mercaptopurine versus thioguanine effects in human leukemic cells. Cancer Res 2001; 61:5810–5816.

[18] Dokmanovic L, Urosevic J, Janic D, Jovanovic N, Petrucev B, Tosic N, Pavlovic S. Analysis of thiopurine S-methyltransferase polymorphism in the population of Serbia and Montenegro and mercaptopurine therapy tolerance in childhood acute lymphoblastic leukemia. Ther Drug Monit 2006; 28:800-806.

[19] Dokmanović L, Janić D, Krstovski N, Zukić B, Tosić N, Pavlović S. Importance of genotyping of thiopurine S-methyltransferase in children with acute lymphoblastic leukaemia during maintenance therapy. Srp Arh Celok Lek 2008; 136:609-616.

[20] Elion GB. Symposium on immunosuppressive drugs. Biochemistry and pharmacology of purine analogues. Federation Proceedings 26:898–904, 1967.

[21] Elion GB. Historical background of 6-mercaptopurine. Toxicol Ind Health 1986; 2:1-9.

[22] Evans WE, Hon YY, Bomgaars L, Coutre S, Holdsworth M, Janco R, Kalwinsky D, Keller F, Khatib Z, Margolin J, Murray J, Quinn J, Ravindranath Y, Ritchey K, Roberts W, Rogers ZR, Schiff D, Steuber C, Tucci F, Kornegay N, Krynetski EY, Relling MV. Preponderance of thiopurine S-methyltransferase deficiency and heterozygosity among patients intolerant to mercaptopurine or azathioprine. J Clin Oncol 2001; 19:2293-2301.

[23] Feng Q, Vannaprasaht S, Peng Y, Angsuthum S, Avihingsanon Y, Yee VC, Tassaneeyakul W, Weinshilboum RM. Thiopurine S-methyltransferase pharmacogenetics: functional characterization of a novel rapidly degraded variant allozyme. Biochem Pharmacol 2010; 79:1053–1061.

[24] Fessing MY, Krynetski EY, Zambetti GP, Evans WE. Functional characterization of the human thiopurine S-methyltransferase (TPMT) gene promoter. Eur J Biochem 1998; 256: 510-517.

[25] Garat A, Cauffiez C, Renault N, Lo-Guidice JM, Allorge D, Chevalier D, Houdret N, Chavatte P, Loriot MA, Gala JL, Broly F. Characterisation of novel defective thiopurine S-methyltransferase allelic variants. Biochem Pharmacol 2008; 76:404-415.

[26] Garrod AE. Inborn factors in disease: an essay. New York: Oxford University, Press, 1931.

[27] Georgitsi M, Zukic B, Pavlovic S, Patrinos GP. Transcriptional regulation and pharmacogenomics. Pharmacogenomics 2011; 12:655-673.

[28] Gurwitz D, Rodríguez-Antona C, Payne K, Newman W, Gisbert JP, de Mesa EG, Ibarreta D. Improving pharmacovigilance in Europe: TPMT genotyping and phenotyping in the UK and Spain. Eur J Hum Genet 2009; 17:991-998.

[29] Haglund S, Lindqvist M, Almer S, Peterson C, Taipalensuu J. Pyrosequencing of TPMT alleles in a general swedish population and in patients with inflammatory bowel disease. Clin Chem 2004; 50:285-294.

[30] Hall AG, Hamilton P, Minto L, Coulthard SA. The use of denaturing high-pressure liquid chromatography for the detectionof mutations in thiopurine methyltransferase. J Biochem Biophys Methods 2001; 47:65-71.

[31] Hamdan-Khalil R, Allorge D, Lo-Guidice JM, Cauffiez C, Chevalier D, Spire C, Houdret N, Libersa C, Lhermitte M, Colombel JF, Gala JL, Broly F. In vitro characterization of four novel non-functional variants of the thiopurine S-methyltransferase. Biochem Biophys Res Commun 2003; 309:1005-1010.

[32] Hamdan-Khalil R, Gala JL, Allorge D, Lo-Guidice JM, Horsmans Y, Houdret N, Broly F. Identification and functional analysis of two rare allelic variants of the thiopurine S-methyltransferase gene, TPMT*16 and TPMT*19. Biochem Pharmacol 2005; 69:525-529.

[33] Hon YY, Fessing MY, Pui CH, Relling MV, Krynetski EY, Evans WE. Polymorphism of the thiopurine S-methyltransferase gene in African-Americans. Hum Mol Genet 1999; 8:371-376.

[34] Honchel R, Aksoy I, Szumlanski C, Wood TC, Otterness DM, Wieben ED, Weinshilboum RM. Human thiopurine methyltransferase: Molecular cloning and expression of T84 colon carcinoma cell cDNA. Mol Pharmacol 1993; 43:878-887.

[35] Hongeng S, Sasanakul W, Chuansumrit A, Pakakasama S, Chattananon A, Hathirat P. Frequency of thiopurine S-methyltransferase genetic variation in Thai children with acute leukemia. Med Pediatr Oncol 2000; 35:410-414.

[36] Katzung B. Basic and clinical pharamcology. 9th Ed. London.: McGraw-Hill, 2004.

[37] Kennedy GC, Matsuzaki H, Dong S, Huang J, Liu G, Su X, Cao M, Chen W, Zhang J, Liu W, Yang G, Di X, Ryder T, He Z, Surti U, Phillips MS, Boice-Jacino MT, Fodor SP, Jones KW. Large-scale genotyping of complex DNA. Nat Biotechnol 2003; 21:1233-1237.

[38] Kham SK, Soh CK, Aw DC, Yeoh AE. TPMT*26 (208F-->L), a novel mutation detected in a Chinese. Br J Clin Pharmacol 2009; 68:120-123.

[39] Kidd KK, Pakstis AJ, Speed WC, Kidd JR. Understanding human DNA sequence variation. J Hered 2004; 95:406-420.

[40] Korbluth A, Sachar DB and the Practice Parameters Committee of the American College of Gastroenterology. Erratum: ulcerative colitis practice guidelines in

adults: American College of Gastroenterology, Practice Paremeters Committee. Ams J Gastroenterol 2010; 105:500-523.

[41] Kroplin T, Weyer N, Gutsche S, Iven H. Thiopurine S-methyltransferase activity in human erythrocytes: A new HPLC method using 6-thioguanine as substrate. Eur J Clin Pharmacol 1998; 54:265–271.

[42] Krynetskaia NF, Krynetski EY, Evans WE. Human RNase H-mediated RNA cleavage from DNA-RNA duplexes is inhibited by 6-deoxythioguanosine incorporation into DNA. Mol Pharmacol 1999; 56:841-848.

[43] Krynetski EY, Krynetskaia NF, Yanishevski Y, Evans WE. Methylation of mercaptopurine, thioguanine, and their nucleotide metabolites by heterologously expressed human thiopurine S-methyltransferase. Mol Pharmacol 1995; 47:1141-1147.

[44] Krynetski EY, Fessing MY, Yates CR, Sun D, Schuetz JD, Evans WE. Promoter and intronic sequences of the human thiopurine S-methyltransferase (TPMT) gene isolated from a human PAC1 genomic library. Pharm Res 1997; 14:1672-1678.

[45] Krynetski E, Evans WE. Drug methylation in cancer therapy: lessons from the TPMT polymorphism. Oncogene 2003; 22:7403-7413.

[46] Kubota T, Chiba K. Frequencies of thiopurine S-methyltransferase mutant alleles (TPMT*2, *3A, *3B and *3C) in 151 healthy Japanese subjects and the inheritance of TPMT*3C in the family of a propositus. Br J Clin Pharmacol 2001; 51:475-477.

[47] Lee D, Szumlanski C, Houtman J, Honchel R, Rojas K, Overhauser J, Wieben ED, Weinshilboum RM. Thiopurine methyltransferase pharmacogenetics: Cloning of human liver cDNA and presence of a processed pseudogene on human chromosome 18q21.1. Drug Metab Dispos 1995; 23:398–405.

[48] Lennard L. The clinical pharmacology of 6-mercaptopurine. Eur J Clin Pharmacol 1992; 43:329–339.

[49] Leung M, Piatkov I, Rochester C, Boyages SC, Leong RW. Normal thiopurine methyltransferase phenotype testing in a Crohn disease patient with azathioprine induced myelosuppression. Intern Med J 2009; 39:121-126.

[50] Lewis JD, Abramson O, Pascua M, Liu L, Asakura LM, Velayos FS, Hutfless SM, Alison JE, Herrinton LJ. Timing of myelosuppression during thiopurine therapy for inflammatory bowel disease: implications for monitoring recommendations. Clin Gastroenterol Hepatol 2009; 7:1195-1201.

[51] Lindqvist M, Almer S, Peterson C, Soderkvist P. Real-time RTPCR methodology for quantification of thiopurine methyltransferase gene expression. Eur J Clin Pharmacol 2003; 59:207–211.

[52] Lindqvist M, Haglund S, Almer S, Peterson C, Taipalensu J, Hertervig E, Lyrenäs E, Söderkvist P. Identification of two novel sequence variants affecting thiopurine methyltransferase enzyme activity. Pharmacogenetics 2004; 14:261-265.

[53] Lindqvist M, Skoglund K, Karlgren A, Söderkvist P, Peterson C, Kidhall I, Almer S. Explaining TPMT genotype/phenotype discrepancy by haplotyping of TPMT*3A and identification of a novel sequence variant, TPMT*23. Pharmacogenet Genomics 2007; 17:891-895.

[54] Ling YH, Chan JY, Beattie KL, Nelson JA. Consequences of 6-thioguanine incorporation into DNA on polymerase, ligase, and endonuclease reactions. Mol Pharmacol 1992; 42:802-807.

[55] Loennechen T, Yates CR, Fessing MY, Relling MV, Krynetski EY, Evans WE. Isolation of a human thiopurine S-methyltransferase (TPMT) complementary DNA with a single nucleotide transition A719G (TPMT*3C) and its association with loss of TPMT protein and catalytic activity in humans. Clin Pharmacol Ther 1998; 64:46-51.

[56] Maybaum J, Mandel HG. Differential chromatid damage induced by 6-thioguanine in CHO cells. Exp Cell Res 1981; 135:465-468.

[57] Maybaum J, Mandel HG. Unilateral chromatid damage: A new basis for 6-thioguanine cytotoxicity. Cancer Res 1983; 43:3852-3856.

[58] McDonald OG, Krynetski EY, Evans WE. Molecular haplotyping of genomic DNA for multiple single-nucleotide polymorphisms located kilobases apart using long-range polymerase chain reaction and intramolecular ligation. Pharmacogenetics 2002; 12:93-99.

[59] McLeod HL, Relling MV, Liu Q, Pui C-H, Evans WE. Polymorphic thiopurine methyltransferase in erythrocytes is indicative of activity in leukemic blasts from children with acute lymphoblastic leukemia. Blood 1995; 85:1897-1902.

[60] McLeod HL, Pritchard SC, Githang'a J, Indalo A, Ameyaw MM, Powrie RH, Booth L, Collie-Duguid ES. Ethnic differences in thiopurine methyltransferase pharmacogenetics: evidence for allele specificity in Caucasian and Kenyan individuals. Pharmacogenetics 1999; 9:773-776.

[61] McLeod HL, Krynetski EY, Relling MV, Evans WE. Genetic polymorphism of thiopurine methyltransferase and its clinical relevance for childhood acute lymphoblastic leukemia. Leukemia 2000; 14:567-572.

[62] Murray JE, Merrill JP, Harrison JH, Wilson RE, Dammin GJ. Prolonged survival of human kidney homografts by immunosuppresssive drug therapy. New Engl J Med 1963; 268:1315-1323.

[63] Nguyen CM, Mendes MAS, Ma JD. Evidence on Genomic Tests: Thiopurine methyltransferase (TPMT) genotyping to predict myelosuppression risk. PLoS Curr 2011; 3:RRN1236.

[64] O'Brien SJ, Menotti-Raymond M, Murphy WJ, Nash WG, Wienberg J, Stanyon R, Copeland NG, Jenkins NA, Womack JE, Marshall Graves JA. The promise of comparative genomics in mammals. Science 1999; 15:458–481.

[65] Oliveira E, Quental S, Alves S, Amorim A, Prata MJ. Do the distribution patterns of polymorphisms at the thiopurine S-methyltransferase locus in sub-Saharan populations need revision? Hints from Cabinda and Mozambique. Eur J Clin Pharmacol 2007; 63:703-706.

[66] Otterness C, Szumlanski C, Lennard L, Klemetsdal B, Aarbakke J, Park-Hah JO, Iven H, Schmiegelow K, Branum E, O'Brien J, Weinshilboum R. Human thiopurine methyltransferase pharmacogenetics: gene sequence polymorphisms. Clin Pharmacol Ther 1997; 62:60-73.

[67] Otterness DM, Szumlanski CL, Wood TC, Weinshilboum RM. Human thiopurine methyltransferase pharmacogenetics. Kindred with a terminal exon splice junction mutation that results in loss of activity. J Clin Invest 1998; 101:1036-1044.

[68] Pan BF, Nelson JA. Characterization of the DNA damage in 6-thioguanine-treated cells. Biochem Pharmacol 1990; 40:1063–1069.

[69] Pavlovic S. TPMT gene polymorphisms: on the doorstep of personalized medicine. Indian J Med Res 2009; 129:478-480.

[70] Pavlovic S, Zukic B. Individualized therapy: role of thiopurine S-methyltransferase protein and genetic variants. JMB 2010; 29:1-5.

[71] Posthuma EF, Westendorp RG, van der Sluys Veer A, Kluin-Nelemans JC, Kluin PM, Lamers CB. Fatal infectious mononucleosis: a severe complication in the treatment of Crohn's disease with azathioprine. Gut 1995; 36:311-313.

[72] Present DH, Meltzer SJ, Krumholz MP, Wolke A, Korelitz BI. 6-mercaptopurine in the management of inflammatory bowel disease: short- and long-term toxicity. Ann Intern Med 1989; 111:641-649.

[73] Relling MV, Altman RB, Goetz MP, Evans WE. Clinical implementation of pharmacogenomics: overcoming genetic exceptionalism. Lancet Oncol 2010; 11:507-509.

[74] Relling MV, Gardner EE, Sandborn WJ, Schmiegelow K, Pui C-H, Yee SW, CM Stein CM, Carrillo M, Evans WE, Klein TE, CPIC. Clinical Pharmacogenetics Implementation Consortium Guidelines for Thiopurine Methyltransferase Genotype and Thiopurine Dosing. Clin Pharmacol Ther 2011a; 89:387-391.

[75] Relling MV, Klein TE, CPIC. Clinical Pharmacogenetics Implementation Consortium of the Pharmacogenomics Research Network. Clin Pharmacol Ther 2011b; 89:474-477.

[76] Remy CN. Metabolism of thiopyrimidines and thiopurines. S-Methylation with S-adenosylmethionine transmethylase and catabolism in mammalian tissues. J Biol Chem 1963; 238:1078-1084.

[77] Roberts RL, Gearry RB, Bland MV, Sies CW, George PM, Burt M, Marinaki AM, Arenas M, Barclay ML, Kennedy MA. Trinucleotide repeat variants in the promoter of the thiopurine S-methyltransferase gene of patients exhibiting ultra-high enzyme activity. Pharmacogenet Genomics 2008; 18:434-438.

[78] Sandborn WJ. Rational dosing of azathioprine and 6-mercaptopurine. Gut 2001; 48:591-592.

[79] Schaeffeler E, Lang T, Zanger UM, Eichelbaum M, Schwab M. High-throughput genotyping of thiopurine S-methyltransferase by denaturing HPLC. Clin Chem 2001; 47:548-555.

[80] Schaeffeler E, Stanulla M, Greil J, Schrappe M, Eichelbaum M, Zanger UM, Schwab M. A novel TPMT missense mutation associated with TPMT deficiency in a 5-year-old boy with ALL. Leukemia 2003; 17:1422-1424.

[81] Schaeffeler E, Fischer C, Brockmeier D, Wernet D, Moerike K, Eichelbaum M, Zanger UM, Schwab M. Comprehensive analysis of thiopurine S-methyltransferase phenotype-genotype correlation in a large population of German-Caucasians and identification of novel TPMT variants. Pharmacogenetics 2004; 14:407-417.

[82] Schaeffeler E, Eichelbaum M, Reinisch W, Zanger UM, Schwab M. Three novel thiopurine S-methyltransferase allelic variants (TPMT*20, *21, *22) – association with decreased enzyme function. Hum Mutat 2006; 27:976.

[83] Schmiegelow K, Forestier E, Kristinsson J, Söderhäll S, Vettenranta K, Weinshilboum R, Wesenberg F; Nordic Society of Paediatric Haematology and Oncology. Thiopurine methyltransferase activity is related to the risk of relapse of childhood acute lymphoblastic leukemia: results from the NOPHO ALL-92 study. Leukemia 2009; 23:557-564.

[84] Schütz E, Gummert J, Mohr F, Oellerich M. Azathioprine-induced myelosuppression in thiopurine methyltransferase deficient heart transplant recipient. Lancet 1993; 341:436.

[85] Schwab M, Schaeffeler E, Marx C, Zanger U, Aulitzky W, Eichelbaum M. Shortcoming in the diagnosis of TPMT deficiency in a patient with Crohn's disease using phenotyping only. Gastroenterology 2001; 121:498–499.

[86] Schwab M, Schäffeler E, Marx C, Fischer C, Lang T, Behrens C, Gregor M, Eichelbaum M, Zanger UM, Kaskas BA. Azathioprine therapy and adverse drug reactions in patients with inflammatory bowel disease: impact of thiopurine S-methyltransferase polymorphism. Pharmacogenetics 2002; 12:429-436.

[87] Slanar O, Chalupná P, Novotný A, Bortlík M, Krska Z, Lukás M. Fatal myelotoxicity after azathioprine treatment. Nucleos Nucleot Nucl 2008; 27:661-665.

[88] Spire-Vayron de la Moureyre C, Debuysere H, Mastain B, Vinner E, Marez D, Lo Guidice JM, Chevalier D, Brique S, Motte K, Colombel JF, Turck D, Noel C, Flipo RM, Pol A, Lhermitte M, Lafitte JJ, Libersa C, Broly F. Genotypic and phenotypic analysis of the polymorphic thiopurine S-methyltransferase gene (TPMT) in a European population. Br J Pharmacol 1998a; 125:879-887.

[89] Spire-Vayron de la Moureyre C, Debuysère H, Sabbagh N, Marez D, Vinner E, Chevalier ED, Lo Guidice JM, Broly F. Detection of known and new mutations in the thiopurine S-methyltransferase gene by single-strand conformation polymorphism analysis. Hum Mutat 1998b; 12:177-185.

[90] Spire-Vayron de la Moureyre C, Debuysere H, Fazio F, Sergent E, Bernard C, Sabbagh N, Marez D, Lo Guidice JM, D'halluin JC, Broly F. Characterization of variable number tandem repeat region in the thiopurine S-methyltransferase gene promoter. Pharmacogenetics 1999; 9:189–198.

[91] Stocco G, Crews KR, Evans WE. Genetic polymorphism of inosine-triphosphate-pyrophosphatase influences mercaptopurine metabolism and toxicity during treatment of acute lymphoblastic leukemia individualized for thiopurine-S-methyl-transferase status Expert Opin Drug Saf 2010; 9:23-37.

[92] Stojiljkovic M, Patrinos GP, Pavlovic S. Clinical Applicability of Sequence Variations in Genes Related to Drug Metabolism. Curr Drug Metab 2011; 12:445-454.

[93] Swen JJ, Nijenhuis M, de Boer A, Grandia L, Maitland-van der Zee AH, Mulder H, Rongen GA, van Schaik RH, Schalekamp T, Touw DJ, van der Weide J, Wilffert B, Deneer VH, Guchelaar HJ. Pharmacogenetics: from bench to byte-an update of guidelines. Clin Pharmacol Ther 2011; 89:662-673.

[94] Szumlanski C, Otterness D, Her C, Lee D, Brandriff B, Kelsell D, Spurr N, Lennard L, Wieben E, Weinshilboum R. Thiopurine methyltransferase pharmacogenetics: human gene cloning and characterization of a common polymorphism. DNA Cell Biol 1996; 15:17-30.

[95] Tai HL, Krynetski EY, Yates CR, Loennechen T, Fessing MY, Krynetskaia NF, Evans WE. Thiopurine S-methyltransferase deficiency: two nucleotide transitions define the most prevalent mutant allele associated with loss of catalytic activity in Caucasians. Am J Hum Genet 1996; 58:694-702.

[96] Tai HL, Krynetski EY, Schuetz EG, Yanishevski Y, Evans WE. Enhanced proteolysis of thiopurine S-methyltransferase (TPMT) encoded by mutant alleles in humans

(TPMT*3A, TPMT*2): mechanisms for the genetic polymorphism of TPMT activity. Proc Natl Acad Sci U S A 1997; 94:6444-6449.

[97] Tay BS, Lilley RM, Murray AW, Atkinson MR. Inhibition of phosphoribosyl pyrophosphate amidotransferase from ehrlich ascitestumour cells by thiopurine nucleotides. Biochem Pharmacol 1969; 18:936–938.

[98] Ugajin T, Miyatani H, Demitsu T, Iwaki T, Ushimaru S, Nakashima Y, Yoshida Y. Severe myelosuppression following alopecia shortly after the initiation of 6-mercaptopurine in a patient with Crohn's disease. Intern Med 2009; 48:693-695.

[99] Ujiie S, Sasaki T, Mizugaki M, Ishikawa M, Hiratsuka M. Functional characterization of 23 allelic variants of thiopurine S-methyltransferase gene (TPMT*2-*24). Pharmacogenet Genomics 2008; 18:887-893.

[100] Van Loon JA, Weinshilboum RM. Thiopurine methyltransferase biochemical genetics: Human lymphocyte activity. Biochem Genet 1982; 20:637–658.

[101] Van Loon JA, Weinshilboum RM. Human lymphocyte thiopurine methyltransferase pharmacogenetics: Effect of phenotype on 6-mercaptopurine-induced inhibition of mitogen stimulation. J Pharmacol Exp Ther 1987; 242:21–26.

[102] Vuchetich JP, Weinshilboum RM, Price RA. Segregation analysis of human red blood cell thiopurine methyltransferase activity. Genet Epidemiol 1995; 12:1-11.

[103] Wang L, Sullivan W, Toft D, Weinshilboum R. Thiopurine S-methyltransferase pharmacogenetics: chaperone protein association and allozyme degradation. Pharmacogenetics 2003; 13:555-564.

[104] Weinshilboum RM, Raymond FA, Pazmiño PA. Human erythrocyte thiopurine methyltransferase: radiochemical microassay and biochemical properties. Clin Chim Acta 1978; 85:323-333.

[105] Weinshilboum RM, Sladek SL. Mercaptopurine pharmacogenetics: monogenic inheritance of erythrocyte thiopurine methyltransferase activity. Am J Hum Genet 1980; 32:651-662.

[106] Weinshilboum R. Thiopurine pharmacogenetics: clinical and molecular studies of thiopurine methyltransferase. Drug Metab Dispos 2001; 29:601-605.

[107] Weinshilboum R. Inheritance and drug response. N Engl J Med 2003; 348:529-537.

[108] Weinshilboum R, Wang L. Thiopurine S-methyltransferase pharmacogenetics: insights, challenges and future directions. Oncogene 2006; 25:1629–1638.

[109] Wolf CR, Smith G, Smith RL. Science, medicine, and the future: Pharmacogenetics. BMJ 2000; 320:987-990.

[110] Yates CR, Krynetski EY, Loennechen T, Fessing MY, Tai HL, Pui CH, Relling MV, Evans WE. Molecular diagnosis of thiopurine S-methyltransferase deficiency: genetic basis for azathioprine and mercaptopurine intolerance. Ann Intern Med 1997; 126:608-614.

[111] Yi L, Tan PL, Hen CK, Huang LQ, Li FY, Quah TC, Yeoh EJ. Arrayed primer extension (APEX): A solid-phase four-color DNA minisequencing to detect the mutations on the human beta-globin and thiopurine methyltransferase (TPMT) genes. Blood 2002; 100: 896.

[112] Zukic B, Radmilovic M, Stojiljkovic M, Tosic N, Pourfarzad F, Dokmanovic L, Janic D, Colovic N, Philipsen S, Patrinos GP, Pavlovic S. Functional analysis of the role of the TPMT gene promoter VNTR polymorphism in TPMT gene transcription. Pharmacogenomics 2010; 11:547-557.

4

S-Adenosylmethionine: A Novel Factor in the Individualization of Thiopurine Therapy

Irena Mlinaric-Rascan, Miha Milek,
Alenka Smid and Natasa Karas Kuzelicki
University of Ljubljana, Faculty of Pharmacy, Ljubljana,
Slovenia

1. Introduction

Individualizing drug therapy by the use of pharmacogenomics offers the opportunity to improve drug efficacy, reduce adverse side effects, and provide cost-effective pharmaceutical care. 6-mercaptopurine (6-MP), 6-thioguanine (6-TG) and azathioprine (AZA) are widely prescribed cytotoxic and immunosuppressive drugs used in the therapy of acute leukaemia, inflammatory bowel diseases, allograft rejections and others.

The efficacy and toxicity of thiopurine drugs has been established to correlate with the extent of their deactivation by S-methylation. The discovery that the activity of thiopurine S-methyltransferase (TPMT) in human tissues depends on the presence of germline single nucleotide polymorphisms (SNPs) led to one of the best examples of the successful clinical application of pharmacogenetic studies (Milek et al., 2006; R. Weinshilboum, 2001; R. M. Weinshilboum&Sladek, 1980). TPMT catalyzes the direct S-methylation of 6-MP to produce the inactive metabolite 6-methylmercaptopurine (6-MMP) leading to the lower toxic potential of the drug. Of more than 20 known polymorphisms in the TPMT gene, the most common variant alleles include TPMT*2, *3A and *3C. In Caucasian populations, individuals with homozygous variant and heterozygous genotypes have, respectively, low and intermediate TPMT activity, while individuals carrying the wild-type gene sequence exhibit a very wide range of high activity values. Patients with decreased TPMT activity are, when treated with standard doses of thiopurine medications, at greater risk of developing thiopurine induced toxicities, such as myelosupression, leucopenia and stomatitis (R. Weinshilboum, 2001).

Homozygous patients with low or absent TPMT activity require a reduction to 10% of the standard dose, while heterozygous individuals should be administered 30-70%, depending on the initial treatment response (Relling et al., 2011). Predictive genotyping for the purpose of optimizing thiopurine treatment represents one of the best clinical applications of pharmacogenetic testing.

In addition to being affected by genotype, TPMT activity is also regulated by a complex metabolic network. We and others have reported on the stabilization of TPMT by its co-factor S-adenosylmethionine (SAM), which represents a candidate biomarker affecting TPMT activity and might to some extent explain the discordance between TPMT genotype and phenotype (Milek et al., 2009; Scheuermann et al., 2004; Tai et al., 1997). In addition, it has been shown that polymorphisms in gene for MTHFR, the enzyme involved in SAM biosynthesis, correlate with the onset of hematotoxic events during the therapy of acute lymphoblastic leukaemia (ALL) (Karas-Kuzelicki et al., 2009).

As the metabolism of SAM is closely related to the methionine cycle and the folate pathway, other endogenous metabolites, such as folates and methionine, as well as enzymes participating in their biosynthesis, might also indirectly influence TPMT activity.

Both the identification and understanding of the factors influencing TPMT activity are crucial for improving the efficacy and safety of thiopurine therapy.

2. Thiopurine drugs

An ingenious idea, the purpose of which was to stop the growth of rapidly growing cells such as bacteria and tumours with modified nucleic acid bases was developed concomitantly with the discovery of DNA structure. A synthetic thiol-analogue of endogenous nucleic bases, thioguanine (6-TG), followed by 6-mercaptopurine (6-MP), and azathioprine (AZA), proved toxic to bacteria and tumours in mice. The initial experiments, conducted in 1948, were followed by clinical trials in 1953 and also present the basis for contemporary thiopurine therapy. Gertrude Elion and George Hitchings were rewarded for this work with the Nobel Prize in Physiology or Medicine in 1988 (Marx, 1988).

2.1 Mode of action

The thiopurines, namely 6-marcaptopurine, azathioprine, and 6-thioguanine are inactive prodrugs which require intestinal absorption, cellular uptake and intracellular metabolism for their cytotoxic activity. The three main metabolic pathways for thiopurines are oxidation by xanthine oxidase (XO), phosphoribosylation by hypoxanthine-guanine phosphoribosyltransferase (HGPRT), and S-methylation by TPMT (R. Weinshilboum, 2001). Oxidation is a purely inactivating pathway, which is relevant only in non-hematopoietic cells, due to the restricted expression of XO in blood cells. Despite the fact that XO activity significantly varies among individuals, a molecular basis has not been completely delineated yet.

The conversion of 6-MP by hypoxanthine phosphoribosyltransferase (HGPRT) yields thioinosine monophosphate (TIMP), which is further metabolized via inosine 5'-monophosphate dehydrogenase (IMPD), guanosine monophosphate synthetase (GMPS), reductase and kinases to active thioguanine nucleotides (TGNs). Alternatively, TIMP can be methylated by thiopurine methyltransferase (TPMT) to 6-methylmercaptopurine ribonucleosides (6-MMPR), namely methylthioinosine monophosphate (MeTIMP), -diphosphate (MeTIDP) and –triphosphate (MeTITP) (Fig.1).

Incorporation of TGNs into DNA and RNA results in S phase arrest and programmed cell death, triggered via the mismatch repair pathway. On the other hand, MeTIMP is a potent inhibitor of de novo purine synthesis (DNPS), causing depletion of purine nucleotides, which results in cell growth arrest and cytotoxicity. DNPS inhibition is thought to be responsible for several adverse effects of thiopurines. Nevertheless, the incorporation of TGNs is considered to be the main mode of action of 6-MP (Relling et al., 1999).

Phosphorylation of TIMP by kinases yields 6-thioinosine triphosphate (TITP), which can be dephosphorylated back to TIMP by inosine triphosphatase (ITPA) (Derijks&Wong, 2010).

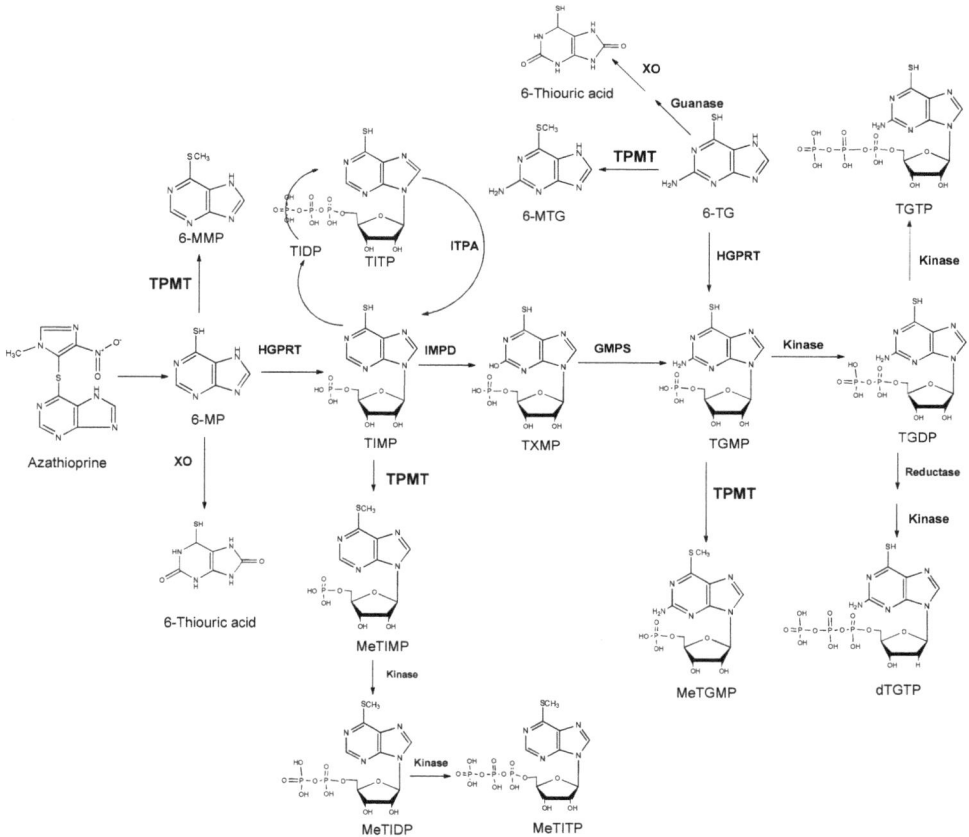

Fig. 1. **Metabolism of thiopurines.** Azathioprine is converted to 6-mercaptopurine (6-MP) by a non-enzymatic process. Both 6-MP and 6-thioguanine (6-TG) are converted by the hypoxanthine–guanine phosphoribosyltransferase (HGPRT) into their respective nucleoside monophosphates (TIMP and TGMP). Thiopurine S-methyltransferase (TPMT) inactivates 6-MP and 6-TG by S-methylation to form 6-methylmercaptopurine (6-MMP) and 6-methylthioguanine (6-TGN), respectively. Xanthine oxidase (XO) inactivates 6-MP by converting it to 6-thiouric acid. TIMP and TGMP are also TPMT substrates, yielding methylated TIMP (meTIMP) and methylated TGMP (meTGMP). TIMP may also be phosphorylated to TIDP and TITP and dephosphorylated to TIMP by ITPA. TIMP that escapes catabolism is further metabolized by inosine monophosphate dehydrogenase (IMPD) and guanine monophosphate synthetase (GMPS) to TGMP. Sequential action of deoxynucleoside kinases and reductase generates the TGTP and dTGTP that are the substrates for incorporation of 6-TG into RNA and DNA, respectively.

The third metabolic pathway, catalyzed by TPMT, is S-methylation of thiopurine to 6-methylmercaptopurine (6-MMP). This pathway is often referred to as being an inactivating pathway, since 6-MMP has no cytotoxic activity (Dervieux et al., 2001) (Fig. 1).

2.2 Efficacy and safety of 6-MP in the treatment of ALL

Acute lymphoblastic leukaemia is the most common malignancy in children. Treatment is stratified on the basis of various combinations of clinical and lymphoblastic characteristics in standard, intermediate and intensive therapy groups. Different therapy protocols have been and continue to be applied, such as USA Pediatric Oncology Group (POG) protocols and German Berlin-Frankfurt-Muenster (BFM) protocols (BFM-83, -86, -90, -95 and IC 2002). Treatment is generally composed of induction, consolidation and maintenance phases along with central nervous system prophylaxis (Moricke et al., 2008).

The induction phase generally lasts 4-6 weeks and involves combinations of drugs including vincristine, prednisone, cyclophosphamide, doxorubicin, and L-asparaginase. This phase is followed by the consolidation phase with multiagent therapy including cytarabine and methotrexate. Maintenance therapy has been included in all protocols. It lasts from 1 to 3 years and consists of 6-MP taken daily per os (50 mg/m²) and low weekly doses of oral methotrexate (MTX) (20 mg/m²) (Karas Kuzelicki et al., 2009).

Due to the narrow therapeutic index, a certain level of side effect manifestations is expected in most patients treated with 6-MP. We have investigated the occurrences of side effects in Slovenian pediatric ALL patients, identified through the national oncology patient registry. These patients had been treated with standard protocols at the University Children's Hospital, University Medical Centre, Ljubljana, Slovenia in the period 1970-2004. The study group consisted of 313 ALL patients. 6-MP and other thiopurines were administered in all phases of ALL treatment. In order to investigate the occurrences of toxic effects and to exclude the influence of other drugs used in ALL treatment, we focused on the maintenance phase of the therapy, because it consisted exclusively of 6-MP and low dose MTX. The doses of 6-MP were calculated on the basis of a patient's body surface (50 mg/m²) and adjusted during the treatment according to desired WBC counts, these being 2000 – 3000 WBC/μL.

Therapy data, such as 6-MP dose reduction and the incidence of toxic effects including hematotoxicity, stomatitis, infections, and secondary tumours were obtained from patients' charts for the maintenance phase of treatment protocols consisting exclusively of 6-MP and low dose MTX. 6-MP dose reduction greater than 10 % for a period longer than 3 months was considered significant. The toxic effect was defined as an event causing one of the following: discontinuation of the therapy for longer than one week, a reduction of over 10 % of 6-MP dose of a duration longer than 3 months, or the hospitalization of the patient. Hematotoxicity corresponded to grade 3 and 4 leukopenia, stomatitis to grade 2 and 3, infections to grade 3 and 4 and secondary tumours to grade 4 adverse events of National Cancer Institute Common Toxicity Criteria (version 2.0) (Karas Kuzelicki et al., 2009).

The incidences of undesirable toxic effects are presented in Table 1. Despite the relatively high safety and efficacy of 6-MP, a dose reduction was determined in 20 % of patients, hematotoxicity in 14 %, stomatitis in 5 %, infections in 21 %, and the incidence of secondary tumours in 4 % of patients. Our observations are also in concordance with other published data (Sanderson et al., 2004).

Side effects % Patients	6-MP DR [†]	HET [‡]	Stomatitis [‡]	Infections[‡]	Secondary TU
Patients with the condition, n (%)	63 (20.2)	44 (14.1)	14 (4.5)	67 (21.4)	13 (4.1)
Patients without the condition, n (%)	249 (79.8)	269 (85.9)	299 (95.5)	246 (78.6)	300 (95.9)

6-MP DR, 6-MP dose reduction; HET, hematotoxicity; TU, tumours; n indicates number of subjects;
[†] More than 10 % 6-MP dose reduction for a period of more than 3 months.
[‡] A 6-MP related toxic effect that caused the discontinuation of the therapy for more than one week, more than 10 % 6-MP dose reduction for a period of more than 3 months or hospitalization of the patient.

Table 1. Analysis of 6-MP related toxic effects in Slovenian ALL patients

2.3 Thiopurines in the immunosuppressive therapy

Azathioprine (AZA) and 6-MP are the most widely used immunosuppressive agents in inflammatory bowel disease (IBD), examples of which being ulcerative colitis and Crohn's disease. AZA is also indicated as an adjunct for the prevention of rejection in renal homotransplantations and for the management of active rheumatoid arthritis. Either alone or, more usually, in combination with corticosteroids and/or other drugs and procedures, AZA has been used in a proportion of patients suffering systemic lupus erythematosus, dermatomyositis and polymyositis, autoimmune chronic active hepatitis, pemphigus vulgaris, polyarteritis nodosa, autoimmune haemolytic anaemia and chronic refractory idiopathic thrombocytopenic purpura (IMURAN® (azathioprine). Product Information). On the other hand, 6-MP has been mostly used in either IBD or acute lymphoblastic leukaemia.

Azathioprine was developed to prolong the half-life of 6-MP; therefore, a 1-methyl-4-nitro-5-imidazole moiety was added to protect the reactive sulphur group from oxidation and hydrolysis. AZA was proven to have better immunomodulatory effects than 6-MP in preventing organ rejection in kidney transplants (Murray et al., 1963). It is postulated that this is associated with an effect of the methyl-nitro-imidazolyl substitute by a currently unknown mechanism. Although both drugs have been extensively used, they have proven ineffective in one-third of patients, while up to one-fifth of patients discontinue thiopurine therapy due to adverse reactions. The observed interindividual differences in therapeutic response and toxicity can, at least partly, be explained by genetic polymorphisms of the genes encoding crucial enzymes in thiopurine metabolism (Derijks&Wong, 2010).

The reported frequencies of dose-dependent and dose-independent adverse effects of AZA and 6-MP are in the ranges of 1.4–5.0 % and 1.0–6.5 %, respectively. Myelotoxicity is considered a dose-dependent adverse effect that can be caused by elevated concentrations of the pharmacologically active 6-TGNs. On the other hand, dose-independent reactions are considered to be immune-mediated, and include rashes, arthralgia, hepatitis, myalgia, flu-like symptoms, gastrointestinal complaints, fever and pancreatitis (de Boer et al., 2007)

3. Individualization of thiopurine therapy

Pharmacogenetic testing has been implemented in clinical practice for selected drugs only. The implementation of pharmacogenetics in the clinical setting was hampered by the recognition that the metabolism of a given drug does not depend solely on a single drug-metabolizing enzyme, but rather on a complex enzymatic network of competing metabolic pathways. It has become apparent that the identification of relevant pharmacogenetic markers is much more complicated than initially believed.

Upon entering the cell, thiopurines are also subject to a complex metabolic network; their metabolic activation thus depends on genetic predisposition as well as nutritional and other environmental factors.

3.1 Thiopurine S-methyltransferase (TPMT)

Although TPMT pharmacogenetics is addressed in detail in a separate chapter of this book, we need to summarize the most relevant facts, since they are the basis for further elaborations.

TPMT plays a pivotal role in thiopurine drug responses, such that decreased TPMT activity correlates with higher cytotoxic thioguanine nucleotide (TGN) levels which may result in life-threatening toxicity. The distribution of TPMT activity in Caucasian populations is trimodal: approximately 89 % of population has normal to high, 11 % intermediate and 0.3 % low or undetectable TPMT activity. Although numerous alleles have been identified, the most prevalent and clinically significant are TPMT*3A (460G>A and 719A>G), TPMT*3B (460G>A) and TPMT*3C (719A>G). TPMT genotyping prior to the initiation of thiopurine therapy represents a quick and reliable pharmacogenetic test. In accordance with advice provided by the FDA in 2004, the recommendation to perform the test before starting therapy with thiopurines has been included in the Summary of Product Characteristics (SmPC) of Purinethol® (6-MP) and Imuran® to highlight the usefulness of TPMT testing in predicting risk for thiopurine toxicity.

TPMT deficient patients tend to be better responders to 6-MP therapy than wild-type patients- due to higher TGN accumulation in cancer cells- but are at greater risk of developing toxic effects such as hematotoxicity, infections, stomatitis and secondary tumours, as a consequence of their accumulation in normal cells. Conversely, ultra-high enzyme activity can lead to superior 6-MP tolerability but also to an increased risk of relapse and hepatic toxicity, which has been related to methylated metabolites of thiopurines (Evans, 2004).

The clinical relevance of 6-MP dose reduction during maintenance therapy is well defined only in patients homozygous for variant TPMT alleles (TPMT*2, *3A, *3C) who exhibit low TPMT activity. Dosing adjustments based on TPMT status is recommended in thiopurine therapy. In the treatment of malignancies, conventional high doses of thiopurines are recommended for homozygous wild-type TPMT patients, while 30-70 % lower-than-normal starting doses should be used in heterozygous deficient patients, and at least 10-fold reduced doses in homozygous deficient patients (Relling et al., 2011).

Due to an incomplete genotype-to-phenotype correlation in heterozygous individuals with variable intermediate activity, the predictive value of TPMT genotyping for the optimization of thiopurine therapy is limited. Therefore, the identification of novel pharmacogenetic and/or biochemical markers is necessary for high prediction. One such factor is S-adenosylmethionine (SAM), which stabilizes the TPMT protein structure by binding to its active site (Scheuermann et al., 2004). Thus, SAM may also modulate TPMT activity in the intercellular setting, possibly by post-translational stabilization. Consequently, the endogenous availability of SAM may influence TPMT activity, the formation of 6-MP metabolites, and the toxicity of thiopurine drugs. In addition, endogenous metabolites (e.g. folates, methionine, ATP) and enzymes participating in the biosynthesis of SAM, (e.g. MTHFR, TYMS), could also influence TPMT activity indirectly.

3.2 The role of SAM in cellular metabolism and disease

S-adenosyl-L-methionine (SAM) is one of the most abundant co-factors in eukaryotic cells and has been initially described as "active methionine" (Cantoni, 1951). It participates in many cellular processes and exerts many biological effects. As a pleiotropic molecule, it is the principal methyl donor in processes such as nucleic acid, protein and phospholipid methylation, acting as a co-substrate for many SAM-dependent methyltransferases (P. K. Chiang et al., 1996). In addition, it is an important regulator of replication, transcription and translation, acting on post-transcriptional and post-translational levels and by epigenetic mechanisms (Finkelstein, 2007). SAM is also involved in polyamine synthesis as well as inhibition of DNA demethylation (Detich et al., 2003), and plays an important role in cell growth, cell cycle progression and apoptosis (Loenen, 2006; Nitta et al., 2002).

Cellular methylation is closely connected to the methionine cycle, methionine recycling pathway, folate metabolism, and polyamine synthesis, as well as transsulfuration and glutathione synthesis (Fig. 2) (Hitchler&Domann, 2007). Active metabolic conversions of the folate pathway and methionine (Met) cycle are ubiquitous, while transsulfuration takes place only in the liver, kidney, pancreas, intestinal tract and brain (Finkelstein, 2007). SAM and SAH act as efficient regulatory molecules in these processes, such that their molar ratio (i.e. methylation potential) determines the activity of many methyltransferases and related enzymes.

SAM is synthesized from Met, the availability of which largely depends on folate pools and dietary intake. Tissue SAM levels thus depend on the expression of methionine adenosyltransferase (MAT), which catalyzes the conversion from Met, and 5,10-methylenetetrahydrofolate reductase (MTHFR) that provides the substrate for the remethylation of homocysteine into Met. Mechanisms of SAM-induced metabolic regulation include the modulation of both tissue expression and kinetic properties of metabolizing enzymes as well as the concentrations of their substrates and products. Vice versa, the modified expression or enzyme activity of some methyltransferases has been shown to impact intracellular SAM and SAH levels, which are most notably determined by the expression of glycine N-methyltransferase (GNMT) (Luka et al., 2009). GNMT degrades excess SAM to SAH and decreases cell methylation capacity. Importantly, GNMT has been described as a key regulator of SAM level and methylation capacity in normal livers, while its expression is diminished in tumour tissue and cultured cells such as HepG2 (Martinez-Chantar et al., 2008).

Moreover, the modified activity of enzymes (e.g. methionine adenosyltransferase, S-adenosylhomocystein hydrolase) that catalyse the afore mentioned metabolic conversions significantly influences the dynamics and concentrations of metabolites; most prominently those of SAM and SAH, which have pleiotropic biological effects. In addition, aberrations in methylation and redox homeostasis have been implicated in several pathologies, such as liver carcinogenesis, hepatocellular carcinoma, chronic steatohepatitis and hyperhomocysteinemia-associated cardiovascular diseases (Martinez-Chantar et al., 2002a).

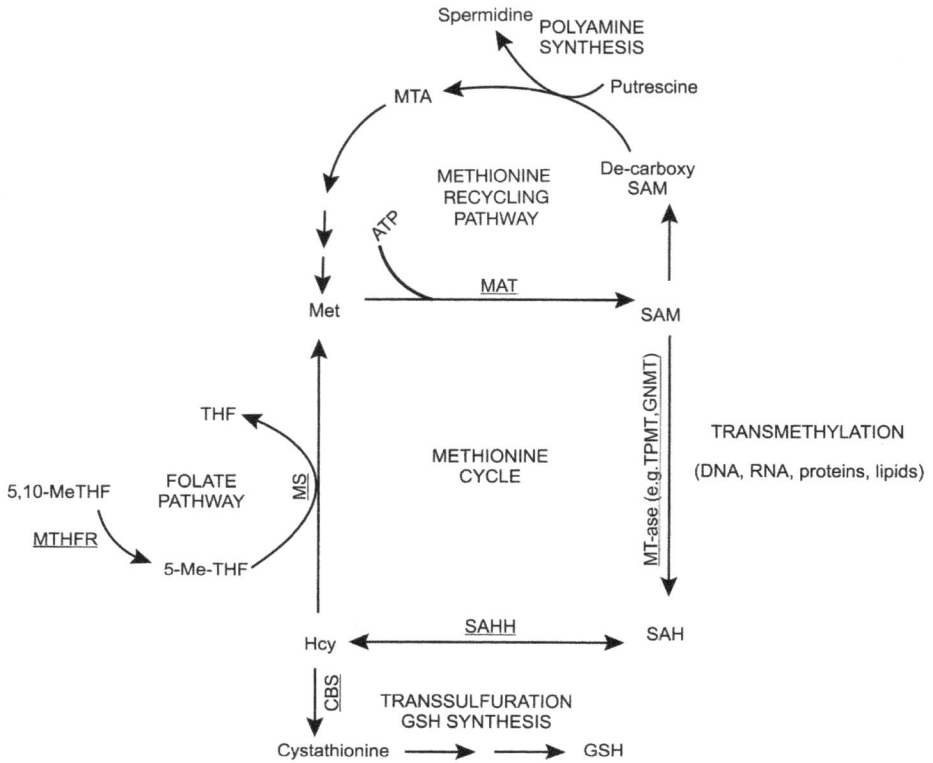

Fig. 2. SAM metabolism, the methionine cycle and related pathways. SAM is consumed in transmethylation reactions catalyzed by SAM-dependent methyltransferases (MT-ases). SAM has many diverse biological effects. Its metabolism is closely connected to homocysteine (Hcy) remethylation and methionine (Met) cycle, the folate pathway, transsulfuration, Met recycling pathway and polyamine synthesis. 5,10-Me-THF, 5,10-methylenetetrahydrofolate; 5-Me-THF, 5-methyltetrahydrofolate; THF, tetrahydrofolate; MS, methionine synthase; MTHFR, 5,10-methylenetetrahydrofolate reductase; CBS, cystathionine-β-synthase; Cys, cysteine; GSH, glutathione; SAHH, S-adenosylhomocysteine hydrolase; MAT, methionine adenosyltransferase; MTA, 5'-methylthioadenosine; MTAP, 5'-methylthioadenosine phosphorylase; Cys, cysteine; SAM, S-adenosylmethionine; SAMDC, SAM decarboxylase; TPMT, thiopurine S-methyltransferase, GNMT, glycine N-methyltransferase.

Unbalanced metabolic conversions in the methionine cycle are most frequently a consequence of a low dietary intake of folic acid, high alcohol consumption, poisoning, or genetic abnormalities. Most commonly, this is observed as hyperhomocysteinemia (i.e. elevated plasma homocysteine, Hcy), as well as SAM depletion, and consequently methionine metabolism related pathogenesis. Consequences of inactivated SAM, Met synthesis and methionine adenosyltransferase activity have been well documented in patients with liver cyrosis and different forms of hyperhomocysteinemia (Martinez-Chantar et al., 2002b).

3.3 The role of SAM in thiopurine metabolism

SAM plays an important role in the intracellular conversions of thiopurines. The metabolism of 6-mercaptopurine and azathioprine results, apart from the synthesis of cytotoxic TGNs, cytosolic, in the production of methylated thiopurine metabolites (methylthioinosine 5'-monofosphate, MeTIMP). These molecules act as antimetabolites by inhibiting phosphoribosyl pyrophosphate amidotransferase, the rate limiting enzyme in de novo purine synthesis (DNPS) pathways, which therefore leads to ineffective ATP production. Non-depleted cellular ATP pools are required for SAM biosynthesis from Met catalyzed by methionine adenosyltransferase (MAT).

The relevance of SAM in thiopurine metabolism has been demonstrated by several in vitro studies. Decreased SAM recycling via the methionine cycle was observed upon the addition of 6-MP or 6-methylmercaptopurine riboside (6-MMPR) to MOLT cells. Due to DNPS inhibition caused by the metabolite MeTIMP (Vogt et al., 1993), endogenous adenine nucleotide pools were depleted, limiting the ATP-dependent synthesis of SAM from methionine (Stet et al., 1994). The depletion of SAM also resulted in DNA hypomethylation (De Abreu et al., 1995). The inhibitory effect of 6-MMPR on the growth of MOLT lymphoblasts was reversed by supplementing adenine nucleotide pools with exogenous adenosine, adenine and inosine (Stet et al., 1995). Finally, exogenous SAM also prevents 6-MP induced programmed cell death via the reduction of intracellular TGN and MeTIMP levels in MOLT cells (Milek et al., 2009).

3.4 Effect of SAM-TPMT interaction on thiopurine drug action

Since TPMT is a SAM-dependent methyltransferase, components of methionine metabolism are closely connected to thiopurine drug action. As in other reactions catalyzed by SAM-dependent methyltransferases, SAM provides the methyl group in the S-methylation of thiopurines, which is catalyzed by TPMT. As a side product in this process, SAM is converted to S-adenosylhomocysteine (Sahasranaman et al., 2008), a potent methyltransferase inhibitor. Apart from its role as a TPMT cofactor, SAM has been shown to exert additional effects on TPMT, in all probability as an efficient post-translational regulator of its activity.

Non-synonymous amino-acid substitutions resulting from common genetic polymorphisms destabilize TPMT protein structure and increase its susceptibility to proteasomal and autophagy-mediated degradation. The tridimensional structure of the yeast TPMT orthologue revealed that sinefungin, a SAM analogue, stabilizes the protein backbone towards a rigid native conformation, very possibly decreasing its susceptibility to proteolytic degradation (Scheuermann et al., 2004; Tai et al., 1999) (Fig. 3).

A similar effect was observed for catechol-O-methyltransferase (COMT), a SAM-dependent methyltransferase, and for cystathionine β–sythase (CBS), the rate limiting enzyme in the transsulfuration pathway (Prudova et al., 2006). In HepG2 cells SAM was found to modulate its own production by destabilizing MAT2A mRNA, thus regulating the activity of MAT, the enzyme catalyzing SAM biosynthesis from Met (Martinez-Chantar et al., 2003).

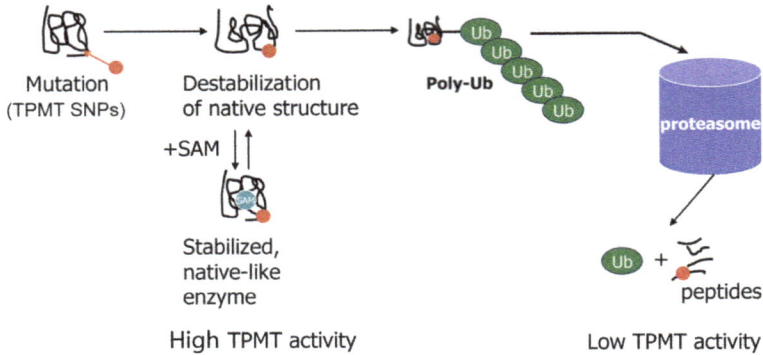

Fig. 3. Role of SAM in TPMT stability and degradation. Decreased tissue TPMT activity is a consequence of the rapid degradation of TPMT variant allozymes via the ubiquitin-proteasome pathway. The binding of SAM to the TPMT protein structure restores intramolecular contacts and shifts the equilibrium towards a highly folded conformation that is less susceptible to intracellular proteolysis. SAM, S-adenosyl-L-methionine; TPMT, thiopurine S-methyltransferase; Ub, ubiquitin.

Molecular and functional studies of TPMT SNPs have shown that non-synonymous amino-acid substitutions in variant TPMT allozymes cause the disruption of intra-molecular van der Waals contacts (Scheuermann et al., 2003). Consequently, such variant proteins are readily degradable via proteasome- and autophagy-mediated proteolysis (Li et al., 2008; Tai et al., 1999). The addition of high concentrations of SAM, the principal cellular methyl donor and a co-substrate in the S-methylation reaction catalyzed by TPMT, resulted in increased TPMT activity in yeast extracts containing recombinant wild-type and TPMT*3C allozymes. The binding of SAM has also been shown to stabilize the 3D structure of the enzyme and shifts the dynamic balance towards the native structure, which prevents the proteolytic degradation of the enzyme. Most recently, exogenous SAM was shown to prevent 6-MP induced programmed cell death via the reduction of intracellular TGN and MeTIMP levels in MOLT cells, possibly by the post-translational stabilisaton of TPMT (Milek et al., 2009). A possible mechanism is indicated in Fig. 4.

The most important evidence of SAM metabolism on TPMT stabilization was presented by two *in vivo* studies, where the presence of low-activity polymorphisms in methylenetetrahydrofolate reductase (MTHFR), the enzyme which catalyzes the formation of 5-methyltetrahydrofolate (5-Me-THF), a rate-determining step in the re-methylation of methionine from homocysteine (Fig. 2), has been found to correlate with decreased TPMT activity in patients with ALL (Arenas et al., 2005). It was postulated that low MTHFR activity results in limited SAM synthesis and, consequently, lower TPMT stability, observed as a modulation of the TPMT phenotype (Karas-Kuzelicki et al., 2009).

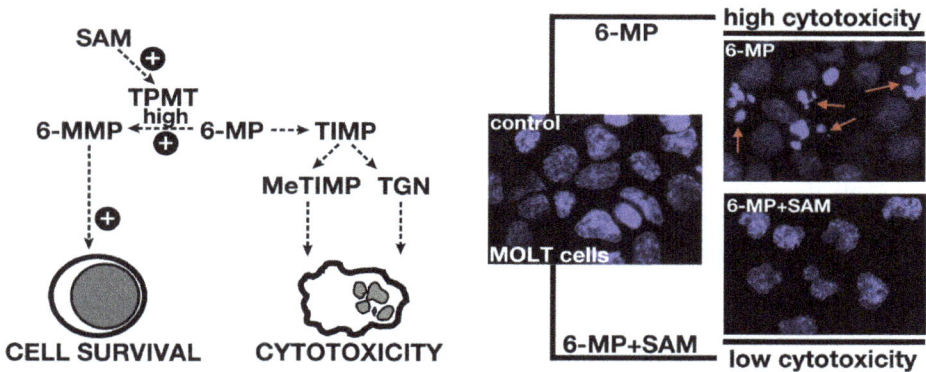

Fig. 4. SAM decreases thiopurine toxicity by stabilizing TPMT protein levels. In TPMT-catalyzed reactions, SAM acts as a methyl donor, but can also stabilize the TPMT 3D structure (indicated by plus, encircled). This results in more extensive deactivation of the drug, i.e. the production of 6-methylmercaptopurine (6-MMP) as opposed to cytotoxic thioguanine nucleotides (TGN) and methylthioinosine monophosphate. Therefore, SAM indirectly decreases the extent of 6-methylmercaptopurine (6-MP) cytotoxicity in MOLT cells. TIMP, thioinosine monophosphate; SAM, S-adenosyl-L-methionine; TPMT, thiopurine S-methyltransferase.

3.5 Synergistic effects of low activity TPMT and MTHFR on 6-MP-induced toxicity

6-MP-induced toxic effects in TPMT heterozygous patients are augmented by a variant methylenetetrahydrofolate reductase (MTHFR) genotype. This is the case as SAM levels depend on the availability of folates, which themselves depend on the activity of MTHFR, the most important folate pathway regulating enzyme.

MTHFR is an enzyme involved in the metabolism of folic acid, through the conversion of 5,10- methylenetetrahydrofolate (5, 10-Me-THF) to 5-methyltetrahydrofolate (5-Me-THF). MTHFR is the rate-determining enzyme of the folate cycle, which plays a major role in methionine and SAM synthesis, and consequently affecting TPMT activity. This is demonstrated in homozygous and heterozygous MTHFR knockout mice (Chen et al., 2001), where decreased MTHFR activity leads to decreased SAM, increased homocysteine and SAH levels, and DNA hypomethylation. In humans, the low activity of MTHFR is coded by two alleles, 677 C>T and 1298 A>C. Homozygosity for 677 C>T and compound heterozygosity for 677 C>T and 1298 A>C is associated with increased blood homocysteine levels, while no apparent discrepancies in biochemical profile are detected in 1298 CC homozygotes (Botto&Yang, 2000; van der Put et al., 1998). These findings reflect enzymatic deficiency due to the presence of polymorphism. MTHFR activity in homozygotes carrying two 677 C>T alleles is 40-50 % of the wild-type enzyme, while in 1298 A>C homozygotes the activity is somewhat higher but still below the normal range. The frequency of 677 T allele is lower in Africans (6-14 %) than in other races (25-43 %), and the highest frequencies have been documented for US Hispanics and Italians. Frequencies of the 1298 C allele are very similar, while the frequencies of compound heterozygosity for both variants range from 15 to 20 % in Caucasian populations (Botto&Yang, 2000).

Individuals with the MTHFR 677 TT genotype have significantly lower serum folate levels (Nishio et al., 2008) and different ratio of methylated to formylated tetrahydrofolates (THF). While only the methylated forms of THF are present in wild-type individuals, up to 59 % of total RBC folates in 677 TT subjects were formyl-THF, as a consequence of lower MTHFR activity and decreased 5,10-Me-THF consumption for the formation of 5-Me-THF (Bagley&Selhub, 1998). Besides genetic predisposition, folate intake is crucial, as sufficient intake may diminish the effect of low-activity alleles. Similarly, the MTHFR 677 TT genotype in transformed human lymphoblasts is most significantly associated with the decreased SAM levels arising from decreased folate-dependent homocysteine re-methylation under conditions of extracellular folate restriction (E. P. Chiang et al., 2007). These data suggest that the effect of genotype-dependent MTHFR status on methionine regeneration and SAM synthesis is also closely related to intracellular folate concentrations.

A correlation between MTHFR and TPMT activity was demonstrated in individuals with intermediate TPMT activity carrying low activity 677 TT MTHFR and wild-type TPMT genotypes (Arenas et al., 2005). The influence of MTHFR activity on TPMT activity is also demonstrated in our recent study addressing the thiopurine toxicity in paediatric ALL patients. The synergistic effect of TPMT and MTHFR variant alleles was observed in patients carrying polymorphisms in both genes, and reflected in severe toxicity. 82 % of these patients experienced hematotoxicity, compared to 4 % of patients with wild-type MTHFR and TPMT genotypes. Similarly, patients carrying polymorphisms in both TPMT and MTHFR genes (59 %) were more likely to have experienced 6-MP dose reductions, as well as stomatitis and infections (Karas-Kuzelicki et al., 2008).

3.6 Other potential pharmacogenetic markers in thiopurine therapy

Individual responses to thiopurine therapy depend beside genetic predisposition, on nutritional and other environmental factors. The genes and their variants identified so far do not suffice to fully justify the variability in drug response. Implementation of novel genetic and metabolomic findings is therefore crucial for the improved prediction of drug efficacy and safety.

Xanthine oxidase (XO) is involved in the first-pass metabolism of 6-MP, and is predominantly expressed in the intestinal mucosa and liver. XO metabolizes 84 % of 6-MP into inactive 6-thiouric acid, resulting in a substantial reduction in 6-MP bioavailability. XO is an alternative name for Xanthine dehydrogenase (XDH), also termed Xanthine oxidoreductase, (XOR). XDH is a molybdenum-containing hydroxylase, readily converted to xanthine oxidase by reversible sulfhydryl oxidation or by irreversible proteolytic modification (http://omim.org/entry/607633). Numerous polymorphisms have been detected either in promoter or coding region of XDH/XO gene. The functional relevance of detected polymorphisms was determined in *in vitro* assays; in the allelic variants tested, a deficiency in enzyme activity was detected in two, low activity in six and high enzymatic activity in two (Kudo et al., 2008). In recent studies, a correlation of two polymorphisms in XO (1936 A>G and 2107 A>G) with the thiopurine therapy outcomes has been addressed; however, due to the small number of patients with myelotoxicity, it was not possible to draw any conclusions (Wong et al., 2007).

Another potential polymorphic enzyme correlating with 6-MP toxicity is inosine triphosphate (ITP) pyrophosphatase (ITPA), which catalyses the pyrophosphohydrolysis of ITP into inosine monophosphate, thereby preventing the accumulation of ITP in normal cells. Decreased ITPA activity leads to the accumulation of the inosine nucleotide, ITP in the cells. Recent studies have shown that the presence of P32T functional polymorphism in ITPA correlates with unwanted thiopurine toxicity in ALL patients. However, studies performed on patients with inflammatory bowel disease or on liver transplant recipients showed no association. Nevertheless, ITPA is emerging as an interesting candidate biomarker, even more so due to relatively high allele frequencies in some populations (Marsh&Van Booven, 2009).

Thymidylate synthase (TYMS) is an enzyme that catalyzes the conversion of dUMP to dTMP by utilizing 5,10-Me-THF and, as such, constitutes a competing pathway for MTHFR-catalyzed 5-Me-THF synthesis. Due to its considerable effect on 5-Me-THF levels and, consequently, on methionine and SAM synthesis, TYMS might, potentially, influence TPMT activity. There is a common tandem repeat polymorphism in the promoter region of TYMS, with the number of tandem repeats affecting TYMS activity levels, mediated through the effects of the repeats on translation efficiency (Kawakami et al., (1999, 2001)). The double repeat (2R) results in lower gene expression than the triple repeat (3R) (Horie et al., 1995). The 3R/3R genotype and high TYMS activity could lead to low 5-Me-THF, methionine and SAM levels and, consequently, low TPMT activity, resulting in higher TGN concentrations and a better therapy response (Karas-Kuzelicki&Mlinaric-Rascan, 2009).

In addition, several other polymorphic genes encoding crucial enzymes of thiopurine metabolism, such as glutathione S-tranferases, hypoxanthine phosphoribosyltransferase, inosine monophosphate dehydrogenase and multidrug resistance proteins, have been described and represent novel pharmacogenetic markers influencing thiopurine therapy (Derijks&Wong, 2010).

4. Future directions and clinical application

The effective stabilization of TPMT by SAM, which prevents thiopurine toxicity, has several clinical implications. An *in vitro* study showed that in patients receiving 6-MP, a decrease in TPMT activity may be expected after 6-MP administration, due to DNPS inhibition and decreased synthesis of the stabilising factor SAM. In patients with wild-type or heterozygous mutant TPMT genotypes, who exhibit high and intermediate TPMT activities respectively, a decrease in the enzyme activity may result in an overproduction of TGNs, increasing the risk of undesirable toxicity. On the other hand, high levels of endogenous SAM, as well as potential compensatory responses to SAM depletion, may contribute to the detoxification of the drug, and, consequently, lead to the wild-type patients being non-responders, by decreasing the production of cytotoxic TGNs. The availability of folate pools may also significantly influence 6-MP related cytotoxic effects, since the metabolic fluxes of homocysteine remethylation and downstream SAM synthesis are folate dependent. The mechanism described in the present study could, therefore, play an important role in patients receiving folates in dietary supplements during thiopurine treatment, modulating the amount of SAM, and, consequently, TPMT activity. Further *in vivo* studies of the correlation of TPMT with the activity of enzymes involved in SAM metabolism, (e.g. methionine adenosyltransferase, S-adenosylmethionine decarboxylase, 5,10-methylenetetrahydrofolate reductase), could reveal additional factors influencing treatment with 6-MP. Moreover, the presence of activity-modulating genetic polymorphisms in these enzymes could explain the poor TPMT genotype-to-phenotype correlations observed in some individuals.

Detailed and relevant understanding of TPMT regulation by SAM in the context of Met metabolism in several cell lines, primary cells, animal models and human samples is a valuable resource for the improved prediction of clinical outcomes. Further studies will have direct consequences in the clinic, by improving the genotype-to-phenotype correlation in heterozygous and wild-type individuals with unexpectedly low TPMT activity. Furthermore, novel factors influencing TPMT activity and thiopurine drug response will enable a much more realistic implementation of existing genetic and biochemical test(s) in clinical practice. In fact, effective antidotes that rapidly decrease thiopurine toxicity by acting as positive regulators of TPMT levels and thiopurine deactivation would be substantially favourable in the clinical setting.

4.1 Methods for measuring SAM

Given the critical role of SAM in many metabolic pathways and its importance in the diagnosis of various pathological manifestations, as well as its potential implication in individualization of thiopurine therapy, the development of an accurate, sensitive and reproducible method for its quantification is very important.

Various methods for the analysis of SAM in different tissues have been developed in the last two decades. Most of the developed methods are HPLC-based and use UV detection (Bottiglieri, 1990; Molloy et al., 1990; Wise et al., 1997) with either ion-pairing or cation exchange chromatography. Some of them use fluorescent detection after conversion of the analytes to fluorescent analogs (Capdevila&Wagner, 1998; Loehrer et al., 1996), others electrochemical detection (Melnyk et al., 2000).

HPLC methods combined with ultraviolet detection are suitable for measuring the concentrations of SAM in tissues, including red blood cells, where SAM can be found in the micromolar range, whereas methods with fluorescent detection show greater sensitivity and can also be used for the detection of SAM in plasma in nanomolar concentrations. In order to enable even better quantification of SAM presented in plasma or cerebrospinal fluid in low nanomolar concentration, some more sensitive LC–MS (Stabler&Allen, 2004) and LC–MS/MS methods (Gellekink et al., 2005; Struys et al., 2000) have also been developed.

A capillary electrophoresis method has been developed for the determination of SAM and SAH in rat liver and kidney as well as in mouse liver, but it can also be used to determine SAM in whole blood (Uthus, 2003).

The stereospecific colorimetric assay for (S,S)-SAM quantification is based on TPMT-catalyzed thiol methylation. All reagents are commercially available and inexpensive, and the necessary enzymes are robust and readily obtainable in large quantities from recombinant sources. The assay can be carried out on UV–visible spectrometers available in most laboratories and can be adapted for batch assay, for example, in a microplate format. The method is linear from 5 µM to at least 60 µM (S,S)-SAM. The higher limits of the assay are restricted by the linear range of individual spectrophotometers at 410 nm, whereas the lower limits are determined by the sensitivity and precision of the spectrophotometer. Although the method was developed to determine SAM concentration in tablets, it could also be applied to measure SAM concentration in physiological fluids (Cannon et al., 2002).

The commercially available assay for SAM determination is a Mediomics Bridge-It® fluorescence assay based on a combination of fluorescence measurement techniques and an assay platform design that utilizes DNA-binding proteins as biosensors for their respective ligands. The affinity of the DNA-binding transcriptional repressor MetJ, labelled with fluorophore, for its DNA-binding site is greatly increased in the presence of its ligand, SAM. This method exhibits a high signal to background ratio, a broad linear dynamic range (0.5 µM – 20 µM), and a detection sensitivity of 0.5 µM; therefore, it is useful for the purpose of quantifying SAM in various samples including biological fluids, cell culture and fermentation medium, and extracts of tissues and cells (www.mediomics.com).

5. S-adenosylmethionine (SAM) in therapy

SAM in the form of its stable p-toluensulphonate or butanedisulfonate salt has been used for more than 20 years in the treatment of depression, liver disorders, and musculoskeletal and joint disorders such as osteoarthritis and fibromyalgia. It has been available as a prescription drug marketed under different brand names (Gumbal, Samyr, Adomet, Heptral and Admethionine) in Italy, Spain, Germany, the Czech Republic, Russia, Argentina and Mexico, whereas in the United States and Canada SAM has been available under the Dietary Supplement and Health Education Act as a nutritional supplement under the marketing name SAM-e.

Depression

Although the mechanism of antidepressant action of SAM is not entirely clear, it is thought that its ability to function as a methyl donor increases brain levels of serotonin, dopamine, and norepinephrine. It has been previously reported that serum and cerebrospinal fluid levels of SAM are low in depressed patients (Bottiglieri 1990; Lakhan 2008) and that increases in serum SAM levels correlate with improved treatment response (Bell 1994). Besides the stimulatory effect of SAM on central monoaminergic neurotransmitters, there may exist alternative mechanisms in which increased or restored membrane phospholipid methylation plays a role in the antidepressant effect. SAM may increase the fluidity of cell membranes by stimulating phospholipid methylation, which has previously been linked to an increase in ß receptor and muscarinic (M1) receptor density (Bottiglieri, 2002).

SAM has been studied for use in various depressive disorders for many decades, with the first clinical trials dating back to as early as 1973 (Fazio et al., 1973). The majority of studies performed since then have reported that SAM is effective for treating depression, the conclusion also drawn later by a meta-analysis (Bressa, 1994) and some other systematic reviews (Williams 2005; Papakostas 2003; Mischoulon 2002). However, due to several quality issues and methodological flaws of the individual studies included in these reviews, the findings should be interpreted with caution. Most studies are quite dated (1970s or 1980s), have short treatment duration and are of small sample size (n < 50). Furthermore, the most appropriate daily dosage for SAM is also not well established. Due to its low oral bioavailability, many of the earlier SAM studies utilized parenteral formulations (intramuscular or intravenous), which may also limit the clinical relevance of those studies (Carpenter, 2011).

Osteoarthritis

SAM has also been studied extensively in the context of the treatment of osteoarthritis. Experimental studies indicate that SAM increases the chondrocyte proteoglycan synthesis and proliferation rate. SAM induces the synthesis of polyamines that might stabilize the polyanionic macromolecules of proteoglycans and protect them from attack by proteolytic and glycotic enzymes. Furthermore, *in vitro* studies show that SAM can antagonize the tumour necrosis factor α–induced decreases in synovial cell proliferation and fibronectin mRNA expression. These findings indicate that SAM restores basal conditions in cultured synovial cells after cytokine-induced cell damage (Bottiglieri, 2002). Many trials have demonstrated that SAM reduces the pain associated with osteoarthritis and is well tolerated in this patient population. However, a systematic review (Rutjes et al., 2009) found that available studies were mainly small and of questionable quality, and that, therefore, the routine use of SAM for osteoarthritis of the knee or hip could not be recommended until such time as further evaluation through larger randomised controlled studies has taken place.

Liver Disease

SAM has been used to treat various types of acute and chronic liver diseases. Although the focus of clinical trials in this area has been diffuse, a number of clinical trials have focused on the effect of SAM on cholestasis arising from a variety of causes, including pregnancy (Almasio et al., 1990; Frezza et al., 1990a; Frezza et al., 1990b). SAM may exert beneficial effects on the liver through a variety of mechanisms. Glutathione, the major anti-oxidant in the liver, plays a key role in detoxification and the limiting of oxidative damage. Studies have shown that abnormal SAM synthesis is associated with chronic liver disease, regardless of its etiology. At customary therapeutic doses, SAM has been shown to increase hepatic glutathione concentrations in patients with chronic liver disease (Chawla et al., 1990). Although some studies have demonstrated clinical improvement in patients with intrahepatic cholestasis, hepatic steatosis and alcoholic liver cirrhosis, a systematic review of 9 randomised placebo-controlled studies could not find evidence to support or refute the claim that SAM has a beneficial effect in patients with alcoholic liver disease (Rambaldi&Gluud, 2006).

Neurological Disorders

Several studies indicate that a CNS methyl group deficiency may play a role in the etiology of Alzheimer disease (AD). Hyperhomocysteinemia, often related to folate or vitamin B 12 deficiency, is a common finding in the elderly and is associated with cognitive impairment and cognitive decline. The association between hyperhomocysteinemia and AD is well established; however, the underlying pathophysiology remains unexplained. Studies in cell culture experiments and mouse models have suggested that 2 metabolites of homocysteine, SAM and S- adenosylhomocysteine (Sahasranaman et al., 2008), may be important in Alzheimer pathogenesis, e.g. by influencing the expression of presenilin 1 and β - secretase, leading to an increase in Aβ production (Linnebank et al., 2010). It is important to note that the use of either SAM or alternative methyl group donors (such as betaine or folate and vitamin B-12) might improve measures of cognitive function. These treatments may be able to restore methyl group metabolism and normalize blood homocysteine concentrations (Bottiglieri, 2002).

6. Conclusions

Prediction of TPMT activity and thiopurine drug response based on TPMT genotyping tests represents one of the most relevant applications of pharmacogenetics. Prediction of TPMT activity and treatment response solely on the basis of presence of mutant TPMT alleles is insufficient, due to the incomplete TPMT phenotype-to-genotype correlation. This problem is most pronounced in heterozygous patients (8-10 % in Caucasian populations), which exhibit a wide range of intermediate enzyme activity, and in those wild-type individuals which do not exhibit high activity. Hence, to improve the prediction of thiopurine therapy outcome, identification of new biomarkers is essential.

One of such candidates is SAM, which, by binding into the active site of TPMT, stabilizes its structure. Several studies suggest that measurement of erythrocyte SAM level, in addition to TPMT genotyping, could serve as an additional predictor of TPMT activity in some thiopurine patient subgroups, and suggest that stabilization of TPMT by SAM has substantial clinical relevance. Some analytical methods for the determination of SAM in biological samples have already been described which are suitable for the implementation into clinical practice.

In addition, SAM, which has been used for more than 20 years in the treatment of depression, liver disorders, and musculoskeletal and joint disorders, may be a promising agent to acutely regulate TPMT activity in order to rapidly decrease excess thiopurine toxicity in some patient subgroups.

In addition to measuring SAM levels in red blood cells, analyses of genes directly or indirectly involved in the folate metabolism (such as MTHFR and TYMS) can add valuable additional information to conventional TPMT genotyping, thus enabling the development of complex diagnostic algorithms, and in turn improving the efficacy and safety of the thiopurine therapy.

7. Acknowledgment

We thank Benedict Dries-Jenkins for proof reading the chapter. The authors were supported by the Slovenian Research Agency grants No. J3-7406 and J3-3615.

8. References

Almasio, P., Bortolini, M., Pagliaro, L., & Coltorti, M. (1990). Role of S-adenosyl-L-methionine in the treatment of intrahepatic cholestasis. *Drugs*, Vol.40 Suppl 3, No. 111-123, 0012-6667

Arenas, M., Simpson, G., Lewis, C.M., Shobowale-Bakre el, M., Escuredo, E., Fairbanks, L.D., Duley, J.A., Ansari, A., Sanderson, J.D., & Marinaki, A.M. (2005). Genetic variation in the MTHFR gene influences thiopurine methyltransferase activity. *Clin Chem*, Vol.51, No. 12, (Dec), pp. 2371-2374, 0009-9147

Bagley, P.J., & Selhub, J. (1998). A common mutation in the methylenetetrahydrofolate reductase gene is associated with an accumulation of formylated tetrahydrofolates in red blood cells. *Proc Natl Acad Sci U S A*, Vol.95, No. 22, (Oct 27), pp. 13217-13220, 0027-8424

Bottiglieri, T. (1990). Isocratic high performance liquid chromatographic analysis of S-adenosylmethionine and S-adenosylhomocysteine in animal tissues: the effect of exposure to nitrous oxide. *Biomed Chromatogr*, Vol.4, No. 6, (Nov), pp. 239-241, 0269-3879

Bottiglieri, T. (2002). S-Adenosyl-L-methionine (SAMe): from the bench to the bedside--molecular basis of a pleiotrophic molecule. *Am J Clin Nutr*, Vol.76, No. 5, (Nov), pp. 1151S-1157S, 0002-9165

Botto, L.D., & Yang, Q. (2000). 5,10-Methylenetetrahydrofolate reductase gene variants and congenital anomalies: a HuGE review. *Am J Epidemiol*, Vol.151, No. 9, (May 1), pp. 862-877, 0002-9262

Bressa, G.M. (1994). S-adenosyl-l-methionine (SAMe) as antidepressant: meta-analysis of clinical studies. *Acta Neurol Scand Suppl*, Vol.154, No. 7-14, 0065-1427

Bridge-It® S-Adenosyl Methionine (SAM) Fluorescence Assay, 11 July 2011, Available from: http://www.mediomics.com/sam.html

Cannon, L.M., Butler, F.N., Wan, W., & Zhou, Z.S. (2002). A stereospecific colorimetric assay for (S,S)-adenosylmethionine quantification based on thiopurine methyltransferase-catalyzed thiol methylation. *Anal Biochem*, Vol.308, No. 2, (Sep 15), pp. 358-363, ISSN 0003-2697

Cantoni, G.L. (1951). Activation of methionine for transmethylation. *The Journal of biological chemistry*, Vol.189, No. 2, (Apr), pp. 745-754, 0021-9258 (Print) 0021-9258 (Linking)

Capdevila, A., & Wagner, C. (1998). Measurement of plasma S-adenosylmethionine and S-adenosylhomocysteine as their fluorescent isoindoles. *Anal Biochem*, Vol.264, No. 2, (Nov 15), pp. 180-184, ISSN 0003-2697

Carpenter, D.J. (2011). St. John's wort and S-adenosyl methionine as "natural" alternatives to conventional antidepressants in the era of the suicidality boxed warning: what is the evidence for clinically relevant benefit? *Altern Med Rev*, Vol.16, No. 1, (Mar), pp. 17-39, ISSN 1089-5159

Chawla, R.K., Bonkovsky, H.L., & Galambos, J.T. (1990). Biochemistry and pharmacology of S-adenosyl-L-methionine and rationale for its use in liver disease. *Drugs*, Vol.40 Suppl 3, No. 98-110, ISSN 0012-6667

Chen, Z., Karaplis, A.C., Ackerman, S.L., Pogribny, I.P., Melnyk, S., Lussier-Cacan, S., Chen, M.F., Pai, A., John, S.W., Smith, R.S., Bottiglieri, T., Bagley, P., Selhub, J., Rudnicki, M.A., James, S.J., & Rozen, R. (2001). Mice deficient in methylenetetrahydrofolate reductase exhibit hyperhomocysteinemia and decreased methylation capacity, with neuropathology and aortic lipid deposition. *Hum Mol Genet*, Vol.10, No. 5, (Mar 1), pp. 433-443, ISSN 0964-6906

Chiang, E.P., Wang, Y.C., & Tang, F.Y. (2007). Folate restriction and methylenetetrahydrofolate reductase 677T polymorphism decreases adoMet synthesis via folate-dependent remethylation in human-transformed lymphoblasts. *Leukemia*, Vol.21, No. 4, (Apr), pp. 651-658, ISSN 0887-6924

Chiang, P.K., Gordon, R.K., Tal, J., Zeng, G.C., Doctor, B.P., Pardhasaradhi, K., & McCann, P.P. (1996). S-Adenosylmethionine and methylation. *FASEB J*, Vol.10, No. 4, (Mar), pp. 471-480, 0892-6638 (Print) 0892-6638 (Linking)

De Abreu, R., Lambooy, L., Stet, E., Vogels-Mentink, T., & Van den Heuvel, L. (1995). Thiopurine induced disturbance of DNA methylation in human malignant cells. *Adv Enzyme Regul*, Vol.35, No. 251-263, 0065-2571 (Print) 0065-2571 (Linking)

de Boer, N.K., van Bodegraven, A.A., Jharap, B., de Graaf, P., & Mulder, C.J. (2007). Drug Insight: pharmacology and toxicity of thiopurine therapy in patients with IBD. *Nat Clin Pract Gastroenterol Hepatol*, Vol.4, No. 12, (Dec), pp. 686-694, ISSN 1743-4386

Derijks, L.J., & Wong, D.R. (2010). Pharmacogenetics of thiopurines in inflammatory bowel disease. *Curr Pharm Des*, Vol.16, No. 2145-154, ISSN 1873-4286

Dervieux, T., Blanco, J.G., Krynetski, E.Y., Vanin, E.F., Roussel, M.F., & Relling, M.V. (2001). Differing contribution of thiopurine methyltransferase to mercaptopurine versus thioguanine effects in human leukemic cells. *Cancer Res*, Vol.61, No. 15, (Aug 1), pp. 5810-5816, ISSN 0008-5472

Detich, N., Hamm, S., Just, G., Knox, J.D., & Szyf, M. (2003). The methyl donor S-Adenosylmethionine inhibits active demethylation of DNA: a candidate novel mechanism for the pharmacological effects of S-Adenosylmethionine. *The Journal of biological chemistry*, Vol.278, No. 23, (Jun 6), pp. 20812-20820, 0021-9258 (Print) 0021-9258 (Linking)

Evans, W.E. (2004). Pharmacogenetics of thiopurine S-methyltransferase and thiopurine therapy. *Ther Drug Monit*, Vol.26, No. 2, (Apr), pp. 186-191, 0163-4356 (Print) 0163-4356 (Linking)

Fazio, C., Andreoli, V., Agnoli, A., Casacchia, M., & Cerbo, R. (1973). [Therapeutic effects and mechanism of action of S-adenosyl-L-methionine (SAM) in depressive syndromes]. *Minerva Med*, Vol.64, No. 29, (Apr 30), pp. 1515-1529, ISSN 0026-4806

Finkelstein, J.D. (2007). Metabolic regulatory properties of S-adenosylmethionine and S-adenosylhomocysteine. *Clinical chemistry and laboratory medicine : CCLM / FESCC*, Vol.45, No. 121694-1699, 1434-6621 (Print) 1434-6621 (Linking)

Frezza, M., Centini, G., Cammareri, G., Le Grazie, C., & Di Padova, C. (1990a). S-adenosylmethionine for the treatment of intrahepatic cholestasis of pregnancy. Results of a controlled clinical trial. *Hepatogastroenterology*, Vol.37 Suppl 2, No., (Dec), pp. 122-125, ISSN 0172-6390

Frezza, M., Surrenti, C., Manzillo, G., Fiaccadori, F., Bortolini, M., & Di Padova, C. (1990b). Oral S-adenosylmethionine in the symptomatic treatment of intrahepatic cholestasis. A double-blind, placebo-controlled study. *Gastroenterology*, Vol.99, No. 1, (Jul), pp. 211-215, ISSN 0016-5085

Gellekink, H., van Oppenraaij-Emmerzaal, D., van Rooij, A., Struys, E.A., den Heijer, M., & Blom, H.J. (2005). Stable-isotope dilution liquid chromatography-electrospray injection tandem mass spectrometry method for fast, selective measurement of S-adenosylmethionine and S-adenosylhomocysteine in plasma. *Clin Chem*, Vol.51, No. 8, (Aug), pp. 1487-1492, ISSN 0009-9147

Heyduk, T., & Heyduk, E. (2002). Molecular beacons for detecting DNA binding proteins. *Nat Biotechnol*, Vol.20, No. 2, (Feb), pp. 171-176, ISSN 1087-0156

Hitchler, M.J., & Domann, F.E. (2007). An epigenetic perspective on the free radical theory of development. *Free radical biology & medicine*, Vol.43, No. 7, (Oct 1), pp. 1023-1036, 0891-5849 (Print) 0891-5849 (Linking)

Horie, N., Aiba, H., Oguro, K., Hojo, H., & Takeishi, K. (1995). Functional analysis and DNA polymorphism of the tandemly repeated sequences in the 5'-terminal regulatory region of the human gene for thymidylate synthase. *Cell Struct Funct*, Vol.20, No. 3, (Jun), pp. 191-197, 0386-7196 (Print)

IMURAN® (azathioprine). Product Information., 7.7.2011, Available from: http://www.accessdata.fda.gov/drugsatfda_docs/label/2005/016324s030,017391s013lbl.pdf

Kager, L., Cheok, M., Yang, W., Zaza, G., Cheng, Q., Panetta, J.C., Pui, C.H., Downing, J.R., Relling, M.V., & Evans, W.E. (2005). Folate pathway gene expression differs in subtypes of acute lymphoblastic leukemia and influences methotrexate pharmacodynamics. *J Clin Invest*, Vol.115, No. 1, (Jan), pp. 110-117, ISSN 0021-9738

Karas Kuzelicki, N., Milek, M., Jazbec, J., & Mlinaric-Rascan, I. (2009). 5,10-Methylenetetrahydrofolate reductase (MTHFR) low activity genotypes reduce the risk of relapse-related acute lymphoblastic leukemia (ALL). *Leuk Res*, Vol.33, No. 10, (Oct), pp. 1344-1348, ISSN 1873-5835

Karas-Kuzelicki, N., & Mlinaric-Rascan, I. (2009). Individualization of thiopurine therapy: thiopurine S-methyltransferase and beyond. *Pharmacogenomics*, Vol.10, No. 8, (Aug), pp. 1309-1322, ISSN 1744-8042

Karas-Kuzelicki, N., Jazbec, J., Milek, M., & Mlinaric-Rascan, I. (2008). Heterozygosity at the TPMT gene locus, augmented by mutated MTHFR gene, predisposes to 6-MP related toxicities in childhood ALL patients. *Leukemia*, No., (Nov 6), pp., 1476-5551 (Electronic)

Karas-Kuzelicki, N., Jazbec, J., Milek, M., & Mlinaric-Rascan, I. (2009). Heterozygosity at the TPMT gene locus, augmented by mutated MTHFR gene, predisposes to 6-MP related toxicities in childhood ALL patients. *Leukemia*, Vol.23, No. 5, (May), pp. 971-974, ISSN 1476-5551

Kudo, M., Moteki, T., Sasaki, T., Konno, Y., Ujiie, S., Onose, A., Mizugaki, M., Ishikawa, M., & Hiratsuka, M. (2008). Functional characterization of human xanthine oxidase allelic variants. *Pharmacogenet Genomics*, Vol.18, No. 3, (Mar), pp. 243-251, ISSN 1744-6872

Li, F., Wang, L., Burgess, R.J., & Weinshilboum, R.M. (2008). Thiopurine S-methyltransferase pharmacogenetics: autophagy as a mechanism for variant allozyme degradation. *Pharmacogenetics and genomics*, Vol.18, No. 12, (Dec), pp. 1083-1094, 1744-6872 (Print) 1744-6872 (Linking)

Linnebank, M., Popp, J., Smulders, Y., Smith, D., Semmler, A., Farkas, M., Kulic, L., Cvetanovska, G., Blom, H., Stoffel-Wagner, B., Kolsch, H., Weller, M., & Jessen, F. (2010). S-adenosylmethionine is decreased in the cerebrospinal fluid of patients with Alzheimer's disease. *Neurodegener Dis*, Vol.7, No. 6373-378, ISSN 1660-2862

Loehrer, F.M., Haefeli, W.E., Angst, C.P., Browne, G., Frick, G., & Fowler, B. (1996). Effect of methionine loading on 5-methyltetrahydrofolate, S-adenosylmethionine and S-adenosylhomocysteine in plasma of healthy humans. *Clin Sci (Lond)*, Vol.91, No. 1, (Jul), pp. 79-86, ISSN 0143-5221

Loenen, W.A. (2006). S-adenosylmethionine: jack of all trades and master of everything? *Biochemical Society transactions*, Vol.34, No. Pt 2, (Apr), pp. 330-333, 0300-5127 (Print) 0300-5127 (Linking)

Luka, Z., Mudd, S.H., & Wagner, C. (2009). Glycine N-methyltransferase and regulation of S-adenosylmethionine levels. *The Journal of biological chemistry*, Vol.284, No. 34, (Aug 21), pp. 22507-22511, 1083-351X (Electronic) 0021-9258 (Linking)

Marsh, S., & Van Booven, D.J. (2009). The increasing complexity of mercaptopurine pharmacogenomics. *Clin Pharmacol Ther*, Vol.85, No. 2, (Feb), pp. 139-141, ISSN 1532-6535

Martinez-Chantar, M.L., Corrales, F.J., Martinez-Cruz, L.A., Garcia-Trevijano, E.R., Huang, Z.Z., Chen, L., Kanel, G., Avila, M.A., Mato, J.M., & Lu, S.C. (2002a). Spontaneous oxidative stress and liver tumors in mice lacking methionine adenosyltransferase 1A. *FASEB J*, Vol.16, No. 10, (Aug), pp. 1292-1294, ISSN 1530-6860

Martinez-Chantar, M.L., Garcia-Trevijano, E.R., Latasa, M.U., Perez-Mato, I., Sanchez del Pino, M.M., Corrales, F.J., Avila, M.A., & Mato, J.M. (2002b). Importance of a deficiency in S-adenosyl-L-methionine synthesis in the pathogenesis of liver injury. *Am J Clin Nutr*, Vol.76, No. 5, (Nov), pp. 1177S-1182S, 0002-9165 (Print) 0002-9165 (Linking)

Martinez-Chantar, M.L., Latasa, M.U., Varela-Rey, M., Lu, S.C., Garcia-Trevijano, E.R., Mato, J.M., & Avila, M.A. (2003). L-methionine availability regulates expression of the methionine adenosyltransferase 2A gene in human hepatocarcinoma cells: role of S-adenosylmethionine. *J Biol Chem*, Vol.278, No. 22, (May 30), pp. 19885-19890, 0021-9258 (Print) 0021-9258 (Linking)

Martinez-Chantar, M.L., Vazquez-Chantada, M., Ariz, U., Martinez, N., Varela, M., Luka, Z., Capdevila, A., Rodriguez, J., Aransay, A.M., Matthiesen, R., Yang, H., Calvisi, D.F., Esteller, M., Fraga, M., Lu, S.C., Wagner, C., & Mato, J.M. (2008). Loss of the glycine N-methyltransferase gene leads to steatosis and hepatocellular carcinoma in mice. *Hepatology*, Vol.47, No. 4, (Apr), pp. 1191-1199, 1527-3350 (Electronic) 0270-9139 (Linking)

Marx, J.L. (1988). The 1988 Nobel Prize for physiology or medicine. *Science*, Vol.242, No. 4878516, ISSN 0036-8075

Melnyk, S., Pogribna, M., Pogribny, I.P., Yi, P., & James, S.J. (2000). Measurement of plasma and intracellular S-adenosylmethionine and S-adenosylhomocysteine utilizing coulometric electrochemical detection: alterations with plasma homocysteine and pyridoxal 5'-phosphate concentrations. *Clin Chem*, Vol.46, No. 2, (Feb), pp. 265-272, ISSN 0009-9147

Milek, M., Karas Kuzelicki, N., Smid, A., & Mlinaric-Rascan, I. (2009). S-adenosylmethionine regulates thiopurine methyltransferase activity and decreases 6-mercaptopurine cytotoxicity in MOLT lymphoblasts. *Biochem Pharmacol*, Vol.77, No. 12, (Jun 15), pp. 1845-1853, ISSN 1873-2968

Milek, M., Murn, J., Jaksic, Z., Lukac Bajalo, J., Jazbec, J., & Mlinaric Rascan, I. (2006). Thiopurine S-methyltransferase pharmacogenetics: genotype to phenotype correlation in the Slovenian population. *Pharmacology*, Vol.77, No. 3105-114, ISSN 0031-7012

Molloy, A.M., Weir, D.G., Kennedy, G., Kennedy, S., & Scott, J.M. (1990). A new high performance liquid chromatographic method for the simultaneous measurement of S-adenosylmethionine and S-adenosylhomocysteine. Concentrations in pig tissues after inactivation of methionine synthase by nitrous oxide. *Biomed Chromatogr*, Vol.4, No. 6, (Nov), pp. 257-260, ISSN 0269-3879

Moricke, A., Reiter, A., Zimmermann, M., Gadner, H., Stanulla, M., Dordelmann, M., Loning, L., Beier, R., Ludwig, W.D., Ratei, R., Harbott, J., Boos, J., Mann, G., Niggli, F., Feldges, A., Henze, G., Welte, K., Beck, J.D., Klingebiel, T., Niemeyer, C., Zintl, F., Bode, U., Urban, C., Wehinger, H., Niethammer, D., Riehm, H., & Schrappe, M. (2008). Risk-adjusted therapy of acute lymphoblastic leukemia can decrease treatment burden and improve survival: treatment results of 2169 unselected pediatric and adolescent patients enrolled in the trial ALL-BFM 95. *Blood*, Vol.111, No. 9, (May 1), pp. 4477-4489, ISSN 1528-0020

Murray, J.E., Merrill, J.P., Harrison, J.H., Wilson, R.E., & Dammin, G.J. (1963). Prolonged survival of human-kidney homografts by immunosuppressive drug therapy. *The New England journal of medicine*, Vol.268, No. 1315, ISSN 0028-4793

Nishio, K., Goto, Y., Kondo, T., Ito, S., Ishida, Y., Kawai, S., Naito, M., Wakai, K., & Hamajima, N. (2008). Serum folate and methylenetetrahydrofolate reductase (MTHFR) C677T polymorphism adjusted for folate intake. *J Epidemiol*, Vol.18, No. 3125-131, ISSN 1349-9092

Nitta, T., Igarashi, K., & Yamamoto, N. (2002). Polyamine depletion induces apoptosis through mitochondria-mediated pathway. *Experimental cell research*, Vol.276, No. 1, (May 15), pp. 120-128, 0014-4827 (Print) 0014-4827 (Linking)

Prudova, A., Bauman, Z., Braun, A., Vitvitsky, V., Lu, S.C., & Banerjee, R. (2006). S-adenosylmethionine stabilizes cystathionine beta-synthase and modulates redox capacity. *Proc Natl Acad Sci U S A*, Vol.103, No. 17, (Apr 25), pp. 6489-6494, 0027-8424 (Print) 0027-8424 (Linking)

PURINETHOL® (mercaptopurine). Product information., 7.7.2011, Available from: http://www.accessdata.fda.gov/drugsatfda_docs/label/2011/009053s032lbl.pdf

Rambaldi, A., & Gluud, C. (2006). S-adenosyl-L-methionine for alcoholic liver diseases. *Cochrane Database Syst Rev*, No. 2CD002235, ISSN 1469-493X

Relling, M.V., Gardner, E.E., Sandborn, W.J., Schmiegelow, K., Pui, C.H., Yee, S.W., Stein, C.M., Carrillo, M., Evans, W.E., & Klein, T.E. (2011). Clinical Pharmacogenetics Implementation Consortium guidelines for thiopurine methyltransferase genotype and thiopurine dosing. *Clin Pharmacol Ther*, Vol.89, No. 3, (Mar), pp. 387-391, 1532-6535 (Electronic) 0009-9236 (Linking)

Relling, M.V., Hancock, M.L., Boyett, J.M., Pui, C.H., & Evans, W.E. (1999). Prognostic importance of 6-mercaptopurine dose intensity in acute lymphoblastic leukemia. *Blood*, Vol.93, No. 9, (May 1), pp. 2817-2823, ISSN 0006-4971

Rutjes, A.W., Nuesch, E., Reichenbach, S., & Juni, P. (2009). S-Adenosylmethionine for osteoarthritis of the knee or hip. *Cochrane Database Syst Rev*, No. 4CD007321, ISSN 1469-493X

Sahasranaman, S., Howard, D., & Roy, S. (2008). Clinical pharmacology and pharmacogenetics of thiopurines. *Eur J Clin Pharmacol*, Vol.64, No. 8, (Aug), pp. 753-767, 0031-6970 (Print) 0031-6970 (Linking)

Sanderson, J., Ansari, A., Marinaki, T., & Duley, J. (2004). Thiopurine methyltransferase: should it be measured before commencing thiopurine drug therapy? *Ann Clin Biochem*, Vol.41, No. Pt 4, (Jul), pp. 294-302, ISSN 0004-5632

Scheuermann, T.H., Keeler, C., & Hodsdon, M.E. (2004). Consequences of binding an S-adenosylmethionine analogue on the structure and dynamics of the thiopurine methyltransferase protein backbone. *Biochemistry*, Vol.43, No. 38, (Sep 28), pp. 12198-12209, ISSN 0006-2960

Scheuermann, T.H., Lolis, E., & Hodsdon, M.E. (2003). Tertiary structure of thiopurine methyltransferase from Pseudomonas syringae, a bacterial orthologue of a polymorphic, drug-metabolizing enzyme. *J Mol Biol*, Vol.333, No. 3, (Oct 24), pp. 573-585, 0022-2836 (Print) 0022-2836 (Linking)

Stabler, S.P., & Allen, R.H. (2004). Quantification of serum and urinary S-adenosylmethionine and S-adenosylhomocysteine by stable-isotope-dilution liquid chromatography-mass spectrometry. *Clin Chem*, Vol.50, No. 2, (Feb), pp. 365-372, ISSN 0009-9147

Stet, E.H., De Abreu, R.A., Bokkerink, J.P., Blom, H.J., Lambooy, L.H., Vogels-Mentink, T.M., de Graaf-Hess, A.C., van Raay-Selten, B., & Trijbels, F.J. (1994). Decrease in S-adenosylmethionine synthesis by 6-mercaptopurine and methylmercaptopurine ribonucleoside in Molt F4 human malignant lymphoblasts. *The Biochemical journal*, Vol.304 (Pt 1), No., (Nov 15), pp. 163-168, 0264-6021 (Print) 0264-6021 (Linking)

Stet, E.H., De Abreu, R.A., Bokkerink, J.P., Lambooy, L.H., Vogels-Mentink, T.M., Keizer-Garritsen, J.J., & Trijbels, F.J. (1995). Reversal of methylmercaptopurine ribonucleoside cytotoxicity by purine ribonucleosides and adenine. *Biochemical pharmacology*, Vol.49, No. 1, (Jan 6), pp. 49-56, 0006-2952 (Print) 0006-2952 (Linking)

Struys, E.A., Jansen, E.E., de Meer, K., & Jakobs, C. (2000). Determination of S-adenosylmethionine and S-adenosylhomocysteine in plasma and cerebrospinal fluid by stable-isotope dilution tandem mass spectrometry. *Clin Chem*, Vol.46, No. 10, (Oct), pp. 1650-1656, ISSN 0009-9147

Tai, H.L., Fessing, M.Y., Bonten, E.J., Yanishevsky, Y., d'Azzo, A., Krynetski, E.Y., & Evans, W.E. (1999). Enhanced proteasomal degradation of mutant human thiopurine S-methyltransferase (TPMT) in mammalian cells: mechanism for TPMT protein deficiency inherited by TPMT*2, TPMT*3A, TPMT*3B or TPMT*3C. *Pharmacogenetics*, Vol.9, No. 5, (Oct), pp. 641-650, 0960-314X (Print) 0960-314X (Linking)

Tai, H.L., Krynetski, E.Y., Schuetz, E.G., Yanishevski, Y., & Evans, W.E. (1997). Enhanced proteolysis of thiopurine S-methyltransferase (TPMT) encoded by mutant alleles in humans (TPMT*3A, TPMT*2): mechanisms for the genetic polymorphism of TPMT activity. *Proc Natl Acad Sci U S A*, Vol.94, No. 12, (Jun 10), pp. 6444-6449, ISSN 0027-8424

Uthus, E.O. (2003). Simultaneous detection of S-adenosylmethionine and S-adenosylhomocysteine in mouse and rat tissues by capillary electrophoresis. *Electrophoresis*, Vol.24, No. 7-8, (Apr), pp. 1221-1226, ISSN 0173-0835

van der Put, N.M., Gabreels, F., Stevens, E.M., Smeitink, J.A., Trijbels, F.J., Eskes, T.K., van den Heuvel, L.P., & Blom, H.J. (1998). A second common mutation in the methylenetetrahydrofolate reductase gene: an additional risk factor for neural-tube defects? *Am J Hum Genet*, Vol.62, No. 5, (May), pp. 1044-1051, ISSN 0002-9297

Vogt, M.H., Stet, E.H., De Abreu, R.A., Bokkerink, J.P., Lambooy, L.H., & Trijbels, F.J. (1993). The importance of methylthio-IMP for methylmercaptopurine ribonucleoside (Me-MPR) cytotoxicity in Molt F4 human malignant T-lymphoblasts. *Biochimica et biophysica acta*, Vol.1181, No. 2, (Apr 30), pp. 189-194, 0006-3002 (Print) 0006-3002 (Linking)

Weinshilboum, R. (2001). Thiopurine pharmacogenetics: clinical and molecular studies of thiopurine methyltransferase. *Drug Metab Dispos*, Vol.29, No. 4 Pt 2, (Apr), pp. 601-605, ISSN 0090-9556

Weinshilboum, R.M., & Sladek, S.L. (1980). Mercaptopurine pharmacogenetics: monogenic inheritance of erythrocyte thiopurine methyltransferase activity. *Am J Hum Genet*, Vol.32, No. 5, (Sep), pp. 651-662, ISSN 0002-9297

Wise, C.K., Cooney, C.A., Ali, S.F., & Poirier, L.A. (1997). Measuring S-adenosylmethionine in whole blood, red blood cells and cultured cells using a fast preparation method and high-performance liquid chromatography. *J Chromatogr B Biomed Sci Appl*, Vol.696, No. 1, (Aug 15), pp. 145-152, ISSN 1387-2273

Wong, D.R., Derijks, L.J., den Dulk, M.O., Gemmeke, E.H., & Hooymans, P.M. (2007). The role of xanthine oxidase in thiopurine metabolism: a case report. *Ther Drug Monit*, Vol.29, No. 6, (Dec), pp. 845-848, ISSN 0163-4356

5

Role of Pharmacogenetics in Gastrointestinal Cancer

Suayib Yalcin
Hacettepe University Institute of Oncology
Turkey

1. Introduction

Worldwide, gastrointestinal (GI) system tumors are the leading group of cancers in terms of incidence and cause of cancer deaths (Parkin, 2005). They are usually diagnosed at an advanced stage which is rarely curable, and even if detected early the rate of recurrence is quite high. Therefore despite improvements in the diagnosis and treatment of GI cancers, 5-year survival rates remain disappointing. Effective new treatments are urgently needed, and existing therapies need to be individualized to determine patients who are likely to respond to a given chemotherapy, as well as to identify patients at risk of developing severe toxicity. This approach will enable clinicians to optimize and personalize cancer treatment. Pharmacogenetics is, perhaps, the most promising method to provide this (Yalcin, 2009). Metabolism of chemotherapy agents varies depending on patient age, gender, diet, concomitant drug use, comorbidities, and hepatic and renal functions and moreover GI functions may be impaired due to surgery, chemotherapy and the disease or existing comorbidities in GI cancer patients.

Pharmacogenetics focuses on the influence of genetic structure on cancer treatment because enzymes that metabolize the drug, proteins that transport the drug and its metabolites, and drug receptors are determined by a patient's genetic profile (Vesell, 1989). However, it is not only the genetics of the patient, but also the genetic alterations of the tumor that are critical (Yong, 2006, Vesell, 1989). Pharmacogenetics may help to decide the most sensitive and least toxic therapy in order to increase survival, reduce treatment related cost and improve patient's quality of life. In this chapter, the most common drugs, combinations thereof, and biological agents used for the treatment of GI tumors are reviewed for their relevant pharmacogenetic aspects.

2. 5-Fluorouracil (5-FU)

The uracil analogue 5-FU has been used in the treatment of GI cancers for over 50 years (Meta-Analysis Group in Cancer, 1998). 5-FU acts in several ways, but principally as a thymidylate synthase (TYMS) inhibitor. Inhibition of this enzyme blocks synthesis of the pyrimidine, thymidine which is a nucleotide required for DNA replication. TYMS methylates deoxyuridine monophosphate (dUMP) into deoxythymidine monophosphate (dTMP). Administration of 5-FU causes a depletion in dTMP, so that rapidly dividing cancer cells undergo cell death.

5-FU itself is a prodrug, which must be activated by entering the pyrimidine synthesis pathway. Although 5-FU can enter the pathway at 3 different points, the key entry point is the conversion of UMP to UDP, which is catalyzed by pyrimidine monophosphate kinase. 5-FU is given intravenously, because oral bioavailability is limited due to high concentrations of dihydropyrimidine dehydrogenase (DPYD) in the gut mucosa. DPYD is an enzyme present in the liver, intestinal mucosa and various other tissues. DPYD catabolizes 5-FU to 5,6-dihydro-5-fluorouracil (DHFU). Capecitabine is an oral analogue of 5-FU which can be used instead of intravenous 5-FU. Capecitabine is converted to 5-FU via a 3 step activation process. The first two steps occur in the liver and the last step is carried out by the enzyme thymidine phosphorylase (TYMP), which is over expressed in a large number of tumors (approximately 3 times more compared to normal tissue). Only a fraction of the administered 5-FU reaches its target cell and is transformed to active metabolites that is converted to 5-fluoro-2'-deoxyuridine-5'-monophosphate (5-FdUMP) within the cell to inhibit TYMS. Eighty-five percent of 5-FU is catabolized to its inactive metabolites via DPYD. Inherited deficiency of DPYD leads to greatly increased drug sensitivity and toxicity (Figure 1) (Daher et al, 1990).

5-Fluorouracil (5-FU)

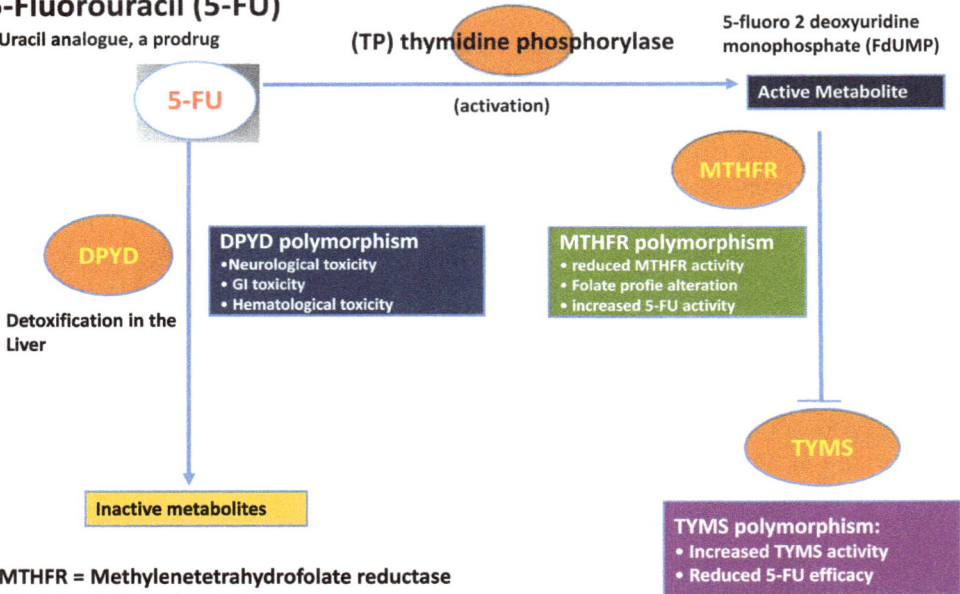

5-FU Uracil analogue, a prodrug

(TP) thymidine phosphorylase

(activation)

5-fluoro 2 deoxyuridine monophosphate (FdUMP)

Active Metabolite

MTHFR

DPYD

Detoxification in the Liver

DPYD polymorphism
•Neurological toxicity
• GI toxicity
• Hematological toxicity

MTHFR polymorphism
• reduced MTHFR activity
• Folate profie alteration
• increased 5-FU activity

TYMS

Inactive metabolites

TYMS polymorphism:
• Increased TYMS activity
• Reduced 5-FU efficacy

MTHFR = Methylenetetrahydrofolate reductase
TP = Thymidilate phosphatase
DPYD = Dihydropyrimidine dehydrogenase
TYMS = Thymidylate syntase

Fig. 1. 5-Fluorouracil metabolism

2.1 Dihydropyrimidine Dehydrogenase (DPYD)

5-FU is primarily degraded by the enzyme DPYD. When DPYD enzyme deficiency is present, blood levels of 5-FU and its active metabolites increase. DPYD enzyme deficiency can result in fatal myelotoxicity, mucositis, neuro and cardiac toxicity such as myocardial infarction, sudden death, unstable angina, hypertension and pulmonary edema (Diasio, 2001, Fleming et al, 1993, Milano et al, 1999). Although technically difficult, determination of DPYD enzyme activity in mononuclear cells may be useful (Lu, Zhang, Diasio, 1993). The gene encoding the DPYD enzyme is located at 1p22 and consists of 23-exons (Wei et al, 1998). The reasons for DPYD deficiency are base substitutions, splicing abnormalities, and frame-shift mutations. More than 40 different DPYD polymorphisms have been reported so far (Ridge et al, 1998). Severe 5-FU toxicity is associated with 17 of these mutations. Homozygote and heterozygote DPYD dysfunction is estimated to be 0.1% and 3% to 5%, respectively in the general population. DPYD*2A is the most common DPYD polymorphism associated with 5-FU toxicity. Partial loss of the enzyme due to heterogeneous G>A transition at the 5′ slicing donor consensus sequence in intron 14 leading to exon 14 skipping is associated with increased 5-FU toxicity due to inactive enzyme formation. The heterozygote form is characterized by severe toxicity while the homozygote form is characterized by mental deficiency. DPYD deficiency was demonstrated in 61% of patients with severe 5-FU toxicity. DPYD*2A polymorphism was identified in 50% of patients with grade 4 neutropenia. P456L (1358C>T) mutation is a novel DPYD variant associated with 5-FU related cardiotoxicity in pancreatic cancer patients (Shahrokni et al, 2009). However, multiple other factors and genes are thought to be involved in 5-FU toxicity because DPYD enzyme activity is normal in most patients with severe 5-FU toxicity (Mattison, Soong, Diasio, 2002, Ridge et al, 1998). Genetic variations of other enzymes particularly TYMS and TYMP involved in 5-FU metabolism are also important.

2.2 Thymidylate Synthase (TYMS)

TYMS is a target of 5-FU. It plays a significant role in folate metabolism. TYMS enables conversion of deoxyuridylate to deoxythymidylate (Miller and McLeod 2007, Johnston et al, 1995). Increased TYMS enzyme expression in tumors has been shown to be associated with resistance to 5-FU and capecitabine (Kidd et al, 2005). In particular, intratumoral TYMS levels in metastatic lesions are indicative of 5-FU resistance. This is a result of differences between TYMS expressions of primary and metastatic lesions (Pullarkat et al, 2001, Marsh et al, 2001, Salonga et al, 2000). The 5′untranslated region of the TYMS (5′-UTR) gene contains a 28-base pair tandem repeat sequence in the promoter region (TSER) which usually hosts double (allele *2) and triple (allele *3) repeats. The *3 allele is associated with a two to four fold increased expression of TYMS compared to *2. In patients with stage III colon cancer treated with adjuvant therapy, the outcome is poor in the presence of a TSER3 polymorphism. While the response rate is 50% in those with *2/*2, it is 8% in those with *3/*3 (Marsh et al, 2001). TYMS polymorphisms also affect survival. Median survival of cases with *2/*2 is 16 months vs. 12 months in cases of *3/*3. (Salonga et al, 2000). TYMS polymorphisms are also relevant in predicting response to neoadjuvant 5-FU treatment in rectal cancer. Cases of *3/*3 are associated with a poor response to the treatment (Salonga et al, 2000, Villafranca et al, 2001).

2.3 Thymidylate Phosphorylase (TYMP)

TYMP mRNA levels in patients not responding to 5-FU were 2.6-fold higher than in responding patients in pretreatment biopsies of patients with colorectal cancer (Metzger et al, 1998). Survival was significantly increased in patients with both TYMS and TYMP under nonresponse cutoff values, and low intratumoral expression of TYMS and TYMP was associated with a response to 5-FU and improved survival (Metzger et al, 1998, Meropol et al, 2006).

2.4 Methylenetetrahydrofolate reductase (MTHFR)

MTHFR generates active folate which is necessary for normal hematopoiesis. Reduced MTHFR activity has been associated with increased sensitivity to 5-FU. Low activity MTHFR variants 677T and 1298C predispose to severe myelotoxicity in patients treated with 5-FU (Robien et al, 2005).

3. Gemcitabine

Chemotherapy has proved of only limited effectiveness in pancreatic cancer. Gemcitabine is a deoxycytidine nucleoside analogue used in the treatment of advanced-stage pancreatic cancer (Burris et al, 1997). It has also proved to be of benefit in the adjuvant treatment of resected pancreatic cancer. Treatment with gemcitabine produces clinical benefit and symptom improvement in 20% to 30% of patients and 1-year survival rate of patients raised from 2% to 18% by gemcitabine. Gemcitabine undergoes metabolic activation by kinases to form a cytotoxic trinucleotide in the cell. Metabolic inactivation of gemcitabine by deamination is catalyzed by cytidine deaminase (CDA) or after phosphorylation by deoxycytidylate deaminase (DCTD) (Plunkett et al, 1995, Gandhi et al, 1990). Gemcitabine is a hydrophilic molecule and therefore does not cross the cell membrane by diffusion. To achieve gemcitabine cytotoxicity functional nucleoside transporters, namely human equilibrative nucleoside (hENT1) and human concentrative nucleoside transporters are needed. Nucleoside-transporter–deficient cells are highly resistant to gemcitabine (Spratlin et al, 2004, Mackey et al, 1998). "SLC29A1" is the most abundant of the nucleoside transporters. Intratumoral SLC29A1 protein expression, was related to prolonged survival in patients with pancreatic carcinoma treated with gemcitabine. Analysis of SLC29A1 mRNA expression revealed a significant correlation with longer survival in these patients following treatment (Sebastiani V et al, 2006, Giovannetti E, 2006).

Deoxycytidine kinase (DCK) deficiency is one of the most common forms of acquired resistance to gemcitabine in vitro (Sebastiani V et al, 2006, Bergman AM, et al, 2002). A correlation has been described between higher levels of DCK activity and increased gemcitabine sensitivity in patients with advanced pancreatic cancer treated with gemcitabine, whereas low tumoral DCK protein expression is associated with a worse overall survival (OS) and progression-free survival (PFS) (Sebastiani V et al, 2002, Kocabas NA et al, 2009). Ribonucleotide reductase (RR) is a target enzyme for gemcitabine (Goan YG et al, 1999). The pharmacology and pharmacogenetics of ribonucleotide reductase subunit M1 (RRM1) is of particular interest due to its potential role in gemcitabine chemosensitivity and synergy with other chemotherapeutic agents, particularly cisplatin (Sebastiani V, et al, Mini E et al, 2006, Ueno H et al, 2007). In genetically modified lung cancer cell lines, RRM1 expression correlated inversely with gemcitabine sensitivity (Bepler G et al, 2006). Deactivating enzymes of gemcitabine include 5′, 3′-nucleotidase, cytosolic (NT5C), deoxycytidylate deaminase (DCTD), and cytidine deaminase (CDA). Upregulation of CDA may play a role in gemcitabine resistance, while impaired activity may result in increased toxicity but not efficacy (Bepler G et al, 2006, Mathijssen RH et al, 2001). In addition to impaired tumor-specific mRNAs'/proteins' expression, a variety of genetic polymorphisms can have an impact on gemcitabine efficacy and toxicity. Tumor-specific expression of ENT1, RRM1 or ERCC1, and some DNA repair genetic polymorphisms appear to be indicators of prognosis in patients receiving gemcitabine chemotherapy. The expression level or genetic polymorphism of CDA seems to be a good predictor of adverse side effects caused by gemcitabine. SNP, CDA 208A4G, or CDA expression level may be used as biomarkers for prediction of gemcitabine-related severe toxicity: germline homozygosity for CDA 208A in a Japanese patient with pancreatic cancer treated with gemcitabine and cisplatinum resulted in severe hematologic and nonhematologic toxicity (Yonemori K et al, 2005). This is an important finding since considerable numbers of homozygote carriers of CDA 208A exist in Japanese and some African populations (Ueno H et al, 2007, Yonemori K et al, 2005).

4. Irinotecan (CPT-11)

Irinotecan is a camptothecin analogue which acts as a topoisomerase I inhibitor (Mathijssen RH et al, 2001). It is used alone or in combination with 5-FU, and folinic acid, in the treatment of colorectal cancer, gastric cancer, and in combination with 5-FU, folinic acid and oxaliplatin in advanced pancreatic cancer. Irinotecan may cause unpredictable severe toxicity such as diarrhea and neutropenia which may lead to either discontinuation or significant dose reduction of the drug. Irinotecan is activated to its cytotoxic metabolite SN-38 that inhibits the nuclear topoisomerase 1 enzyme, which is critical for DNA replication. Activation, transportation, and deactivation of irinotecan are complex and involve several enzymes, including carboxylesterase (CE), "CYP3A4", and uridine diphosphate glucuronosyltransferase (UGT1A1). Irinotecan is converted to its active metabolite, SN38, by the CE present in the gastrointestinal tract (Figure 2) (Charasson et al, 2004, Khanna et al, 2000). This enzyme has many allelic variants and genotypes. SN38 is primarily inactivated in the liver by UGT1A1 via glucuronidation. Mild hereditary deficiency of UGT1A1 leads to Gilberts syndrome which is characterized by intermittent hyperbiliribunemia (Innocenti et al, 2004, Iyer et al, 2002). Since patients with Gilbert's syndrome experienced severe toxicity in early phase studies, the association of irinotecan toxicity and the UGT1A1 polymorphism has been under thorough investigation (Wasserman et al, 1997). UGT1A1 inactivates SN38 via a phase II reaction. The wild type UGT1A1 is designated as UGT1A1*1. More than 50 genetic variations of UGT1A1 have been identified up to now (Tukey et al, 2002). Each of these leads to different degrees of functional variations. Among them UGT1A1*6, UGT1A1*28, UGT1A1*36 and UGT1A1*37 are functionally important polymorphisms. The UGT1A1*28 polymorphism is associated with reduced UGT1A1 expression and, as a result, decreased glucuronidation of SN38. This, in turn, increases blood levels of active metabolites resulting in increased toxicity (Khanna et al, 2000, Innocenti 2004, Iyer 2002, Hoskins et al, 2007). The pharmacokinetics of irinotecan is poorly associated with body surface area. Since SN38 undergoes glucuronidation to a lesser extent in patients with Gilbert and Crigler Najjar syndromes, irinotecan toxicity increases in these patients, because of reduced or deficient expression levels of UGT1A1. Gilbert syndrome results from the UGT1A1*28 homozygote transition of a promoter polymorphism caused by seven TA repetitions. In the presence of the UGT1A1*28 polymorphism, transcription is decreased by 70% and toxicity is increased. Patients with the 7/7 genotype (homozygous for seven TA repetitions) exhibit a

9.3-fold increase in risk of grade 4 neutropenia, and irinotecan is associated with severe side effects in this population (Iyer et al, 2002, Hoskins et al, 2007; McLeod et al, 2003). In an early study the UGT1A1*28 allele increased the risk of leukopenia and/or diarrhea, however most of the later studies found only increased risk of hematological toxicity such as neutropenia (Ando et al, 2000). In fact, in a meta-analysis of 10 studies assessing the irinotecan induced toxicity in UGT1A1*28 patients, irinotecan dose, and overall toxicity, risk of experiencing irinotecan induced hematologic toxicity for homozygous UGT1A1*28 patients was found to be a function of the dose of irinotecan administered, and genotyping was recommended at only high doses (> 200 mg/m2) of irinotecan (Hoskins et al, 2007). Genotyping has limited benefit at intermediate doses, such as 180mg/m^2 used in the FOLFIRI (folinic acid/5-FU/irinotecan) regimen. Unless administered concomitantly with another myelotoxic agent, UGT1A1*28 testing is not recommended at doses < 150 mg/m^2.

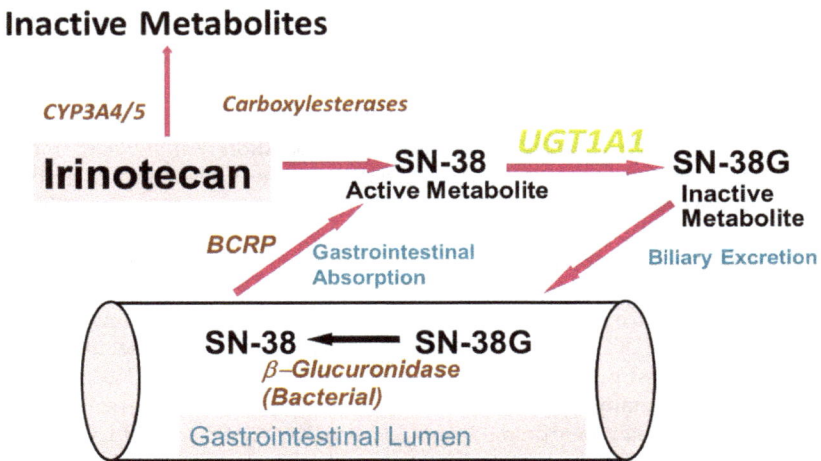

Fig. 2. Irinotecan Metabolism

Transport proteins that excrete irinotecan and metabolites have also been investigated for their potential association with irinotecan response and toxicity. P-glycoprotein represents one of these proteins, and it is encoded by the ATP binding B1 (ABCB1 or MDR1) gene. However, the pharmacogenetic results regarding ABCB1 and irinotecan are conflicting to date. Genetic variation in ABCB1 was associated with early toxicity and lower response to treatment. Specifically, carriers of the ABCB1 1236T-2677T-3435T haplotype responded to treatment less frequently with shorter survival (Glimelius et al, 2011).

5. Platinum compounds (Cisplatin and Oxaliplatin)

Cisplatin and oxaliplatin are commonly used in gastrointestinal cancers (Vermorken et al, 1984, Raymond et al, 1998, Levi et al, 2000) Platinum analogues block DNA replication by forming different DNA adducts, through intra-strand and inter-strand crosslinks. Platin resistance occurs due to detoxification or efficient repair of DNA by the nucleotide excision repair system. DNA repair enzymes "ERCC1" and "ERCC2" — also known as "XPD" and glutathione S transferase π (GSTP) enzymes — are involved in the activity of these agents (Levi et al, 2000). GSTπ is a phase II metabolic enzyme that inactivates platinum derivatives by adding a glutathione to its electrophile group. High expression of the genes that code for these enzymes is inversely correlated with therapeutic response in colorectal and gastric cancer (Ruzzo et al, 2007). Preclinical models of oxaliplatin resistance have also been studied in colorectal cancer cell lines. In these cell lines a total of 6 target genes were identified: AKT1, CDK5, RGS11, GARP, TRIP, and UGCGL1. Three of these genes (AKT1, CDK5 and TRIP) were shown to be involved in NF-κβ pathway regulation. It was suggested that low levels of TRIP and high levels of AKT1 and CDK5 could contribute to NF-κβ activation and consequently cell antiapoptotic activity and oxaliplatin acquired resistance. These findings show that the NF-κβ pathway plays a pivotal role in mechanisms of acquired oxaliplatin resistance (Martinez-Cardus et al, 2009).

6. Combination chemotherapy

6.1 Folfox (Oxaliplatin/5-FU/folinic acid)

Many chemotherapy combinations are used in the treatment of gastrointestinal cancers. However, strong evidence of pharmacogenetics is available only in a minority of the reference studies (Stoehlmacher et al, 2004; Goldberg et al, 2006). The N9741 trial is a randomized phase III trial designed to compare the efficacy of FOLFOX (folinic acid/5-FU/oxaliplatin), IROX (irinotecan/oxaliplatin), and IFL (irinotecan/bolus 5-FU/folinic acid) in patients with metastatic colorectal cancer (Goldberg et al, 2006). The pharmacogenetic evaluation of this study revealed that both the objective response rate and incidence of grade ¾ side effects, particularly diarrhea, were lower in black patients. The low response rate in black patients was especially marked in the FOLFOX arm. Overall, the rate of response was 41% and 30% in white and black patients, respectively (P = .015). The rate of severe toxicity was 48% in whites and 34% in black patients in the FOLFOX arm (P = .047). Despite the lack of significant median survival difference between these two patient groups in the FOLFOX arm, median survival was lower in black patients in both the IFL and IROX groups. In all arms, black patients experienced less toxicity, particularly less diarrhea, compared to white patients. The UGT1A1 7/7 polymorphism was identified at a rate of 21% and 9% in black and white patients, respectively, in this study. However, the role of the UGT1A1 polymorphism with respect to response and toxicity could not be demonstrated. Significant differences were also detected between white and black patients in the prevalence of other pharmacogenetic variances such as CYP3A, MDR (multidrug resistance), ERCC1, ERCC2, and GSTP. These genes are important in the metabolism and detoxification of irinotecan and oxaliplatin (Grothey et al, 2005). Of note, the type of GSTP polymorphism was shown to be associated with early development of oxaliplatin neuropathy in patients receiving FOLFOX.

The polymorphism that causes a single nucleotide change of C to T, at codon 118, converts a codon of common usage (AAC) to a less used codon (AAT), both coding for asparagine. This change results in decreased ERCC1 gene expression, which impairs repair activity. A small study showed that the ERCC1 codon 118 polymorphism predicted response to oxaliplatin/5-FU chemotherapy in patients with advanced colorectal cancer (Viguier et al, 2005). In this retrospective study including 91 patients, response rate was 61.9%, 42.3%, and 21.4% in T/T, C/T, and C/C groups, respectively (P= 0.018). However, the results of the studies regarding the ERCC1 codon 118 polymorphism are somewhat contradictory, likely due to a variety of factors such as ethnicity, environment (smoking or diet), the number of patients enrolled and/or linkage to other polymorphisms (Ryu, 2006). A SNP in codon 751 of the ERCC2 gene which leads to glutamine instead of lysine, was associated with a reduced response rate (Park et al, 2001, Stoehlmacher et al, 2004). Additionally, patients with the GSTπ 105 Val/Val genotype had a better progression free survival (PFS) and overall survival (OS) than patients carrying the GSTπ 105 Ile allele (Stoehlmacher et al, 2004). In a more recent study analyzing the pharmacogenetic factors in patients with advanced colorectal cancer treated with FOLFOX chemotherapy PFS was related only to genes involved in oxaliplatin pharmacodynamics, with a tendency for a better outcome in patients bearing the GSTπ 105 Val/Val genotype or the XPD 751Lys allele (Etienne-Grimaldi et al, 2010). Lymphocytic activity of GSTπ has been shown to be significantly reduced in GSTπ 105 Val/Val patients compared with GSTπ 105 Ile/Ile patients (Dusinská et al, 2001). However, the functional impact of XPD 751 Lys→Gln at the protein level is not clearly established.

6.2 Cisplatin/5-fluorouracil

Combination of cisplatin and 5-FU (CF) constitutes the backbone of chemotherapy regimens commonly used for upper gastrointestinal system tumors including gastric and hepatobiliary cancer (Kilickap et al, 2011). In gastric cancer TYMS and ERCC gene expression has been studied individually as the predictors of chemoresistance (Lenz et al, 1996, Metzger et al, 1998). In another study although TYMS and ERCC1 expression associated with poor prognosis, it did not reach statistical significance ($P = 0.076$) (Metzger et al, 1998). Kim et al, developed a three gene predictor of clinical outcome for metastatic gastric cancer patients treated with cisplatin and 5-FU (Kim et al, 2010). The combined expression of MYC, epidermal growth factor receptor (EGFR) and fibroblast growth factor receptor 2 (FGFR2) was found to be an independent predictor of decreased OS of CF treated metastatic gastric cancer patients (Kim et al, 2010). The findings of the study showed that over expression of these 3 genes was associated with chemoresistance and the results were consistent with the experimental studies showing that inhibitors of EGFR act synergistically with cisplatin and 5-FU, while an FGFR2 inhibitor acts synergistically with 5-FU and MYC over expression is associated with cisplatin resistance (Kim et al, 2010). Taken together, combined expression of MYC, EGFR and FGFR2 is predictive of poor survival in patients with metastatic gastric cancer treated with CF chemotherapy.

The xCT gene, which codes for part of the plasma membrane cysteine/glutamate transporter, contributes to tumor cell protection against immune defense mechanisms (Huang et al, 2010). The plasma membrane xc-cysteine/glutamate transporter mediates cellular uptake of cysteine in exchange for intracellular glutamate and is highly expressed by pancreatic cancer cells. In advanced pancreatic cancer Huang et al, looked at the prognostic significance of SNPs in the xCT gene in patients treated with a combination of gemcitabine and platinum (Huang et al, 2010). The xCT gene, encodes the cysteine-specific xCT protein subunit of xc-, which is important in regulating intracellular glutathione levels, critical for cancer cell protection against oxidative stress, tumor growth and resistance to chemotherapeutic agents. A statistically significant correlation was noted between the 3' UTR xCT SNP rs7674870 and OS: Median survival time (MST) was 10.9 and 13.6 months, respectively, for the TT and TC/CC genotypes (P = 0.027). In another study Pacetti *et al*, investigated polymorphisms in genes involved in activity and resistance to drugs, mainly DNA repair gene polymorphisms, in an effort to link them to treatment response. The substitution of glutamine for lysine in position 751 of the XPD gene (Figure 2) led to increased overall survival from 262 days to 446 days (Pacetti et al, 2010). These studies suggest that genetic polymorphisms in xCT gene may serve as a predictor of treatment outcome in advanced pancreatic cancer.

7. Biologic agents

7.1 Overview

Biologic agents used in GI cancers alone or in combination with chemotherapy include bevacizumab (Avastin, Roche), cetuximab (Erbitux, KGaA), panitumumab (Vectibix, Amgen), and erlotinib (Tarceva, Roche), sunitinib (Sutent, Pfizer), imatinib (Glivec, Gleevec, Novartis). These drugs do not act only through different mechanisms of action but also demonstrate differences in their pharmacokinetics and pharmacodynamics. Meanwhile, data on their pharmacogenetics are only now emerging.

7.2 Bevacizumab

Bevacizumab is a humanized monoclonal antibody (MoAB) that binds the vascular endothelial growth factor (VEGF). Increased VEGF expression is involved in tumoral angiogenesis and associated with poor prognosis. Bevacizumab prevents receptor binding of VEGF, and inhibits VEGF signaling pathways, thus stops angiogenesis and tumor growth. The therapeutic benefit of bevacizumab has been shown in the treatment of patients with advanced-stage colorectal cancer. Thus far, however, adequate pharmacogenetic data have not been produced to predict toxicity, response, or resistance.

7.3 EGFR monoclonal antibodies (Cetuximab and Panitumumab)

Cetuximab and panitumumab are MoAB used as single agents or in combination with chemotherapy for the treatment of advanced colorectal cancer. Cetuximab is a MoAB that binds to the EGFR and blocks EGF signaling pathway and tumor growth. Panitumumab is the anti-EGFR MoAB similar to cetuximab, binds EGFR and inhibits downstream of EGF signaling. Panitumumab is a fully human MoAB in contrast to cetuximab which is chimeric. The pioneering studies of BOND trials, showed that cetuximab may provide benefit in patients with chemotherapy refractory advanced colorectal cancer (Saltz et al, 2007). In the BOND 2 trial metastatic colorectal cancer patients progressing after irinotecan-based chemotherapy were randomized to receive irinotecan plus bevacizumab plus cetuximab (CBI) or bevacizumab and cetuximab (CB) (Lenz et al, 2007). In this trial, germline polymorphisms of the genes involved in angiogenesis (VEGF, interleukin-8 [IL-8], transforming growth factor [TGF]-β), the EGFR pathway (EGFR, cyclooxygenase-2, E-cadherin), DNA repair (ERCC1, ERCC2, XRCC1, XPD), and drug metabolism pathway (GSTP, UGT1A1) were investigated. Genomic DNA was extracted for genotyping from 65 patients (31: CBI arm and 34: CB arm). Thirty five patients had tissue samples available for the gene expression assay (18: CBI arm and 17: CB arm). High intratumoral gene expression levels of EGFR, VEGFR2 and NRP1 were associated with longer OS in patients receiving combined monoclonal antibodies with or without irinotecan. The FCGR3A V158F, cyclinD1 A870G and EGFR R497K polymorphisms were associated with clinical outcome in patients receiving the cetuximab and bevacizumab combination independent of KRAS mutation status (Lenz et al, 2007, Zhang et al, 2007). Patients with high intratumoral EGFR gene expression levels had a median survival time of 21.8 (range, 9.6-28.2) months, compared to patients with low EGFR gene expression levels, whose median survival was 10.2 (range, 8.3-13.6) months (P = 0.033). In the RP analysis, the EGFR gene expression level was found to be the best single determinant of survival (Zhang et al, 2007)

Initially anti-EGFR antibodies were tested in patients with metastatic colorectal cancer which showed elevated EGFR expression, as determined by immunohistochemistry. However, response to EGFR MoAB was not found to be correlated to EGFR expression. Retrospective data suggested that the severity of skin rash might be positively correlated with tumor response to anti-EGFR MoAB, but only in patients with tumors expressing wild type K-RAS. In the NCIC CTG CO17 study a rash of grade 2 or higher was strongly associated with improved survival in patients treated with cetuximab (Jonker et al, 2007). A correlation between K-RAS mutation and resistance to the EGFR antibodies cetuximab and panitumumab has been demonstrated. K-RAS mutations account for approximately 30% to 40% of patients with mCRC. (Van Cutsem et al, 2008, Amado et al, 2008, Bokemeyer et al, 2008). Patients with a K-RAS mutation in codons 12, 13 and 61 in their tumor tissue have lower rates of response to cetuximab and panitumumab and shorter PFS time. The benefit of anti-EGFR MoAB monotherapy is limited to only the patients with K-RAS wild type CRC except patients with the codon 13 D13G K-RAS mutation benefit from the therapy similar to the wild type tumors (De Roock et al, 2010). Therefore, K-RAS mutation analysis is required before prescribing EGFR MoAB therapies.

The B-type Raf kinase BRAF V600E mutation was detected in 11 of 79 patients who had wild type K-RAS (Di Nicolantonio et al, 2008). This BRAF mutation is associated with resistance to cetuximab and panitumumab with significantly shorter PFS and OS compared to wild type patients (Di Nicolantonio et al, Di Fiore et al, 2008). Mutations of genes other than K-RAS and BRAF, such as the phosphatase and tensin homologue (PTEN), and phosphatidylinositol 3-kinase (PI3K) were also associated with shorter survival of MCRC patients receiving EGFR antagonists (Karapedis et al, 2008). Thus, these mutations may serve as additional biomarkers to predict resistance of EGFR antagonists.

7.4 Erlotinib

Erlotinib belongs to a group of drugs called EGFR tyrosine kinase inhibitors. EGF has receptors on cancer cell surfaces. Stimulation of this receptor activates the tyrosine kinase enzyme inside the cell. The drugs that inhibit this enzyme, and stop the growth factor receptor are known as tyrosine kinase inhibitors (TKIs). Erlotinib is a small-molecule TKI targeting EGFR (Hidalgo et al, 2001; Li et al, 2007). Erlotinib, similarly to other EGFR-directed therapies, is associated with toxicity involving skin rash and diarrhea. The molecular basis of these side effects is under investigation. Basal layers of both the epidermis and the GI mucosa express EGFR, and EGFR signaling has been implicated in the physiological regulation of these tissues. Inhibition of this physiological pathway is implicated in toxicity. Erlotinib is metabolized predominantly by CYP3A4, so inhibitors of this enzyme would be expected to increase systemic availability and inducers would be expected to decrease it (Moore et al, 2007a). Potent inducers of CYP3A4 may reduce the efficacy of erlotinib, whereas potent inhibitors of CYP3A4 may lead to increased toxicity (Hidalgo et al, 2001, Li et al, 2007, Rudin et al, 2008). For example, concomitant use of ketacanozole, a CYP3A4 and ABCB1 inhibitor, increases the AUC of erlotinib by 66% which will result in increased erlotinib toxicity. Meanwhile pre- or co-treatment with rifampicin, a CYP3A4 inducer, increases erlotinib clearance by three-fold and reduces AUC by 66%, which will result in the loss of clinical activity. Therefore concomitant use of inhibitors and inducers of CYP3A4 should be avoided.

Besides CYP genes the inhibition of glucuronidation may also cause interactions between erlotinib and substrates of UGT1A1. Patients with low expression of UGT1A1 or genetic glucuronidation disorders may have hyperbilirubinemia (Rudin et al, 2008). In advanced pancreatic cancer, erlotinib in combination with gemcitabine showed statistically superior overall survival compared with gemcitabine alone (6.4 months vs. 5.9 months, respectively) (Moore MJ et al, 2007). In this study, patients responded equally well to treatment with erlotinib regardless of whether their tumors expressed abnormal levels of EGFR. In a subgroup of analyses in this study the mutation status of the K-RAS and EGFR gene copy number (GCN) were evaluated as predictive markers in 26% of patients who had tumor samples available for analysis. The K-RAS mutation status was evaluated by direct sequencing of exon 2, and EGFR GCN was determined by fluorescence in situ hybridization (FISH) analysis. The results were correlated with survival, which was the primary endpoint of the trial. K-RAS mutations were identified in 78.6% of the patients and EGFR amplification or high polysomy (FISH-positive results) was identified in 46.7% of the patients. The hazard ratio of death between gemcitabine/erlotinib and gemcitabine/placebo was 0.66 (95% confidence interval [CI], 0.28-1.57) for patients with wild type K-RAS and 1.07 (95% CI, 0.68-1.66) for patients with mutant K-RAS (P value for interaction = .38), and the hazard ratio was 0.6 (95% CI, 0.34-1.07) for FISH-negative patients and 0.90 (95% CI, 0.49-1.65) for FISH-positive patients (P value for interaction = .32). Although survival was longer in patients with wild type K-RAS in comparison to K-RAS mutated patients, in this molecular subset analysis of patients from NCIC CTG PA.3, EGFR GCN and K-RAS mutation status were not identified as markers predictive of a survival benefit from the combination of erlotinib with gemcitabine for the first-line treatment of advanced pancreatic carcinoma (da Cunha Santos et al, 2010, Moore MJ et al, 2007b).

In the AViTA study, patients with advanced stage pancreatic cancer were treated with gemcitabine plus erlotinib with or without bevacizumab. In this study, although no molecular pharmacogenetic marker has been identified yet, survival was positively correlated with severity of erlotinib induced skin rash (Verslype C et al, 2009). Therefore, reassessment of erlotinib treatment is recommended in patients who do not develop rash within the first 4 to 8 weeks of treatment.

7.5 Imatinib

Imatinitib mesylate is approved for the treatment of advanced and also resected high risk patients with cKIT or platelet derived growth factor receptor alpha (PDGFRA) activating mutation positive gastrointestinal stromal tumors (GIST). Sensitivity of imatinib in GIST correlates to exon mutations of cKIT and PDGFRA. The outcome of patients with cKIT exon 11 mutations are more favorable compared to exon 9 mutations and to wild type tumors.

Approximately 80% of GISTs harbor an activating mutation in the cKIT gene and another 5% to 7% have a PDGFRA gene mutation (Heinrich MC et al, 2008). These mutations are not only important in tumorigenesis, but also predict treatment response to imatinib, and provide prognostic information. If the tumors have a c-KIT exon 11 mutation the response rate is 69% to 86%, but only 17% to 48% in patients with tumors harboring a c-KIT exon 9 mutation (Heinrich MC et al, 2008). These patients respond better to the dose of 800 mg imatinib compared to the standard 400 mg dose. Most of PDGFRA gene mutations are associated with imatinib response, with the most notable exception of D842V. In wild type GIST without any c-KIT and PDGFRA mutations, the response rate to imatinib is only 0% to 45% (Heinrich MC et al, 2008). Median time to progression (TTP) is 25, 17, and 13 months for patients with tumor mutations in c-KIT exon 11, c-KIT exon 9, and neither c-KIT nor PDGFRA genes, respectively (Heinrich et al, 2008). Median OS is 60, 38, and 49 months, respectively. Although patients may experience prolonged disease control while on imatinib, most patients will develop imatinib resistance within 2-3 years on therapy. Lowered plasma levels of imatinib over time is often responsible for disease progression. This phenomenon is called as "acquired pharmacokinetic drug resistance". This may be because of an altered expression pattern or activity of drug transporters such as efflux transporters (ATP-binding cassette transporters, such as ABCB1 and ABCG2) and uptake transporters [solute carriers such as organic cation transporter 1 (OCT1) and organic anion transporting polypeptide 1A2 (OATP1A2)]. ABCB1 and ABCC1 expression was shown in GIST, whereas ABCB1, ABCG2, and OCT1 were found in mononuclear cells in CML patients. Despite increasing accumulation of preclinical data, clinical studies on imatinib pharmacogenetics are still insufficient and the results are somewhat contradictory.

7.6 Sunitinib

Sunitinib is an oral, multitargeted TKI. It inhibits VEGF receptors (VEGFRs) 1, 2, and 3, PDGFR α and β KIT, Fms-like tyrosine kinase 3 receptor (FLT3), and the receptor encoded by the RET proto-oncogene. Among the GI tumors sunitinib is approved for first-line treatment of metastatic pancreatic neuorendocrine tumours (PNET) and in imatinib-resistant metastatic GIST. In a multicenter study including patients with GIST, metastatic renal cell cancer or other cancers, genetic markers in the pharmacokinetic and pharmacodynamic pathways of sunitinib that predispose to development of toxicity were investigated (van Erp et al, 2009). The study was performed in 219 patients treated with single-agent sunitinib. A total of 31 SNPs in 12 candidate genes were analyzed for a possible association with toxicity. The risk for leukopenia was increased when the G allele in CYP1A1 2455A/G (odds ratio (OR), 6.24; P = .029) or the T allele in FLT3 738T/C (OR, 2.8; P = .008) were present or CAG in the NR1I3 (5719C/T, 7738A/C, 7837T/G) haplotype (OR, 1.74; P = .041) was absent. Any toxicity higher than grade 2 prevalence was increased when the T allele of VEGFR2 1191C/T (OR, 2.39; P = .046) or a copy of TT in the ABCG2 (-15622C/T, 1143C/T) haplotype (OR, 2.63; P = .016) were present. The risk for mucosal inflammation was increased in the presence of the G allele in CYP1A1 2455A/G (OR, 4.03; P = .021) and the prevalence of hand-foot syndrome was increased when a copy of TTT in the ABCB1 (3435C/T, 1236C/T, 2677G/T) haplotype (OR, 2.56; P = .035) was present. This study suggested that polymorphisms in specific genes encoding for metabolizing enzymes, efflux transporters, and drug targets are associated with sunitinib-related toxicity. The response of patients with advanced GIST to sunitinib is related to the type of primary mutation. Patients with original (pre-imatinib) exon 9 mutant or wild type tumor had a significantly longer duration of response compared to patients with exon 11 mutations. The median time to progression was 14.3 months for patients with original exon 9 mutations, 13.8 months for patients with wild type cKIT and PDGFRA, and 5.1 months for patients whose original mutation was in exon 11 (Heinrich MC et al, 2008).

8. Conclusion

Despite progress in the development of new chemotherapy agents and targeted therapies, and the improved outcome in patients with GI cancers, there is still need for development of more efficacious treatments. Meanwhile, individualization of management of cancer patients is also crucial because only a portion of patients respond to a given treatment, usually with a low complete response rate. Therefore oncologists are seeking ways to predict whether a selected chemotherapy will be effective and tolerable in patients prior to treatment. Coupled with the complexity and diversity of each individual patient and the disease, each case should be handled uniquely and treatment should be tailor made. At this point pharmacogenetic plays a pivotal role. Recent progress in our understanding of carcinogenesis and molecular biology led to development of sophisticated pharmacogenetic assays to facilitate the delivery of more effective, less toxic chemotherapy regimens by individualizing treatments for patients with relatively resistant tumors of the GI tract. Based on the results of pharmacogenetic studies of clinical trials new tests are on the horizon and, data from these tests will enable cancer physicians to treat their patients better and save more lives. In this chapter recent pharmacogenetic studies relevant to the treatment of patients with GI cancer are reviewed. Genetic polymorphisms and tumor gene expression patterns are discussed. Many of the trials reviewed herein are expected to result in approval of new pharmacogenetic tests.

9. References

Aksoy S, Karaca B, Dincer M, et al: Common etiology of capecitabine and fluorouracil-induced coronary vasospasm in a colon cancer patient. Ann Pharmacother 39:573–74, 2005.

Amado RG, Wolf M, Peeters M, et al: Wild type KRAS is required for panitumumab efficacy in patients with metastatic colorectal cancer. J Clin Oncol 26:1626–34, 2008

Ando Y, Saka H, Ando M et al: Polymorphisms of UDP-glucuronosyl transferese. Gene and irinotecan toxicity: a pharmacogenetic analysis. Cancer Res 60:6971-26, 2000

Bepler G, Kusmartseva I, Sharma S, et al: RRM1 modulated in vitro and in vivo efficacy of gemcitabine and platinum in non-small-cell lung cancer. J Clin Oncol 24:4731–37, 2006

Bergman AM, Pinedo HM, Peters GJ: Determinants of resistance to 2′,2′-difluorodeoxycytidine (gemcitabine). Drug Resist Update 5:19–33, 2002

Bokemeyer C, Bondarenko I, Hartmann J, et al: KRAS status and efficacy of first-line treatment of patients with metastatic colorectal cancer (mCRC) with FOLFOX with or without cetuximab: The OPUS experience. J Clin Oncol 26 (15S):178s, 2008 (abstr 4000)

Burris HA 3rd, Moore MJ, Andersen J, et al: Improvements in survival and clinical benefit with gemcitabine as first-line therapy for patients with advanced pancreas cancer: a randomized trial. J Clin Oncol 15(6):2403–2413, 1997

Charasson V, Bellott R, Meynard D, et al: Pharmacogenetics of human carboxylesterase 2, an enzyme involved in the activation of irinotecan into SN-38. Clin Pharmacol Ther 76:528–535, 2004

da Cunha Santos, G., Dhani, N., Tu, D., Chin, K., et al: Molecular predictors of outcome in a phase 3 study of gemcitabine and erlotinib therapy in patients with advanced pancreatic cancer. Cancer, 116: 5599–5607, 2010

Daher GC, Harris BE, Diasio RB: Metabolism of pyrimidine analogues and their nucleosides. Pharmacol Ther 48:189–222, 1990.

De Roock W, Jonker DJ, Di Nicolantonio F et al: Association of KRAS p.G13D mutation with outcome in patients with chemotherapy-refractory metastatic colorectal cancer treated with cetuximab. JAMA, 304:1812-20, 2010.

Diasio RB: Clinical implications of dihydropyrimidine dehydrogenase on 5-FU pharmacology. Oncology 15:21–26, 2001.

Di Nicolantonio F, Martini M, Molinari F, et al: Wild type BRAF is required for response to panitumumab or cetuximab in metastatic colorectal cancer. J Clin Oncol 26:5705–5712, 2008

Dusinská M, Ficek A, Horská A, et al: Glutathione S-transferase polymorphisms influence the level of oxidative DNA damage and anti-oxidant protection in humans. Mutat Res 482:47–55, 2001.

Etienne-Grimaldi MC, Milano G, Maindrault-Gœbel F et al: Methylenetetrahydrofolate reductase (MTHFR) gene polymorphisms and FOLFOX response in colorectal cancer patients. Br J Clin Pharmacol 69: 58–66; 2010.

Fleming RA, Milano GA, Gaspard MH, et al: Dihydropyrimidine dehydrogenase activity in cancer patients. Eur J Cancer 29A:740–44, 1993

Gandhi V, Plunkett W: Modulatory activity of 2',2'-difluorodeoxycytidine on the phosphorylation and cytotoxicity of arabinosyl nucleosides. Cancer Res 50:3675–80, 1990

Giovannetti E, Mey V, Nannizzi S, et al: Pharmacogenetics of anticancer drug sensitivity in pancreatic cancer. Mol Cancer Ther 5:1387–95, 2006

Glimelius B, Garmo H, Berglund A et al: Prediction of irinotecan and 5-fluorouracil toxicity and response in patients with advanced colorectal cancer. The pharmocogenomics journal 11:61-71, 2011

Goan YG, Zhou B, Hu E, et al: Overexpression of ribonucleotide reductase as a mechanism of resistance to 2,2 diflouorodeoxycytidine in the human KB cancer cell line. Cancer Res 59; 4204-4207, 1999

Goldberg RM, McLeod HL, Sargent DJ, et al: Genetic polymorphisms, toxicity, and responserate in African Americans (AA) with metastatic colorectal cancer (MCRC) compared to Caucasians(C) when treated with IFL, FOLFOX or IROX in Intergroup N9741. J Clin Oncol 24(18S):2006 (abstr 3503)

Grothey A, McLeod HL, Green EM, et al: Glutathione S-transferase P1 I105V (GSTP1 I105V) polymorphism is associated with early onset of oxaliplatin-induced neurotoxicity. J Clin Oncol 23 (16S):2005 (abstr 3509)

Heinrich MC, Owzar K, Corless CL, et al: Correlation of kinase genotype and clinical outcome in the North American Intergroup Phase III Trial of imatinib mesylate for treatment of advanced gastrointestinal stromal tumor: CALGB 150105 Study by Cancer and Leukemia Group B and Southwest Oncology Group. J Clin Oncol, 26:5360-7, 2008.

Heinrich MC, Maki RG, Corless CL, et al: Primary and secondary kinase genotypes correlate with the biological and clinical activity of sunitinib in imatinib-resistant gastrointestinal stromal tumor. J Clin Oncol; 26:5352-9, 2008.

Hidalgo M, Siu LL, Nemunaitis J, et al: Phase I and pharmacologic study of OSI-774, an epidermal growth factor receptor tyrosine kinase inhibitor, in patients with advanced solid malignancies. J Clin Oncol 19:3267–3279, 2001

Hoskins J, Goldberg R, Qu P, et al: UGT1A1*28genotype and irinotecan induced neutropenia: dose matters. J Natl Cancer Inst 99:1290–1295, 2007

Huang TJ, Li D, Weatherly J, Tang H, et al: Prognostic significance of xCT gene single nucleotide polymorphisms (SNPs) in patients (pts) with advanced pancreatic cancer (PC) treated with gemcitabine (GEM) plus platinum analogues (PLTA). J Clin Oncol; 28 (15 Suppl):4065, 2010.

Innocenti F, Undevia SD, Iyer L, et al: Genetic variants in the UDP-glucuronosyltransferase 1A1 gene predict the risk of severe neutropenia of irinotecan. J Clin Oncol 22:1382, 2004

Iyer L, Das S, Janisch L, et al: UGT1A1*28 polimorphism as a determinant of irinotecan disposition and toxicity. Pharmacogenomics J 2:43–47, 2002

Johnston PG, Lenz HJ, Leichman CG, et al: Thymidylate synthase gene and protein expression correlate and are associated with response to 5-fluorouracil in human colorectal and gastric tumors. Cancer Res 55(7):1407–12, 1995.

Jonker DJ, O'Callaghan CJ, Karapetis CS, et al: Cetuximab for the treatment of colorectal cancer. N Engl J Med; 357:2040-8, 2007.

Karapetis CS, Khambata-Ford S, Jonker DJ, et al: K-ras mutations and benefit from cetuximab in advanced colorectal cancer. N Engl J Med 359:1757-65, 2008

Khanna R, Morton C, Danks MK, et al: Proficient metabolism of irinotecan by a human intestinal carboylesterase. Cancer Res 60:4725–28, 2000

Kidd EA, Yu J, Li X, et al: Variance in the expression of 5-fluorouracil pathway genes in colorectal cancer. Clin Cancer Res 11:2612–19, 2005

Kilickap S, Yalcin S, Ates O, Tekuzman G: The first line systemic chemotherapy in metastatic gastric carcinoma: A comparison of docetaxel, cisplatin and fluorouracil (DCF) versus cisplatin and fluorouracil (CF); versus epirubicin, cisplatin and fluorouracil (ECF) regimens in clinical setting. Hepatogastroenterology 58 :208-12, 2011.

Kim HK, Choi IJ, Kim CG et al: Three gene predictor of clinical outcome for gastric cancer patients treated with chemotherapy. The pharmacogenomics Journal doi 10.1038/tpj.2010.

Kocabas NA, Aksoy P, Pelleymounter LL et al: Gemcitabine pharmacogenomics: deoxycytidine kinase and cytidylate kinase genes resquencing and functional genomics. Drug metabolism and disposition 36:1951-59, 2009

Lenz HJ, Leichman CG, Danenberg KD et al: Thymidylate synthase mRNA level in adenocarcinoma of the stomach: a predictor for primary tumor response and overall survival. J Clin Oncol 14:176-182, 1996

Lenz H, Zhang W, Yang D, et al: Pharmacogenomic analysis of a randomized phase II trial (BOND 2) of cetuximab/bevacizumab/irinotecan (CBI) versus cetuximab / bevacizumab (CB) in irinotecan-refractory colorectal cancer. 2007 Gastrointestinal Cancers Symposium (abstr 401)

Levi F, Metzger G, Massari C, et al: Oxaliplatin: pharmacokinetics and chronopharmacological aspects. Clin Pharmacokinet 5:1–21, 2000

Li J, Zhao M, He P, et al: Differential metabolism of gefitinib and erlotinib by human cytochrome P450 enzymes. Clin Cancer Res13:3731–3737, 2007

Lu Z, Zhang R, Diasio RB: Dihydropyrimidine dehydrogenase activity in human peripheral blood mononuclear cells and liver: population characteristics newly identified deficient patients and clinical implications in 5-fluorouracil in cancer patients. Cancer Res 53:5433–5438, 1993.

Mackey JR, Mani RS, Selner M, et al: Functional nucleoside transporters are required for gemcitabine influx and manifestation of toxicity in cancer cell lines. Cancer Res 58:4349–4357,1998

Marsh S, McKay JA, Cassidy J, et al: Polymorphism in the thymidylate synthase promoter enhancer region in colorectal cancer. Int J Oncol 19:383–386, 2001

Martinez-Cardús A, Martinez-Balibrea E, Bandrés E et al: Pharmacogenomic approach for the identification of novel determinants of acquired resistance to oxaliplatin in colorectal cancer. Mol Cancer Ther. 8:194-202, 2009.

Mathijssen RH, van Alphen RJ, Verweij J, et al: Clinical pharmacokinetics and metabolism of irinotecan (CPT-11). Clin Cancer Res 7:2182–2194, 2001

Mattison L, Soong R, Diasio R: Implications of dihydropyrimidine dehydrogenase on 5FU pharmacogenetics and pharmacogenomics. Pharmacogenomics 3:485–491, 2002

McLeod, HL, Sargent DJ, Marsh S, et al: Pharmacogenetic analysis of systemic toxicity and response after 5-fluorouracil (5FU)/CPT-11,5FU/oxaliplatin (oxal), or CPT-11/oxal therapy for advanced colorectal cancer (CRC): Results from an intergroup trial. Proc Am Soc Clin Oncol 22:2003 (abstr 1013)

Meta-Analysis Group in Cancer Toxicity of fluorouracil in patients with advanced colorectal cancer: effect of administration schedule and prognostic factors. J Clin Oncol 16:3537–3541, 1998

Meropol NJ, Gold PJ, Diasio RB, et al: Thymidine phosphorylase expression is associated with response to capecitabine plus irinotecan in patients with metastatic colorectal cancer. J Clin Oncol 24(25):4069–4077, 2006

Metzger R, Danenberg K, Leichman CG, et al: High basal level gene expression of thymidine phosphorylase (platelet-derived endothelial cell growth factor) in colorectal tumors is associated with nonresponse to 5-fluorouracil. Clin Cancer Res 4:2371–2376, 1998

Metzger R, Leichman CG, Danenberg KD et al: ERCC1 mRNA levels complement thymidylate synthase mRNA levels in predicting response and survival for gastric cancer patients receiving cisplatin and 5-fluorouracil chemotherapy. J Clin Oncol 16: 309-316, 1998.

Milano G, Etienne MC, Pierrefite V, et al: Dihydropyrimidine dehydrogenase deficiency and fluorouracil-related toxicity. Br J Cancer 79:627–630, 1999

Miller CR, McLeod HL: Pharmacogenomics of cancer chemotherapy-induced toxicity. Support Oncol 5:9–14, 2007.

Mini E, Nobili S, Caciagli B, et al: Cellular pharmacology of gemcitabine. Ann Oncol 17 (suppl 5):v7–v12, 2006

Moore MJ, da Cunha Santos G, Kamel-Reid S: The relationship of K-ras mutations and EGFR gene copy number to outcome in patients treated with erlotinib on National Cancer Institute of Canada Clinical Trials Group trial study PA.3. J Clin Oncol 25(18S):2007 (abstr 4521)

Moore MJ, Goldstein D, Hamm J, et al: Erlotinib plus gemcitabine compared with gemcitabine alone in patients with advanced pancreaticcancer: a phase III trial of the National Cancer Institute of Canada Clinical Trials Group. J ClinOncol 25:1960–1966, 2007

Pacetti P, Giovannetti E, Reni M, et al: Association between DNA repair polymorphisms and survival in pancreatic cancer patients treated with combination chemotherapy. J Clin Oncol 28(15 Suppl):4098, 2010

Park DJ, Stoehlmacher J, Zhang W, et al: A Xeroderma pigmentosum group D gene polymorphism predicts clinical outcome to platinum-based chemotherapy in patients with advanced colorectal cancer. Cancer Res 61:8654–8, 2001

Parkin MD, Bray F, Ferlay J, et al: Global Cancer Statistics, 2002. CA Cancer J Clin 55:74 – 108, 2005

Plunkett W, Huang P, Xu YZ, et al: Gemcitabine: metabolism, mechanisms of action, and self potentiation. Semin Oncol 22:3–10, 1995

Pullarkat ST, Stoehlmacher J, Ghaderi V, et al: Thymidylate synthase gene polymorphism determines response and toxicity of 5-FU chemotherapy. Pharmacogenomics J 1:65–70, 2001

Raymond E, Faivre S, Woynarowski JM, et al: Oxaliplatin: mechanism of action and antineoplastic activity. Semin Oncol 25(2 suppl 5):4–12, 1998

Ridge S, Sludden J, Wei X, et al: Dihydropyrimidine dehydrogenase pharmacogenetics in patients with colorectal cancer. Br J Cancer 77:497, 1998

Robien K, Boynton A, Ulrich CM: Pharmacogenetics of folate related drug targets in cancer treatment. Pharmacogenomics; 6:673-689, 2005

Rudin CM, Liu W, Desai A, et al: Pharmacogenomic and pharmacokinetic determinants of erlotinib toxicity. J Clin Oncol 26:1119–1127, 2008

Ruzzo A, Graziano F, Loupakis F, et al: Pharmacogenetic profiling in patients with advanced colorectal cancer treated with first-line FOLFOX-4 chemotherapy. J Clin Oncol 25:1247–1254, 2007

Ryu JS: Genetic Effect of ERCC1 codon 118 polymorphism and confounding factors. Clin Cancer Res 12; 4784, 2006

Salonga D, Danenberg KD, Johnson M, et al: Colorectal tumors responding to 5-fluorouracil have low gene expression levels of dihydropyridine dehydrogenase, thymidylate synthase, and thymidine phosphorylase. Clin Cancer Res 6:1322–1327, 2000

Saltz LB, Lenz HJ, Kindler HL, et al: Randomized phase II trial of cetuximab, bevacizumab, and irinotecan compared with cetuximab and bevacizumab alone in irinotecan-refractory colorectal cancer: the BOND-2 study. J Clin Oncol, 25:4557-61, 2007. Epub 2007 Sep 17.

Sebastiani V, Ricci F, Rubio-Viqueira B, et al: Immunohistochemical and genetic evaluation of deoxycytidine kinase in pancreatic cancer: relationship to molecular mechanisms of gemcitabine resistance and survival. Clin Cancer Res 12:2492-2497, 2006

Shahrokni A, Rajebi MR, Harold L et al: Cardiotoxicity of 5-fluorouracil and capecitabine in pancreatic cancer patients with a novel mutation in the dihydropyrimidine dehydrogenase gene. JOP; 10:215-20, 2009

Spratlin J, Sangha R, Glubrecht D, et al: The absence of human equilibrative nucleoside transporter 1 is associated with reduced survival in patients with gemcitabine-treated pancreas adenocarcinoma. Clin Cancer Res 10:6956–6961, 2004

Stoehlmacher J, Park DJ, Zhang W, et al: A multivariate analysis of genomic polymorphisms: Prediction of clinical outcome to 5-fluorouracil/oxaliplatin combination chemotherapy in refractory colorectal cancer. Br J Cancer 91:344–354, 2004

Tukey RH, Strassburg CP, and Mackenzie PI: Pharmacogenomics of human UDP-Glucuronosyl transferases and irinotecan toxicity. Mol Pharmacol 62:446–450, 2002

Ueno H, Kiyosawa K, Kaniwa N: Pharmacogenomics of gemcitabine: can genetic studies lead to tailor-made therapy? Br J Cancer 97:145–151, 2007

Uetake H, Ichikawa W, Takechi T, et al: Relationship between intratumoral dihydropyrimidine dehydrogenase activity and gene expression in human colorectal cancer. Clin Cancer Res 5:2836–2839, 1999

van Erp NP, Eechoute K, van der Veldt AA, et al: Pharmacogenetic pathway analysis for determination of sunitinib-induced toxicity. Clin Oncol 27:4406-4412, 2009

Van Cutsem E, Lang I, D'haens G, et al: KRAS status and efficacy in the first-line treatment of patients with metastatic colorectal cancer (mCRC) treated with FOLFIRI with or without cetuximab: The CRYSTAL experience. J Clin Oncol 26 (15S) :5s, 2008 (abstr 2)

Vermorken JB, van der Vijgh WJF, Klein I, et al: Pharmacokinetics of free and total platinum species after short infusion of cisplatin. Cancer Treat Rep 68:505–513, 1984

Verslype C, Vervenne W, Bennouna J, et al: Rashas a marker for the efficacy of gemcitabine plus erlotinib-based therapy in pancreatic cancer: Results from the AViTA Study. Rash as a marker for the efficacy of gemcitabine plus erlotinib based therapy in pancreatic cancer: Results from the AViTA Study. J Clin Oncol 27(15S):2009 (abstr 4532)

Vesell ES: Pharmacogenetic perspectives gained from twin and family studies. Pharmacol Ther 41:535–552, 1989

Villafranca E, Okruzhnov Y, Dominguez MA, et al: Polymorphisms of the repeated sequencesin the enhancer region of the thymidylate synthase gene promoter may predict down staging after preoperative chemoradiation in rectal cancer. J Clin Oncol 19:1779–1786, 2001

Viguier J, Boige V, Miquel C, et al: ERCC1 codon118 polymorphism is a predictive factor for the tumor response to oxaliplatin/5-fluorouracil combination chemotherapy in patients with advanced colorectal cancer. Clin Cancer Res 11:6212–6217, 2005

Wasserman E, Myara A, Lokiec F et al: Severe CPT 11 toxicity in patients with Gilbert's syndrome: Two case reports. Ann Oncol 8:1049-1051, 1997

Wei X, Elizondo G, Sapone A, et al: Characterization of the human dihydropyrimidine dehydrogenase gene. Genomics 51:391–400, 1998.

Yalcin S: Increasing role of pharmacogenetics in gastrointestinal cancers. Gastrointest Cancer Res 3:197–203, 2009.

Yalcin S, Oksuzoglu B, Tekuzman G, et al: Biweekly irinotecan (CPT-11) plus bolus 5-fluourouracil (5-FU) and folinic acid in patients with advanced stage colorectal cancer (ACRC). Jpn J Clin Oncol 33:580–583, 2003

Yonemori K, Ueno H, Okusaka T, et al: Severe drug toxicity associated with a single-nucleotide polymorphism of the cytidine deaminase gene in a Japanese cancer patient treated with gemcitabine plus cisplatin. Clin Cancer Res 11:2620–2624, 2005

Yong WP, Innocenti F, Ratain MJ: The role of pharmacogenetics in cancer therapeutics. Br J Clin Pharmacol 62:35–46, 2006

Zhang W, Vallböhmer D, Yang D, et al: Genomic profile associated with clinical outcome of EGFR-expressing metastatic colorectal cancer patients treated with epidermal growth factor receptor (EGFR) inhibitor cetuximab. J Clin Oncol 23(16S):2005 (abstr 3557)

Zhang W, Yang D, Capanu M, et al: Pharmacogenomic analysis of a randomized phase II trial (BOND 2) of cetuximab/bevacizumab/irinotecan (CBI) versus cetuximab/bevacizumab (CB) in irinotecan-refractory colorectal cancer. J Clin Oncol 25(18S):2007 (abstr 4128)

Part 3

Pharmacogenetics in Cardiovascular Disease

6

Clinical Implications of Genetic Admixture in Hispanic Puerto Ricans: Impact on the Pharmacogenetics of *CYP2C19* and *PON1*

Jorge Duconge[1], Odalys Escalera[1], Mohan Korchela[2] and Gualberto Ruaño[2]
*[1]University of Puerto Rico School of Pharmacy, Medical Sciences Campus,
Pharmaceutical Sciences Department, San Juan,
[2]Genetic Research Center, Hartford Hospital, Hartford,
[1]Puerto Rico
[2]USA*

1. Introduction

Antiplatelet therapy with clopidogrel (Plavix®) is now considered a cornerstone of cardiovascular medicine. Clopidogrel resistance is an emerging clinical entity with potentially severe consequences such as recurrent myocardial infarction (MI), stroke, or death. Since its initial description, multiple investigators have confirmed the phenomenon of clopidogrel resistance (Dziewierz et al., 2005; Gurbel & Tantry, 2007; Mega et al., 2009; Mobley et al., 2004; Müller et al., 2003). The prevalence of clopidogrel non-responsiveness has been reported at 5–44% in other populations (Gurbel & Tantry, 2007). Although the occurrence of clopidogrel resistance is multi-factorial, it has been associated with a *CYP2C19*- and *PON1*-mediated[1] patient's metabolic inability to generate sufficient active metabolite to arrest platelet reactivity. Rapid and accurate detection of clopidogrel resistance in Hispanic Puerto Rican patients remain unsolved as new bedside genetic tests are developed.

In a recent GWAS analysis, it was estimated that up to 83% of individual variance in response to clopidogrel might be attributable to genetic effects (Shuldiner et al., 2009), but the gene variants investigated thus far explain only a minor proportion of such response variability (Holmes et al., 2010; Hulot et al., 2010). The high heritability of clopidogrel response but relatively weak prediction by existing proposed genetic markers argues for the involvement of some as yet undiscovered genetic factors. The *CYP2C19*2* allele was reported to account for only 12% of the variability in ADP-stimulated platelet response to clopidogrel (Shuldiner et al., 2009). The *PON1* Q192R polymorphism explained 72.5% of clopidogrel response variability in individuals of European ancestry (Bouman et al., 2011). However, a previous GWAS in a cohort of related healthy subjects of Amish descent provided no evidence for an association of the *PON1* gene region with the platelet response to clopidogrel (Shuldiner et al., 2009).

Due to its remarkable heterogeneity and trichotomous ancestral genetic admixture, the Puerto Rican population may significantly differ from other earlier pharmacogenetically

---

[1] *CYP2C19* stands for Cytochrome P450 isoform 2C19 (family 2, subfamily C, polypeptide 19) gene; *PON1* stands for Paraoxonase 1 gene.

characterized populations with respect to the frequency, distribution and combination of allelic variants in genes associated with drug response and diseases (González-Burchard et al., 2005; Suarez-Kurtz et al., 2006). We have published a physiogenomic analysis to infer structure and ancestry in the Puerto Rican population. The Puerto Rican sample was found to be broadly heterogeneous, with three main clusters reflecting the historical admixture from Taino Amerindians, West-Africans, and Iberian European ancestors (Ruaño et al., 2009). Our results matched previously published estimations of Puerto Rican admixture that were ascertained using more traditional ancestral genetic markers (Bertoni et al., 2003; Bonilla et al., 2004a, 2004b; Choudhry et al., 2006; Hammer et al., 2006; Hanis et al., 1991; Martinez-Cruzado et al., 2001, 2005). The study provided a set of 384 physiologically informative SNPs from 222 cardio-metabolic and neuro-endocrine genes that can be used to facilitate the translation of genome diversity into personalized medicine and control for admixture in Puerto Ricans. The observed large variance in admixture proportions suggested that this population is ideal for admixture matching studies.

Admixture is of great relevance to the clinical application of pharmacogenetics and personalized medicine, but unfortunately these studies have been scarce. As physiogenomic-guided multi-gene models are developed to predict drug response, the range of possible allelic combinations in the Puerto Rican population is certain to exceed that in populations without admixture. In addition, the allele frequencies for both the CYP2C19 and PON1 candidate genes in this population have not been fully characterized. Accordingly, we investigated whether a correlation between overall genetic similarity and CYP2C19 and PON1 genotypes could be established in the study population. This chapter also provides valuable evidence on the importance of controlling for admixture in pharmacogenetic studies of admixed populations like Puerto Ricans. Indeed, we will discuss how known or cryptic population stratification can have a strong confounding effect on further clinical association analysis. Finally, the necessity to utilize results of our admixture analysis to parameterize population structure appropriately and account for it as a covariate in the corresponding association studies will also be considered.

2. Methods

2.1 Specimens

100 human genomic DNA samples (40-60 ng/μL) were extracted and purified from existing dried blood spots on Guthrie cards supplied by the Puerto Rico Newborn Screening Program (PRNSP), where >95% of Puerto Rican newborns are screened for common hereditary diseases. Accordingly, sample analysis in this survey (*protocol #A4070107*) was exempt from IRB review under FDA and OHRP guidelines based on category 4, 45CFR46.118. A controlled stratified-by-region random sampling protocol was followed, taking into consideration the percentage of birth at each region across the Island of Puerto Rican based on the 2004 national register of total births. Two samples were discarded from final analysis due to poor quality.

2.2 Array

The extracted genomic DNA samples were genotyped on a physiogenomic (PG) array detecting 384 SNPs from 222 cardio-metabolic and neuro-endocrine genes spanning their entire genome (Ruaño et al., 2005a; Ruaño & Windemuth, 2006). Since the PG-array was constructed such that it covers all common variations in the general population for pharmacologically relevant cardio-metabolic pathways, virtually any set of candidate genes within these pathways can be tested from the resulting dataset without any further assay. Consequently, genotypes associated with the clinically relevant CYP2C19*2 (rs4244285; splicing defect G681A SNP) and nonsynonymous PON1 (rs662; p.Q192R) polymorphisms were loaded from the derived database. Instead, array translation was used to impute genotyping related to CYP2C19*3 (rs4986893; stop codon G636A SNP) with high accuracy, given its strong linkage disequilibrium with SNP rs3758581. Wild-types were assigned as a result of the absence of such SNPs. The PG array has been tested on nearly 5,000 patients and has been successfully applied in cardiovascular and neuropsychiatric pharmacogenetic research, resulting in ten publications (de Leon et al., 2008; Liu et al., 2009; Ruaño et al., 2005b, 2007a, 2007b, 2008, 2009, 2010; Seip et al., 2008; Windemuth et al., 2008). Careful manual analysis was performed on the alignments underlying the genotype calls using GenCall 6.1.3.24 and 50 SNPs with even a slight degree of uncertainty about calling accuracy were not included in the analysis, leaving 332 SNPs from 196 genes. Genotyping was accomplished using Illumina® BeadArray™ technology (Oliphant et al., 2002).

2.3 Clustering and statistical analysis

Analysis of the results using the STRUCTURE v2.2 software package was used to cluster those subjects with similar genetic profiles (Falush et al., 2007; Pritchard et al., 2000). Hierarchical clustering algorithm was blind as to ethno-geographic ancestry. A detailed explanation of the analytics underlying the clustering of the samples and the hierarchical stratification by allelic dissimilarities to infer population structure, as well as a full list of the genes and SNPs in the PG array, is provided elsewhere in our physiogenomic analysis study (Ruaño et al., 2009). Allele frequencies, f, linkage disequilibrium (LD), and haplotype structure were individually determined for all loci. Wright's F-statistic was calculated for each locus from the observed total heterozygosity $H_T=N_{hz}/N$ and the subpopulation heterozygosity $H_S=2f \cdot (1-f)$, assumed under Hardy-Weinberg equilibrium (HWE), as $F_{ST}=(H_T-H_S)/H_T$. A t-test was performed to see whether the average Fst across all loci is different from zero. Departure from HWE were estimated under the null hypothesis of the predictable segregation ratio of specific matching genotypes (p>0.05) by use of χ^2 goodness-of-fit test with one degree of freedom. In addition, χ^2 test was also used to compare observed allele frequencies within each sector in the corresponding dendrogram with expected frequencies given the overall allelic ratios, at 5% of significance.

3. Results

Results are presented in **Table 1**, and graphically in **Figure 1** by hierarchical dendrograms to illustrate the population structure as represented by allelic dissimilarity (i.e., genetic distance). There appear to be three main sectors, from left to right: PR126–PR341; PR321–PR69 and PR97–PR175. There are also two smaller sectors between the three main sectors. One pair of samples (PR26 and PR92) shows an unusually low allelic dissimilarity, suggesting relatedness. However, due to anonymousness of collected samples, we were unable to further investigate this issue. Those individuals who shared many polymorphisms were grouped together in one "sector" while those with whom they had much more genetic dissimilarities lie on the other side of the "phylogenetic tree' map; thus greater distances denoting lesser degrees of common ancestry.

Gene	SNP	Ch	Location	Nᵃ	Allelesᵇ	MAF (%)	Genotypes			Fst
							WT	HET	MUT	
CYP2C19	rs4244285 (CYP2C19*2)	10	96541616	98	G A	14.8	52	17	2	0.042
CYP2C19	rs3758581 (CYP2C19*3)	10	96602623	95	G A	3.5	66	5	0	0.017
PON1	rs662	7	94937446	96	A G (T/C)	45.1	22	34	15	0.174

Table 1. Genes, allele and genotype frequency distributions of clopidogrel-associated polymorphisms in the representative sample of Puerto Ricans analyzed by PG-array. Ch column display the chromosome on which the SNP can be found. Location column contains the chromosome location for each SNP given by the NCBI Entrez SNP database, build 36.3 reference assembly. MAF stands for minor allele frequency. ᵃTotal number of samples analyzed by PG-array ranged between 95 to 98. However, only 71 samples were used for STRUCTURE clustering analysis due to incomplete combinatorial genotyping data. Only those samples having a strong association with one of the three clusters were finally included in the superimposition analysis. ᵇAncestral allele in bold. First allele is the reference one.

To determine if there are relationships between genetic clusters defined by STRUCTURE analysis and clopidogrel-related genotypes, we superimposed the individual genotypes for CYP2C19 and PON1 on the dendrogram. **Figures 1**, panel A and B, show less than 98 cases (i.e., some lanes in the genetic distance map do not have identified ancestry) due to incomplete combinatorial genotyping data during the initial PG array analysis or because the individual residing in the site did not meet a categorical criterion of proximity (> 0.20), which precluded definitive assignment to any of the three STRUCTURE clusters (ancestry). Furthermore, only those samples having a strong association with one of the three clusters were included in the superimposition analysis, yielding 71 total subjects. Notice that only 52 out of these 71 analyzed cases were actually located within any of the three identified sectors in the genetic distance dendrograms seen in **Figures 1**. The other 19 cases, although located outside the sectors, were also included in the analysis because they all had a significant contribution from one of three ancestries (i.e., Taino Amerindians, Iberian Caucasians or West-Africans), as denoted by their ancestral coefficients. To this purpose, each of these 19 individual was allocated to the sector that best matched with his/her greater ancestral coefficient. The distribution of samples by sectors in the corresponding genetic distance dendrograms was then as follows: 20 samples in sector 1; 27 in sector 2 and 24 in sector 3.

Clinical Implications of Genetic Admixture
in Hispanic Puerto Ricans: Impact on the Pharmacogenetics of CYP2C19 and PON1

125

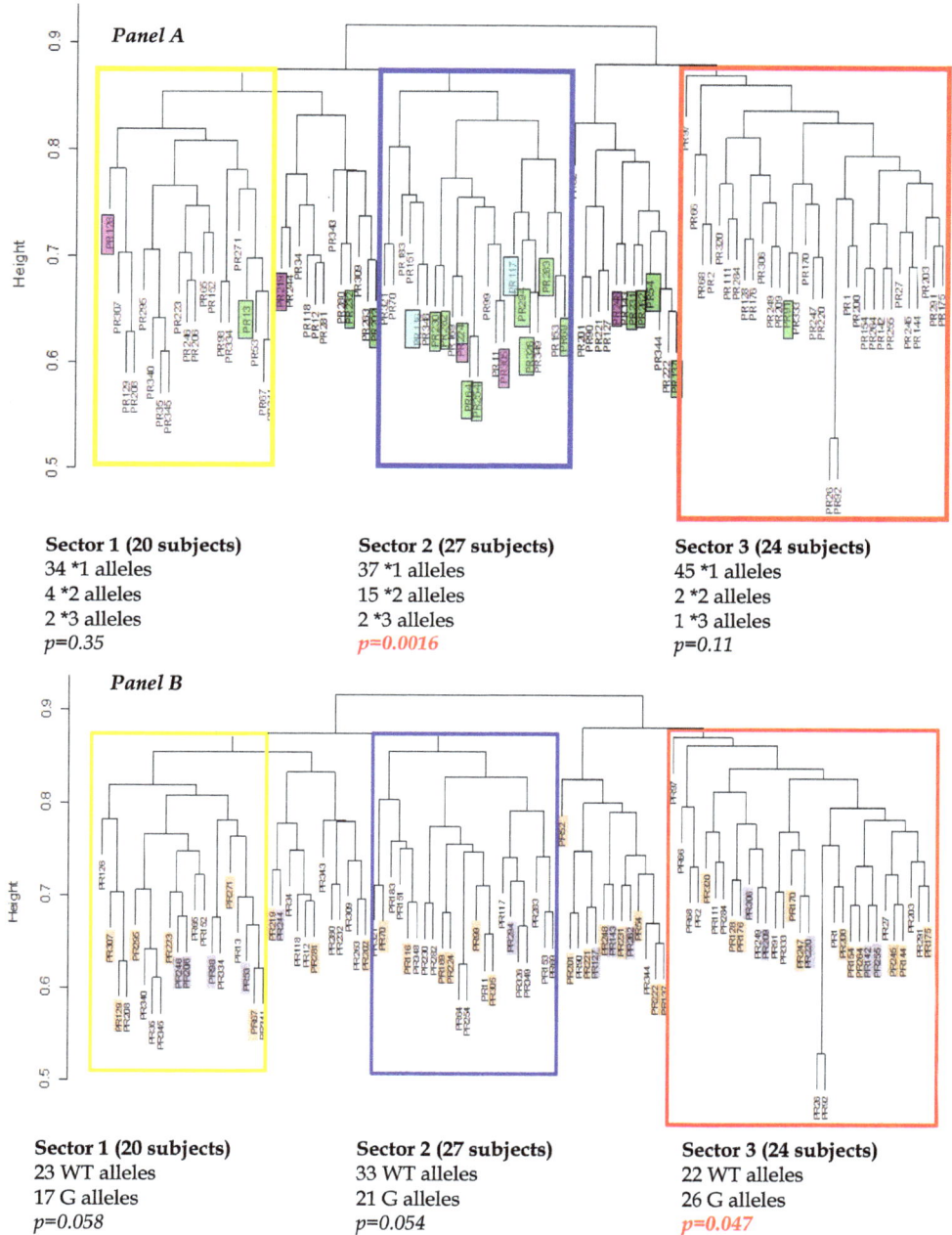

Sector 1 (20 subjects)
34 *1 alleles
4 *2 alleles
2 *3 alleles
p=0.35

Sector 2 (27 subjects)
37 *1 alleles
15 *2 alleles
2 *3 alleles
p=0.0016

Sector 3 (24 subjects)
45 *1 alleles
2 *2 alleles
1 *3 alleles
p=0.11

Sector 1 (20 subjects)
23 WT alleles
17 G alleles
p=0.058

Sector 2 (27 subjects)
33 WT alleles
21 G alleles
p=0.054

Sector 3 (24 subjects)
22 WT alleles
26 G alleles
p=0.047

Fig. 1. **Panel A**. Individual CYP2C19*2 and *3 genotypes overlaid on the genetic distance dendrogram for the samples from the Puerto Rican population (dendrogram taken from previously published physiogenomic population analysis [21]). Green boxes are depicting those individuals having a single *CYP2C19**2 polymorphism (G/A); Blue-colored boxes represent double carriers for *CYP2C19**2 (A/A); whereas, purple-colored rectangles indicate single carriers of *CYP2C19**3 (A/G). Double-colored rectangle (subject PR224) highlights the one having the *2/*3 genotype. The *CYP2C19**3 G→A polymorphism is in high linkage disequilibrium with *rs3758581*, which has been associated with a significant decrease in clopidogrel activation per allele and, therefore, resistance phenotype (non-responder) to standard dose. **Panel B**: Individual *PON1* Q192R genotypes overlaid on the genetic distance dendrogram for the samples from the Puerto Rican population. Yellow color represents single carriers; purple color denotes double carriers of this polymorphism (G allele). *p*-values were calculated by a $\chi 2$ test comparing observed allele frequencies with expected frequencies given the overall allelic ratios.

By previous STRUCTURE clustering analyses, the dendrogram sectors 1, 2 and 3 in **Figure 1** correspond to Taino Amerindian, Iberian Caucasian, and West-African heritage, respectively (Ruaño et al., 2009). Indeed, sector 1 bears a concentration of samples assigned to cluster 2 (Amerindians) in the STRUCTURE plot. Sector 2, in the middle, is disproportionately rich in samples corresponding to cluster 3 (Europeans). Sector 3, to the right, is clearly enriched with cluster 1 samples (Africans). For the 71 cases with complete genotypes, the *CYP2C19**2 allele frequency was 14.8%, whereas the *3 allele frequency was 3.5%. Although slightly higher, these findings are consistent with early reports in 22 Latin Americans (Mexicans and Puerto Ricans) from the 1,000 Genomes Phase I selection, where the *CYP2C19**2 and *3 minor allele frequencies were 13.6% and 1.7%, respectively. Regarding to *CYP2C19**2 polymorphism, we identified 52 homozygous for the wild-type allele G, 17 heterozygous and 2 double carriers of the variant allele A. However, the analysis for *CYP2C19**3 revealed 66 wild-types, 5 single carriers of the variant allele, but none double carrier of this polymorphism in the study population. Sectors 1 and 3 in Figure 1, panel A, show *CYP2C19**2 allele frequencies of 10% (4 out of 40) and 4.16% (2 out of 48), respectively, as compared to 27.8% (15 out of 54) in sector 2. Statistical analyses to compare each sector to the overall allelic ratios, revealed that sector 2 (in the middle of the genetic distance dendrogram, **Figure 1**-panel A), showed a frequency of *CYP2C19**2 that was 4-fold higher than the rest of the population (*p*=0.0016). Likewise, carrier prevalence in sector 2 (48.15%) was significantly greater than that observed in the other two sectors (i.e., 20 and 8.3%, respectively).

Sector 2 is associated with Iberian European heritage (Ruaño et al., 2009). According to the HapMap project dataset (International HapMap Consortium, 2005), the minor allele frequency for *CYP2C19**2 is 14.3% in 223 Caucasians who are Utah residents with Northern and Western European ancestry from the CEPH collection (HapMap-CEU; data release#28, Phase II + III). Similarly, the *CYP2C19**2 allele frequency was 13% for 261 Europeans in the 1,000 Genomes Phase I selection (Amigo et al., 2008). The present study reports a relatively inflated minor allele frequency of 27.8% for the *CYP2C19**2 variant in sector 2 (primarily Caucasian), consistent with the possible interpretation that Puerto Ricans in this sector reflect an increased admixture with Asians (i.e., Taino Amerindians). The link between Amerindians and Asians originates with the "Bering Strait" theory (Jennings, 1979). According to previous reports, there seems to be a very high frequency for the *CYP2C19**2 variant in East Asian populations, ranging from 27-32.5% (Amigo et al., 2008).

Likewise, the observed minor allele frequency of 4.16% in sector 3 is lower than expected for a population of purely African ethno-geographic origin, no surprise given the heterogeneity of the Puerto Rican population. The reported *CYP2C19*3* allele frequencies of 5% for sector 1, 3.7% for sector 2 and 2.1% for sector 3 compare to the expected HapMap values of 5.6%, 1.7% and 0.3%, respectively. The higher than expected frequencies observed in sector 2 and 3 seem to be a direct consequence of significant admixture with Asian ancestry in individuals assigned to these clusters. Interestingly, the NCBI webpage reports a *CYP2C19*3* minor allele frequency of 2.1% in 24 individuals of self-described African-American heritage (AFR1, SNP500Cancer project, this database is an integral component of the NCI Cancer Genome Anatomy Project, available at http://cgap.nci.nih.gov), which is a population with certain genetic admixture (Packer et al., 2006). This value matched the observed allele frequency in sector 3, a cluster of majorly African ancestry.

With respect to the *PON1* gene (**Table 1**), the overall allele frequency was 45.1% (34 heterozygous and 15 homozygous for the variant allele), which is stratified by clusters as 42.5%, 38.9% and 54.2% in sectors 1, 2 and 3, respectively (**Figure 1**-Panel B). The observed prevalence for this variant is consistent with early reports in both 22 Latin America inhabitants (Mexicans and Puerto Ricans; 1,000 Genomes Phase I selection) and 58 Mexican descendants who reside in Los Angeles, California (HapMap-MEX; HapMap project dataset, release#28, Phase II + III), where the *PON1* minor allele frequencies were estimated to be 47.7% and 50%, respectively. The minor allele frequency in the general population ranges from 42.2 to 47.9%. However, when comparing observed allele frequencies in each of the three sectors (i.e., 1=Amerindian; 2=Caucasian; 3=West African) with the HapMap and 1,000 Genomes Phase I project values, the results are showing a significantly higher than expected prevalence of this *PON1* polymorphism. In sector 1, there was a minor allele frequency of 42.5% as compared with the HapMap report of about 36% for the Han Chinese of Beijing (International HapMap Consortium, 2005) and the 36.2% in East Asians from 1,000 Genomes Phase I selection (Amigo et al., 2008).

Furthermore, the allele frequency in sector 2 was 38.9% (13 heterozygous and 4 double carriers), considerably higher than the reported 29% for Caucasian residents of Utah, documented in the HapMap database (International HapMap Consortium, 2005), and the 28.4% presented by the 1,000 Genomes Phase I selection for Europeans (Amigo et al., 2008). Additionally, in sector 3 the allele frequency was 54.2% (12 heterozygous and 7 double carriers), which is by far a higher prevalence versus the HapMap allele frequency of 27.9% for the Nigerian YRI population or the 23.4% in Africans of the 1,000 Genomes Phase I selection (Amigo et al., 2008; International HapMap Consortium, 2005). Statistical analyses to compare each sector to the overall allelic ratios, revealed that sector 3 (right-most portion of the genetic distance dendrogram, **Figure 1**-panel B), showed a frequency of *PON1* Q192R that was only marginally different than the rest of the population (*p*=0.047).

Greater admixture and heterogeneity in the Puerto Rican population as compared to the African-American population or certainly the Yoruba population allow for the presence of the twenty-six *PON1* variant allele observed in the twenty-four individuals in sector 3 (**Figure 1**-Panel B) to have come from partial Amerindian ancestry, as no individual in that sector was of purely West-African descent (Ruaño et al., 2009). The observed trends may also be an artifact of chance given the relatively small sample size. No statistically significant deviations from HWE were found with respect to the distribution frequencies of either *PON1* or *CYP2C19* polymorphisms. Since no departures from HWE were observed and considering that our study cohort is island-wide, chosen by a controlled, stratified-by-region, representative sampling from the Puerto Rican population, we can expect the observed frequencies of the *PON1* and *CYP2C19* polymorphisms to be representative for the rest of this population.

4. Discussion

In this work, we examined two clinically relevant *CYP2C19* gene polymorphisms (i.e., *CYP2C19*2* and *CYP2C19*3*) and the emerging *PON1* variant in a representative sample of the Puerto Rican population. Our findings suggest a significant burden of loss-of-function *CYP2C19* and *PON1* carriers within the Puerto Rican population. Based on observed prevalence of functional *CYP2C19* and *PON1* polymorphisms in Puerto Ricans, and the postulated role of the enzymes encoded by these genes in the clopidogrel activation (Bouman et al., 2011; Mega et al., 2009; Shuldiner et al., 2009), we hypothesized that about 30-40% of Puerto Ricans may be non-responders to clopidogrel and such resistant patients may be at particular risk for short-term thrombo-ischemic complications including periprocedural infarction and early stent thrombosis.

Because thromboembolism is a major risk of cardiovascular disease, genotyping for clopidogrel's response-associated gene *CYP2C19*, and *PON1* to a lesser extent, have been advanced as desirable in Caucasians to improve patient's clinical outcomes (Bouman et al., 2011; Holmes et al., 2010; Hulot et al., 2010; Mega et al., 2009; Shuldiner et al., 2009). However, heterogeneity and admixture may preclude their full application in other populations such as Puerto Ricans. Accordingly, there is an urgent need for ascertaining admixture adjustments that may prove clinically useful in Puerto Ricans and other Hispanic groups. Indeed, the richer genetic variation in Puerto Ricans is likely to contribute substantially to a wider variation in response to clopidogrel treatment, a component that will be missed by traditional studies in homogeneous populations. This addressable oversight is of great concern, since it will tend to exacerbate the healthcare disparity already experienced by Hispanics in USA.

The population of the Americas carries a genomic legacy resulting from the continents' native inhabitants, European colonization and African slavery. In those parts of the Americas where admixture took hold, the populations manifest the combined anthropological heritage in their genomes, lifestyle, diet, and even socioeconomic status. Admixture is of great relevance to the clinical application of the pharmacogenetic-guided personalized medicine paradigm, but unfortunately these studies have been scarce in Puerto Ricans. We have performed pivotal physiogenomic studies on the Puerto Rican population by using an array of 384 SNPs in 222 cardio-metabolic and neuro-endocrine genes coding for relevant pharmaceutical targets. According to our findings, the Puerto Rican population represents different admixtures of 3 major ethno-geographic groups (i.e., Taino-Amerindians, Iberian-Europeans and West-Africans). Notably, each subject in the study population was a 'genetic mosaic', with contributions from each of these three clusters, but in widely different proportions.

Consequently, admixture in the Puerto Rican population exists in the form of a continuous gradient with varying levels of mixture that results in a rich repertoire of combinatorial genotypes for key pharmacological pathways such as the one associated with CYP2C9 and PON1 activity in humans. This phenomenon may explain discrepancies between observed and expected genotype and allele frequencies across the three sectors in the genetic distance dendrograms (**Figure 1**-panel A and B), particularly with respect to other homogeneous (parental) populations previously characterized through the HapMap, SNP500Cancer and 1,000 Genomes projects. Moreover, the diversity observed in the genetic structure within African populations from varying regions of this continent (Tishkoff et al., 2009) may also contribute to explain the higher than expected prevalence of *PON1* variant allele at sector 3 (**Figure 1**-panel B) in our study population, which is an Afro-Caribbean population, as compared to continental Africans like Yoruba from Nigeria (HapMap-YRI). Overall, our findings further substantiate the argument for including admixture as a critical covariant in predicting clopidogrel response within heterogeneous populations, but also render the Puerto Rican population a good resource to develop DNA-guided systems for clinical management of thromboembolic disorders, an urgent medical need not only in Hispanics but also in the population at large.

Recently, we provided valuable evidence on the importance of controlling for admixture when conducting pharmacogenetic studies of warfarin (Coumadin®) in the Puerto Rican population and stressed the argument for incorporating admixture-matching in order to probe variations in warfarin response across different stratum within the population (Villagra et al., 2010). In this study we postulated that interindividual variations in ancestral contributions of Puerto Ricans may help explain the observed poor performance and low predictability of DNA-guided warfarin dosing algorithms derived in other populations. Admixture introduces distinct levels of population sub-structure or stratum, with marked variations in individual ancestry among the members of a particular population or ethnic group, depending on the dynamics of the process. Accordingly, any extrapolations of clinically relevant pharmacogenetic data from non-admixed to admixed groups will be plagued with uncertainty as exemplified by Suarez-Kurtz (Suarez-Kurtz, 2005). Consequently, the predictive power of previously published DNA-guided algorithms for admixed populations like Puerto Ricans is expected to be inaccurate, if not inadequate.

A previous study by Perini and co-workers (Perini et al., 2008) stated that self-reported race, using labels defined by skin color as a proxy for ethnicity, was not a reliable indicator of effective anticoagulation therapy in admixed Brazilians. What proved useful, instead, was a precise knowledge of individual ancestral proportions so as to place the patient on a continuum between "black" and "white". The utility of this model was verified later on a separate cohort in the same population (Vargens et al., 2008). To control for possible marginal effects of ancestry on drug response, investigators of the GALA and SAGE projects included genetic ancestry as an independent variable in the regression model used to test association between *IL6R* SNPs and bronchodilator effect. Interestingly, the mean bronchodilator response for the pharmacogenetic interaction increased with increasing amounts of Native American ancestry; whereas, the drug response among asthmatic patients for the same pharmacogenetic interaction decreased with increasing amounts of European ancestry (Corvol et al., 2009). Differences observed among Mexican, Puerto Ricans and African-Americans were thus explained by the different proportions of Native American and European ancestries in these three ethnically diverse populations. Recently, Bryc and co-workers found evidence of a significant sex bias in admixture proportions of Hispanics that is consistent with disproportionate contribution of European male and Amerindian or African female ancestry to present populations (Bryc et al., 2010). These authors also suggested that future genome-wide association studies in Hispanics will require correction for local genomic ancestry at a sub-continental scale.

Population stratification by admixture is a well-known confounder in pharmacogenetic association studies of candidate gene to complex traits, including drug response (e.g., clopidogrel). In this context, it might be difficult to find a matching control for an individual with diverse ethnic origins; therefore, we will be forced to rely on multivariate adjustment models. That is, rather than allocate the subject to a single stratum in the analysis, we recommend to construct a covariate for each stratum, giving the corresponding ancestral proportion derived from our admixture-driven clustering analysis, and then include these covariates as adjustment factors in a multiple regression model for clopidogrel association studies in Puerto Ricans. In doing so, we will be able to parameterize admixture-derived population structure appropriately and account for it as a covariate in the corresponding association studies in order to minimize the effect of population stratification.

We call these covariates "admixture indexes", which we believe are indispensable to assure that pharmacogenetic research can be pursued in Hispanic populations. From a key methodological perspective, the wider genetic variation found in our population for these markers broaden the reach and enhance the statistical sensitivity of tests for the effects of that variation on clopidogrel response. At the same time, the admixture index could become indispensable for the globalization of patho- and pharmacogenetic research beyond the Americas, to Africa, Asia and Europe, the continents whose populations contributed to the admixture in the first place.

In the context of admixture matching, if a resistant allele is more common in one of the ancestral populations, then non-responders to clopidogrel will share a greater level of ancestry from that population around the locus as compared with responders. In future studies, we expect to generate a detailed admixture map in the Puerto Rican population at very high resolution using all 1.2 million SNPs from a total genome (TG) array. Admixture studies at this resolution afford delineation of candidate genes for pharmacogenetic traits related not only to clopidogrel, but also to other drugs commonly used to treat cardiovascular conditions of high prevalence in Hispanics.

A major advance in healthcare would be a transition from the current empirical approaches in drug therapy to a genetically predictive framework for determining the individual patient's response to medicines. Accordingly, an understanding of how human genetic diversity and admixture in Hispanics is structured is not only of anthropological importance, but also of medical relevance. In addition, it is important to recognize that some minority groups in the U.S. (e.g., Hispanics) might be underrepresented in typical clinical pharmacogenetic trials with respect to the real impact of these groups on the current U.S. population. Because of the heterogeneity and extensive admixture of the Puerto Rican population, extrapolation on a global scale of data derived from well-defined ethnic groups (i.e., Caucasians) is clearly not applicable to the majority of Puerto Ricans.

5. Conclusion

In conclusion, we have established clinical correlations between overall genetic similarities and both CYP2C19 and PON1 genotypes in a representative sample of the Puerto Rican population. To this purpose, the major CYP2C19 and PON1 polymorphisms were interrogated in 98 genomic DNA specimens using the physiogenomic (PG)-array that also inferred population structure and admixture pattern. Individual *CYP2C19* and *PON1* genotypes were visually overlaid atop three major sectors of a genetic distance dendrogram that was constructed by clustering subjects with similar genetic profiles. Results suggest that the observed inter-individual variations in ancestral contributions will have significant implications for the way each Puerto Rican responds to antiplatelet therapy with clopidogrel. Our findings also provided valuable evidence on the importance of parameterizes the population structure in order to account for admixture as a covariate in pharmacogenetic association studies for clopidogrel in Hispanic Puerto Ricans.

Rather than ignoring admixture, pharmacogeneticists should consider it as starting point for better understanding the underlying basis of the observed wider variability in drug responses among patients of mixed populations. Such understanding provides the opportunity to develop strategies for leapfrogging the healthcare standards in these populations.

6. Acknowledgement

This investigation was supported, in part, by a Research Centers in Minority Institution Award G12RR-03051 from the National Center for Research Resources, NIH and by the Puerto Rico Newborn Screening Program and Genomas internal research and development funds. The authors want to thank Dr. Pedro J Santiago-Borrero for kindly supplying the samples for this work; MSc. Jessicca Y Renta, Mrs. Yolanda Rodriguez, Dr. Carmen L Cadilla, Dr. Andrea Windemuth, Mr. David Villagra and Mrs. Krystyna Gorowski for their support in collecting and processing the samples.

7. Statement

A glossary of genetic terminology is maintained by the National Human Genome Research Institute at www.genome.gov/glossary.cfm.

8. Keywords

Admixture; Puerto Ricans; Pharmacogenetics; Clopidogrel; *CYP2C19*; *PON1*

9. Disclosure

Dr Ruaño is founder and President of Genomas, Inc. Mr. Kocherla is full-time employee of Genomas, Inc. The rest of the authors have no potential conflicts of interest to disclose.

10. References

Amigo, J., Salas, A., Phillips, C., & Carracedo, A. (2008). SPSmart: adapting population based SNP genotype databases for fast and comprehensive web access. *BMC Bioinformatics*, 9, pp. 428

Bertoni, B., Budowle, B., Sans, M., Barton, S.A., & Chakraborty, R. (2003). Admixture in Hispanics: distribution of ancestral population contributions in the Continental United States. *Hum Biol*, 75, pp. 1-11

Bonilla, C., Parra, E.J., Pfaff, C.L., et al. (2004a). Admixture in the Hispanics of the San Luis Valley, Colorado, and its implications for complex trait gene mapping. *Ann Hum Genet*, 68, pp. 139-53

Bonilla, C., Shriver, M.D., Parra, E.J., Jones, A., & Fernandez, J.R. (2004b). Ancestral proportions and their association with skin pigmentation and bone mineral density in Puerto Rican women from New York City. *Hum Genet*, 115, pp. 57-68

Bouman, H.J., Schömig, E., van Werkum, J.W., Velder, J., Hackeng, C.M., Hirschhäuser, C., Waldmann, C., Schmalz, H.G., ten Berg, J.M., & Taubert, D. (2011). Paraoxonase-1 is a major determinant of clopidogrel efficacy. *Nature Med*, 17, pp. 110-6

Bryc, K., Velez, C., Karafet, T., Moreno-Estrada, A., Reynolds, A., et al. (2010). Colloquium paper: genome-wide patterns of population structure and admixture among Hispanic/Latino populations. *Proc Natl Acad Sci USA*, 107, pp. 8954-8961

Choudhry, S., Coyle, N.E., Tang, H., et al. (2006). Population stratification confounds genetic association studies among Latinos. *Hum Genet*, 118, pp. 652-64

Corvol, H., De Giacomo, A., Eng, C., Seibold, M., Ziv, E., et al. (2009). Genetic ancestry modifies pharmacogenetic gene-gene interaction for asthma. *Pharmacogenet Genomics*, 19, pp. 489-496

de Leon, J., Correa, J.C., Ruaño, G., Windemuth, A., Arranz, M.J., & Díaz, F.J. (2008). Exploring genetic variations that may be associated with the direct effects of some antipsychotics on lipid levels. *Schizophr Res*, 98, pp. 40-6

Dziewierz, A., Dudek, D., Heba, G., Rakowski, T., Mielecki, W., & Dubiel, J.S. (2005). Inter-individual variability in response to clopidogrel in patients with coronary artery disease. *Kardiol Pol*, 62, pp. 108-17

Falush D, Stephens M, Pritchard JK. Inference of population structure using multilocus genotype data: dominant markers and null alleles. Mol Ecol Notes 2007;7:574-8

González-Burchard, E., Borrell, L.N., Choudhry, S., Naqvi, M., Tsai, H.J., Rodriguez-Santana, J.R., Chapela, R., Rogers, S.D., Mei, R., Rodriguez-Cintron, W., Arena, J.F., Kittles, R., Perez-Stable, E.J., Ziv, E., & Risch, N. (2005). Latino populations: a unique opportunity for the study of race, genetics, and social environment in epidemiological research. *Am J Public Health*, 95, pp. 2161-8

Gurbel, P.A., & Tantry, (2007). U.S. Clopidogrel resistance? *Thromb Res*, 120, pp. 311-321

Hammer, M.F., Chamberlain, V.F., Kearney, V.F., et al. (2006). Population structure of Y chromosome SNP haplogroups in the United States and forensic implications for constructing Y chromosome STR databases. *Forensic Sci Int*, 164, pp. 45-55

Hanis, C.L., Hewett-Emmett, D., Bertin, T.K., & Schull, W.J. (1991). Origins of U.S. Hispanics. Implications for diabetes. *Diabetes Care*, 14, pp. 618-27

Holmes, D.R. Jr., Dehmer, G.J., Kaul, S., Leifer, D., O'Gara, P.T., & Stein, C.M, (2010). Society for Cardiovascular Angiography and Interventions; Society of Thoracic Surgeons; Writing Committee Members. ACCF/AHA clopidogrel clinical alert: approaches to the FDA "boxed warning": a report of the American College of Cardiology Foundation Task Force on Clinical Expert Consensus Documents and the American Heart Association. *Circulation*, 122, pp. 537–557

Hulot, J.S., Collet, J.P., Silvain, J., Pena, A., Bellemain-Appaix, A., Barthélémy, O., Cayla, G., Beygui, F., & Montalescot, G. (2010). Cardiovascular risk in clopidogrel-treated patients according to cytochrome P450 2C19*2 loss-of-function allele or proton pump inhibitor co-administration: a systematic meta-analysis. *J Am Coll Cardiol*, 56, pp. 134–143

Jennings, J. (1979). Across an arctic bridge. In: *The World of the American Indian*. Billard J, editor, National Geographic Society, Washington, DC

Liu, J., Pearlson, G., Windemuth, A., Ruaño, G., Perrone-Bizzozero, N.I., & Calhoun, V. (2009). Combining fMRI and SNP data to investigate connections between brain function and genetics using parallel ICA. *Hum Brain Mapp*, 30, pp. 241-55

Martinez-Cruzado, J.C., Toro-Labrador, G., Ho-Fung, V., et al. (2001). Mitochondrial DNA analysis reveals substantial Native American ancestry in Puerto Rico. *Hum Biol*, 73, pp. 491-511

Martinez-Cruzado, J.C., Toro-Labrador, G., Viera-Vera, J., et al. (2005). Reconstructing the population history of Puerto Rico by means of mtDNA phylogeographic analysis. *Am J Phys Anthropol*, 128, pp. 131-55

Mega, J.L., Close, S.L., Wiviott, S.D., et al. (2009). Cytochrome P-450 polymorphisms and response to clopidogrel. *N Engl J Med*, 360, pp. 354-362

Mobley, J.E., Bresee, S.J., Wortham, D.C., Craft, R.M., Snider, C.C., & Carroll, R.C. (2004). Frequency of non-response antiplatelet activity of clopidogrel during pretreatment for cardiac catheterization. *Am J Cardiol*, 93, pp. 456-8

Müller, I., Besta, F., Schulz, C., Massberg, S., Schönig, A., & Gawaz, M. (2003). Prevalence of clopidogrel non-responders among patients with stable angina pectoris scheduled for elective coronary stent placement. *Thromb Haemost*, 89, pp.783–7

Oliphant, A., Barker, D.L., Stuelpnagel, J.R., & Chee, M.S. (2002). BeadArray technology: enabling an accurate, cost-effective approach to high-throughput genotyping. *Biotechniques*, 56, pp. 60-1

Packer, B.R., Yeager, M., Burdett, L., Welch, R., Beerman, M., Qi, L., Sicotte, H., Staats, B., Acharya, M., Crenshaw, A., Eckert, A., Puri, V., Gerhard, D.S., & Chanock, S.J. (2006). SNP500Cancer: a public resource for sequence validation, assay development, and frequency analysis for genetic variation in candidate genes. *Nucleic Acids Res*, 34(Database issue), pp. D617-21

Perini, J.A., Struchiner, C.J., Silva-Assuncao, E., et al. (2008). Pharmacogenetics of warfarin: development of a dosing algorithm for Brazilian patients. *Clin Pharmacol Ther*, 84, pp. 722–8

Pritchard, J.K., Stephens, M., & Donnelly, P. (2000). Inference of population structure using multilocus genotype data. *Genetics*, 155, pp. 945-59

Ruaño, G., Windemuth, A., & Holford, T. (2005a). Physiogenomics: Integrating Systems Engineering and Nanotechnology for Personalized Medicine, In: *The Biomedical Engineering Handbook*, J. Bronzino, ed., pp. 281-289, CRC Press

Ruaño G, Thompson PD, Windemuth A, et al. (2005b). Physiogenomic analysis links serum creatine kinase activities during statin therapy to vascular smooth muscle homeostasis. *Pharmacogenomics*, 6, pp. 865-72

Ruaño G, Windemuth A. (2006). Physiogenomic Method for Predicting Clinical Outcomes of Treatments in Patients. 20060278241, USA patent

Ruaño G, Thompson PD, Windemuth A, et al. (2007a). Physiogenomic association of statin-related myalgia to serotonin receptors. *Muscle Nerve*, 36, pp. 329-35

Ruaño, G., Goethe, J.W., Caley, C., et al. (2007b). Physiogenomic comparison of weight profiles of olanzapine- and risperidone-treated patients. *Mol Psychiatry*, 12, pp. 474-82

Ruaño, G., Bernene, J., Windemuth, A., et al. (2008). Physiogenomic comparison of edema and BMI in patients receiving rosiglitazone or pioglitazone. *Clin Chim Acta*, 400, pp. 48-55

Ruaño, G., Duconge, J., Windemuth, A., Cadilla, C.L., Kocherla, M., Villagra, D., Renta, J., Holford, T., & Santiago-Borrero, P.J. (2009). Physiogenomic Analysis of the Puerto Rican Population. *Pharmacogenomics*, 10, pp. 565-577

Ruaño, G., Thompson, P.D., Kane, J.P., Pullinger, C.R., Windemuth, A., Seip, R.L., Kocherla, M., Holford, T.R., & Wu, A.H. (2010). Physiogenomic analysis of statin-treated patients: domain-specific counter effects within the ACACB gene on low-density lipoprotein cholesterol? *Pharmacogenomics*, 11, pp. 959-71

Seip, R.L., Volek, J.S., Windemuth, A., et al. (2008). Physiogenomic comparison of human fat loss in response to diets restrictive of carbohydrate or fat. *Nutr Metab*, 5, p. 4

Shuldiner, A.R., O'Connell, J.R., Bliden, K.P., et al. (2009). Association of cytochrome P450 2C19 genotype with the antiplatelet effect and clinical efficacy of clopidogrel therapy. *JAMA*, 302, pp. 849–857

Suarez-Kurtz, G. (2005). Pharmacogenomics in admixed populations. *Trends Pharmacol Sci*, 26, pp. 196-201

Suarez-Kurtz, G., & Pena, S.D. (2006). Pharmacogenomics in the Americas: the impact of genetic admixture. *Curr Drug Targets*, 7, pp. 1649–58

The International HapMap Consortium. (2005). A haplotype map of the human genome. *Nature*, 437, pp. 1299-1320

Tishkoff, S.A., Reed, F.A., Friedlaender, F.R., et al. (2009). The genetic structure and history of Africans and African Americans. *Science*, 324, pp. 1035–44

Vargens, D.D., Almendra, L., Struchiner, C.J., & Suarez-Kurtz, G. (2008). Distribution of the GNB3 825CNT polymorphism among Brazilians: impact of population structure. *Eur J Clin Pharmacol*, 64, pp. 253–6

Villagra, D., Duconge, J., Windemuth, A., Cadilla, C.L., Kocherla, M., et al. (2010). CYP2C9 and VKORC1 genotypes in Puerto Ricans: A case for admixture matching in clinical pharmacogenetic studies. *Clin Chim Acta*, 411, pp. 1306-1311

Windemuth, A., Calhoun, V.D., Pearlson, G.D., Kocherla, M., Jagannathan, K., & Ruaño, G. (2008). Physiogenomic analysis of localized FMRI brain activity in schizophrenia. *Ann Biomed Eng*, 36, pp. 877-88

7

Current Status of Pharmacogenetics in Antithrombotic Drug Therapy

Eva Gak* and Rivka Inzelberg
Sagol Neuroscience Center (JSNC), Sheba Medical Center
Sackler Faculty of Medicine, Tel Aviv University
Israel

1. Introduction

"Personalized medicine" represents a conceptual change in pharmacotherapeutics, where an individual's genetic profile will determine the appropriate drug and/or dose the patient should receive. Currently, medicine is addressing this challenge through the lens of genomic technologies. In the domain of anthithrombotic therapy, warfarin, clopidogrel and aspirin are still the most relevant drugs for treatment of thromboembolic cardiovascular disorders and prevention of stroke. Incorporation of pharmacogenetic approaches, particularly in the antithrombotic drug therapy, may lead to better understanding of what stands behind the individual differences in drug efficacy and adverse drug effects, with the aim of increasing benefits and reducing risks on individual level. For now, two antithrombotics, warfarin and clopidogrel are emerging as the leading examples for pharmacogenetically-guided therapeutic optimization. Several recent randomized and controlled trials have demonstrated a number of improved clinical outcomes in warfarin-treated patients undertaking pharmacogenetic testing, particularly in patients with exceptionally low or high warfarin dose requirements (outliers). In addition, there were significant achievements in identification of genetic markers of reduced clopidogrel pharmacokinetics, which can partially explain inefficiency of clopidogrel response. The American Food and Drug Association (FDA) acted quickly on these developments in approving additional labeling for warfarin and clopidogrel package inserts to include relevant genetic testing, and called for further large-scale studies on the effectiveness of pharmacogenetic approaches to therapies using these drugs. However, there is still a considerable debate on the quality, quantity, and type of evidence that are needed to encourage such changes in clinical practice. There are also pertinent questions regarding which genetic markers should be used to ensure overall population benefits from genetic testing on a population level. It is also important to establish the relationship between genetic and non-genetic factors, particularly the effects of drug-drug interactions, and also the most appropriate pharmacogenetically-based dosing algorithm designed for clinical use. This review provides an update on the most significant pharmacogenetic studies on the commonly used oral anticoagulants and antiplatelet drugs, summarizing knowledge on the known genetic polymorphisms, their therapeutic effects

---

* Corresponding Author

and utility of pharmacogenetic approaches in various world populations, with special emphasis on current gaps of knowledge and challenges for future research. Most recently, a new oral warfarin alternative, a direct thrombolytic dabigatran, has been approved by the FDA. This new drug is particularly relevant for warfarin dose outliers and un-stabilized patients, making warfarin pharmacogenetics especially relevant for selection of safe and efficient antithrombotic therapy for each patient.

2. Antithrombotic therapy

Cardiovascular disease (CVD) remains the leading cause of death in the modern Western societies, despite scientific and technological advancements. According to the American Heart Association (AHA) statistical update 2009, an estimated 80 million American adults (approximately 1 in 3) have one or more types of CVD (Lloyd-Jones et al., 2009). Arterial and venous thrombotic complications closely accompany CVD in contexts of myocardial infarction (MI) and stroke (Mackman, 2008). Venous thromboembolitic disorders (VTE), including deep venous thrombosis and pulmonary embolism, are considered the third leading cause of CVD-related death after MI and stroke (Cushman, 2007), particularly in patients with cancer (Heit, 2005). Antithrombotic therapies with anticoagulant and antiplatelet agents have been the most important means for prevention and treatment of CVD, with validity established in a wide range of clinical conditions, including acute coronary syndrome (ACS) (Anderson et al., 2007a), ischemic stroke (Sacco et al., 2006), peripheral vascular disease (Hirsch et al., 2006), atrial fibrillation (AF) (Fuster et al., 2006), and symptomatic and asymptomatic VTE (Hirsh et al., 2008). Over the past decades, increasing resources have been devoted to the improvement of antithrombotic therapy, specifically focusing on development and validation of new antithrombotic agents. A series of anticoagulants and antiplatelet drugs with already known or totally new mechanisms of action have been developed and tested in randomized controlled clinical trials (Table 1). However, although providing support for improved clinical outcomes in a population defined by explicit clinical criteria, these trials generally did not address the issue why some patients do not respond to the antithrombotic treatment, while others have excessive pharmacologic responses and distinctive patterns of adverse effects. This broad inter-patient variability in drug response in terms of both, pharmacological efficacy and toxicological adverse effects, imposes a major concern with the use of antithrombotic drugs. In common clinical practice, physicians cope with this variability by "trial and error" approach in ruling out inappropriate types of drug or dosage for each patient. The best example over the past 50 years is warfarin (coumadin) and its derivatives, in which to avoid drug over- or under-dosing and risks of bleedings or drug insufficiency, individual dose is determined by frequent monitoring of the International Normalized Ratio (INR), especially at the initial phase of treatment. Furthermore, intermitted medical conditions and subsequent changes in concomitant medications and their interaction with warfarin produce additional difficulties in the daily management of warfarin-treated patients. In the same way, there are growing concerns over inter-individual variability in drug response to antiplatelet drugs, which have been given so far in a universal dose estimated as effective in clinical trials (Steinhubl et al., 2002; Yusuf et al., 2001). Specifically, there is an increasing awareness of the need for individualized dosing of the high-profile antiplatelet clopidogrel (Bonello et al., 2008), to which this review dedicates special discussion.

Drug class	Drug	Administration	Mechanisms of action	Metabolizing enzyme	Limitations	References
Vitamin K antagonists	Warfarin	Oral	Inhibits VKOR	Predominantly CYP2C9	Frequent INR monitoring; Sensitivity or resistance	(Mackman, 2008) (Kamali & Wynne, 2010)
Heparins	Low Molecular Weight Heparins (LMWH)/ Clexan	Intravenous	Inhibit factor Xa and thrombin	Not metabolized by CYP450 enzymes	Thrombocytopenia; Antibodies for heparin-platelet factor complex	(Mackman, 2008)
Antiplatelet agents	Aspirin	Oral	Irreversibly acetylates COX1	Not metabolized by CYP450 enzymes	Weak antiplatelet agent; Gastric ulceration Aspirin resistance	(Michelson, 2010)
	Clopidogrel/Plavix	Oral	Active metabolite irreversibly inhibits P2Y$_{12}$ receptor	CYP2C9 and CYP3A4 Pro-drug activated by CYP2C19	Inter-patient variability; Clopidogrel resistance	(Michelson, 2010) (Giorgi et al. 2011)
	Prasugrel	Oral	Active metabolite irreversibly inhibits P2Y$_{12}$ receptor	CYP3A4-5 and CYP2B6	Bleedings; Superior to clopidogrel in TRITON-TIMI 38 trial	(Michelson, 2010) (Giorgi et al., 2011)
	Ticagrelor	Oral	Reversibly inhibits P2Y$_{12}$ receptor	CYP3A4-5	Bleedings; Superior to clopidogrel in Phase III PLATO trial	(Wallentin et al., 2009) (Giorgi et al., 2011)
	Integrin αIIbβ3 anatagotists	Intravenous	Interfere with platelet activation	Not metabolized by CYP450 enzymes	Bleedings; Thrombocytopenia	(Michelson, 2010)
Direct thrombin inhibitors (DTIs)	Dabigatran/ Pradaxa	Oral	Reversibly inhibits free and clot-bound thrombin	Neither metabolized nor induced by CYP450 enzymes	Superior to warfarin in Phase III RE-LY trial	(Galanis et al., 2011); (Wallentin et al., 2010b)
	Rivaroxaban	Oral	Reversibly inhibits Factor Xa	CYP3A4	Phase III ROCKET-AF trial	(Galanis et al., 2011)
	Apixaban	Oral	Reversibly inhibits Factor Xa	CYP3A4	Phase III ARISTOTLE trial	(Galanis et al., 2011)

Abbreviations: VKORC1 vitamin K epoxide reductase; CYP2C9, CYP3A4-5 and CYP2C19 cytochrome P450 enzymes; COX1 cyclooxygenase-1; P2Y$_{12}$ platelet plasma membrane receptor; INR International Normalized Ratio.

Table 1. Antithrombotic drugs including generic, FDA approved and currently tested anticoagulants and antiplatelet agents

While the phenomenon of individual drug response variability has been well-recognized, its causes are not well-defined and are likely to be multifactorial, in which patient's age, sex, weight, nutrition, infections, concomitant medications and genetics play an important role (Sadee & Dai, 2005). Pharmacogenetic point of view, essentially referred to as "personalized medicine", suggests that in parallel to the development of new drugs improvement of known drugs efficacy and safety should be pursued and can be achieved by taking into account an individual's genetic make up (Aspinall & Hamermesh, 2007). Pharmacogenetics suggests that knowing more about genes implicated in drug mechanisms, drug pharmacokinetics (drug metabolic enzymes and transporters) and pharmacodynamics (target enzymes or receptors), and genetic variations with meaningful biological and population impacts, could potentially lead to more intelligent clinical decisions on therapeutic doses and risks of adverse events for individual patients. Pharmacogenetic approaches, using only a limited number of genetic variations, are currently emerging across broad classes of antithrombotic drugs. For warfarin in particular, it has been recently demonstrated that incorporation of a pharmacogenetic rationale into the clinical decision making may hold promise for better optimization of drug benefit-to-risk outcomes (Klein et al., 2009). In the near future, pharmacogenetics together with advanced diagnostic technologies such as molecular imaging may enable to shift from the study of single genes to more comprehensive paradigms focusing on functions and interactions of multiple genes and gene products, among themselves and with an environment. The information gained from such analyses, in combination with clinical data will improve individual risk assessments, eventually guiding clinical management and decision-making to improved use of antithrombotic drugs for prevention and treatment of CVD.

This review provides an update on the most significant pharmacogenetic studies on the commonly used oral anticoagulants and antiplatelet drugs, principally including warfarin, clopidogrel and aspirin. It summarizes knowledge on the known genetic polymorphisms, their therapeutic effects and utility in pharmacogenetic approaches in various world populations, with special emphasis on current gaps of knowledge and challenges for future research. There is an ongoing debate over the utility of pharmacogenetic diagnostics in the routine clinical practice (Woodcock, 2010). This review tackles on these unresolved issues in the context of antithrombotic drug, specifically whether implementation of pharmacogenetic testing indeed improves therapy benefits, damage reduction and clinical outcomes. In a broader sense, this review relates to the place of genetics among traditional approaches to personalized clinical care, which rely on knowledge of patient's behavior, diet, social circumstances and environment, and if in the future physicians could use genetics to "personalize" treatment.

3. Pharmacogenomics

The conceptual basis of pharmacogenetics was laid more that 50 years ago (Motulsky, 1965). Since then, the science behind pharmacogenetics has contributed a great deal to basic understanding of molecular mechanisms responsible for variation in drug response and to translation of that understanding to the drug development process (Weinshilboum & Wang, 2006). Clinically relevant pharmacogenetic examples, mainly involving drug metabolism, have been recognized. With the completion of the Human Genome Project and advancement of genotyping technologies, both genomic science and its application to drug response have undergone major advances (Feero et al., 2010). The field of pharmacogenetics has evolved into "pharmacogenomics", involving a shift from candidate gene approach to whole genome studies that now can be performed with more precision in a lot more samples. Former analyses of genetic variations using lower density chromosomal markers, such as tandem nucleotide repeats (VNTRs and STRs), are now mostly focus on more ubiquitous and informative variations - single-nucleotide polymorphisms (SNPs). More efficient and accurate platforms are now adapted for ever smaller DNA samples to detect

SNPs, gene copy variations (CNV) and insertion/deletion (INDEL) mutations, and also for analyses of gene expression (RNA/protein microarrays) and DNA chemical modifications (epigenomics). The HapMap project, launched in 2002, now includes a remarkable number of common human genetic variations. Most notably, new methods have dramatically increased the rates and lowered costs of DNA sequencing (Collins, 2010; Venter, 2010), facilitating the discovery of new genetic variations. More advanced bioinformatic and statistical tools have enabled genome-wide association studies (GWAS) that transformed the search for genetic factors in complex traits (Manolio, 2010), although applicability of GWAS to drug response has been hampered by the complexity and multifactorial nature of this phenotype.

It is not uncommon that drugs have a narrow therapeutic index. Warfarin and clopidogrel, the most widely prescribed antithrombotic drugs, have narrow therapeutic indexes that are influenced by genetic variations, a hallmark of drugs for which pharmacogenetic/genomic approaches can potentially provide substantial clinical benefits (Wang et al., 2011). Pharmacogenetic studies of these drugs illustrate the rapid evolution of our understanding regarding the relationships between genetic variations and drug efficacy and safety. For both these drugs, the classical candidate gene approach provided identification of important genetic markers of inter-individual variability in drug response. Additional data supporting pharmacogenetic testing for both these drugs are rapidly accumulating, among them a recent GWAS confirming the principal genetic determinants of warfarin response (Takeuchi et al., 2009) and most recent studies supporting the significance of the only known genetic factor in clopidogrel response (Mega et al., 2010b; Pare et al., 2010). Despite only partial resolution of clopidogrel pharmacogenetics, the American Food and Drug Association (FDA) acted quickly on these data by re-labeling warfarin and adding a warning on the clopidogrel label to include relevant genetic testing prior to drug use. In addition, the FDA approved several diagnostic kits for genetic testing of warfarin dosing markers, specifically those associated with warfarin sensitivity and related risk of bleedings. It is not surprising that dosing markers of warfarin and clopidogrel include variants of cytochrome P450 (CYP) enzymes that are responsible for drug metabolism or pro-drug activation. Distinct CYP polymorphisms related to reduced enzyme activity have been demonstrated as significant determinants of warfarin and clopidogrel responses and toxicity effects (Higashi et al., 2002; Mega et al., 2009b). As CYPs are responsible for metabolism of many other types of drugs (Sadee & Dai, 2005), we can presume that inclusion of genetic data on CYP polymorphisms in drug package labels is only starting to emerge. While these developments represent relative success of pharmacogenetics in the antithrombotic drug therapy, they also raised some pressing questions regarding clinical utility of pharmacogenetic testing, especially in the general population of patients (Woodcock, 2010). One problem is that the pharmacogenetic puzzle for clopidogrel is far from being complete (Fuster & Sweeny, 2010), and even more so for prasugrel, the third generation antiplatelet drug acting by the same mechanism, in addition evaluation of relative effects of genetic and non-genetic factors is still limited (Zhang et al., 2008). From an evolutionary point of view, pharmacogenetically meaningful inherited variations have most probably evolved and persisted in the human population due to ancient natural stressors such as nutrition and parasites, understanding of which may provide yet unknown and unexpected insights into the etiopathology and mechanisms of human diseases and evolutionary adaptations.

On the way towards personalize medicine, pharmacogenetics ultimately aims to replace "one drug fits all" or "trial and error" methods in choosing an optimal drug at the most advantageous dose for each patient. Even if pharmacogenetics is still unable to achieve accurate predictions of therapeutic dose at an individual level, it can assist in identifying patients who are likely to benefit from a drug from those who are prone to adverse reactions that could lead to toxicity and death ("outliers"). Perhaps the most promising advances in implementation of pharmacogenetics have been made so far in the field of oncology, using a patient's genetic profile to predict the need and the choice of chemotherapy (Huang et al., 2003; Kroese et al., 2007). Adverse drug reactions are a major problem with current antithrombotic drugs and are the major cause of hospitalizations in the US today (Lloyd-Jones et al., 2009). Reducing the number of failed drug attempts and number hospitalizations due to adverse events, are all reasons why the implementation of pharmacogenetics could be beneficial and cost effective, and overall could potentially lead to decreased costs of health care (Ginsburg et al., 2005).

4. Warfarin pharmacogenetics

The most complete pharmacogenomic picture is presently available on the anticoagulant warfarin. Warfarin (coumadin), originally patented as rat poison, was introduced into the clinical practice in the 40s as an anticoagulant inhibiting the vitamin K cycle and thereby the action of vitamin K-dependent factors of the coagulation cascade, specifically factors II, VII, IX, and X (Figure 1). Warfarin and other coumarin derivatives are indicated in a wide range of clinical conditions, including prevention and treatment of venous thrombosis (VTE) and arterial thromboembolism in patients with AF and mechanical heart valves. Maintenance on warfarin most often persists for years or lifetime. Warfarin is still the most commonly prescribed oral anticoagulant in the North America and much of Europe (phenprocoumon and acenocoumarol) (Daly & King, 2003). Every year, two million patients start warfarin therapy in the US alone (Melnikova, 2009). One problem with warfarin is a narrow therapeutic index resulting in serious risks of adverse reactions at both ends of the dosing scale: low-responders to warfarin are at increased risk for embolic events and high-responders can develop intracranial hemorrhages or gastrointestinal bleeds. The other problem is an extensive variability in warfarin dose response, reflected in more than 20-fold inter-individual differences in warfarin dosing. All patients receiving warfarin are closely monitored using INR, a universal laboratory test for anticoagulation efficiency (prothrombin time). Frequent INR monitoring is especially crucial in naive patients at the beginning of warfarin administration. For most clinical indications, the therapeutic range for target INR is between 2.0 and 3.5, while INRs below or above this range are indicative of under-anticoagulation (risk of thrombosis) or over-anticoagulation (risk of bleeding), respectively. Although therapeutic control, i.e. achieving and maintaining target INR within the therapeutic range, is considered an important predictor of adverse events, it is still insufficient even in clinical trials settings, in which the average time spent in the therapeutic INR is only 50-70% (Ansell et al., 2008). Thus, it is not surprising that warfarin still ranks among the five top most "hazardous" drugs that are most often responsible for emergency room visits (Budnitz et al., 2007; Wysowski et al., 2007), making it a leading candidate for genetic testing before starting any patient on warfarin therapy.

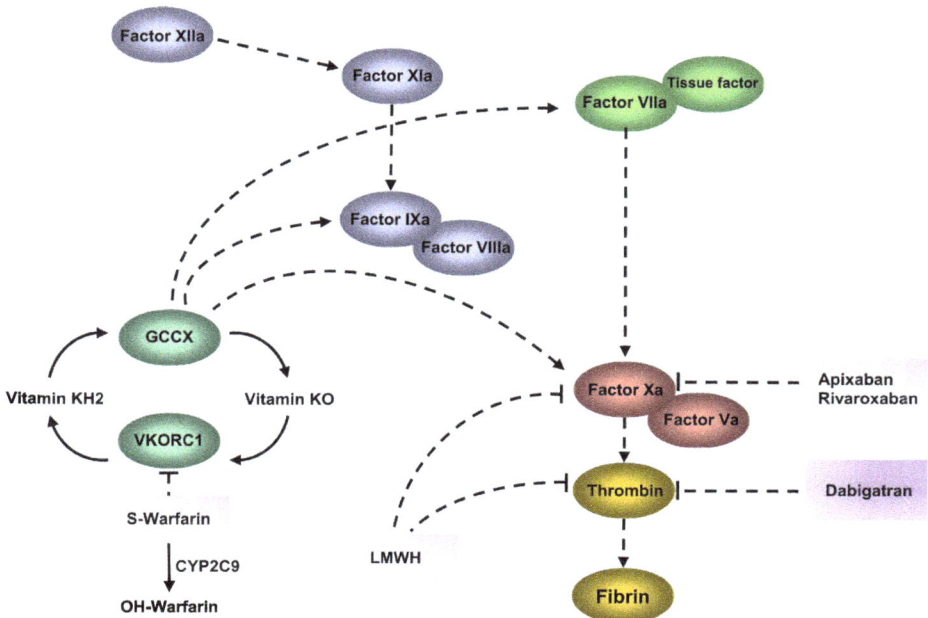

Abbreviations: VKORC1 vitamin K epoxide reductase; GCCX γ-glutamyl carboxylase; CYP2C9 cytochrome P450 enzyme; OH-Warfarin inactive hydroxylated warfarin metabolites; LMWH low molecular weigh heparins; arrows indicate activation and blocked lines inhibition.

Fig. 1. Targets of anticoagulants and direct thrombin inhibitors (DTIs)

Warfarin pharmacokinetics is predominantly determined by the hepatic CYP2C9 enzyme responsible for its metabolism. Warfarin is a racemic mixture of S and R enantiomers, S-warfarin is the main CYP2C9 substrate, has a shorter half-life and is 3-5 times more potent anticoagulant. Other drugs interfering with CYP2C9 activity and warfarin clearance (Holbrook et al., 2005), as well as age and weight (Dobrzanski et al., 1983; Wynne et al., 1995), can have significant effects on the efficacy of warfarin therapy, and also nutritional factors affecting the vitamin K cycle (Greenblatt & von Moltke, 2005). A number of genetic variants of CYP2C9 have been identified in various world populations (http://www.cypalleles.ki.se/), the two most important due to occurrence and functional implications are Arg144Cys (*2) and Ile359Leu (*3). CYP2C9*2 and *3 have been related to approximately 30% and 80% respective reductions in enzymatic activity *in vitro* (Rettie et al., 1994; Takahashi et al., 1998) and to reduced S-warfarin clearance *in vivo*, comparing wild type allele homozygotes *1/*1 to mutation carriers *1/*2 or *1/*3 (40-45% reduced clearance) or homozygotes *2/*2 and *3/*3 (70-85%) (Kaminsky & Zhang, 1997). Following key study (Aithal et al., 1999) suggested that a patient's CYP2C9 genetic composition is indicative of his warfarin dose requirement, in showing that hypofunctional *2 and *3 alleles were more common among patients with significantly lower steady-state doses, and that *2, *3 carriers and homozygotes had greater INR instability and more bleeding complications at warfarin induction. Gene-dose relationship between hypofunctional *2 and *3 alleles and reduced warfarin requirements was subsequently reproduced and refined in numerous studies. A retrospective study representing an unselected patients population (Higashi et al., 2002) investigated whether patients with CYP2C9*2,*3 genotypes also demonstrate increased time to therapeutic INR, time taken to achieve stable dosing, incidence of supra-therapeutic INR and risk of serious or life-threatening bleeding events. The investigators found that carriers of *2,*3 required more time to achieve stable dosing (hazard ratio HR=0.65 [95% confidence interval CI: 0.45-0.94] with a median difference of 95 days (p=0.004), had higher risk of supra-therapeutic INR (HR=1.4 [1.03–1.90]) and moreover were more prone to bleedings at warfarin initiation (HR=3.94 [1.29–12.06]) and over the entire study (HR=2.39 [1.18–4.86]). While deciphering the relationship between patient's CYP2C9 genotype and warfarin therapeutic dose, this study suggested an optimistic perspective that the use of genotype-guided dosing can reduce the time to reach stable therapeutic dose, risk of above-range INR's and incidence of bleeding events. A recent meta-analysis (Lindh et al., 2009) summarizing data for almost 8,000 patients from 39 studies estimated that compared to patients with the wild type *1/*1 genotype, the steady-state warfarin maintenance dose was reduced by 20% [17-22%] and 34% [29-38%] for *1/*2 and *1/*3 carriers, and by 36% [30-42%], 57% [49-64%] and 78% [72-84%] for *2/*2, *2/*3 and *3/*3 homozygotes and compound heterozygotes, respectively. It is worth mentioning that CYP2C9*2,*3 have been similarly associated with reduced S-acenocoumarol clearance, lower steady state acenocoumarol dose requirements and higher risk for supra-therapeutic INRs, but not of bleeding complications (Stehle et al., 2008; Teichert et al., 2009).Thus, significant contribution of common hypofunctional CYP2C9 variants to warfarin sensitivity has been well-established, although accurate estimates of their contribution varies between studies and is dependent on inclusion of other factors.

Despite these advances, robust estimates of bleeding risks for specific CYP2C9 genotypes are still ambiguous, due to the rarity of severe bleeding events and the need of large cohort studies. In order to circumvent this limitation, most studies use grouping of CYP2C9 genotypes. For instance, a 365 patients study (Sanderson et al., 2005) reported relative bleeding risk RR=2.26 [1.36-3.75] for carriers of *2 or *3 variants, while a 446 patients study (Limdi et al., 2008) a reported hazard ratio HR=3.0 [1.1-8.0] for major bleeding that was highest during induction (5.3-fold) but remained increased (2.2-fold) after stabilization. A large prospective Swedish Warfarin Genetics (WARG) cohort of 1496 patients (Wadelius et al., 2009) reported that 1 of 8 (12.5%) patients homozygous for *3 experienced a serious bleeding event, compared to 4 of 1482 (0.27%) with other CYP2C9 genotypes (p=0.066). Judging from these and other observations, it was clear that CYP2C9 polymorphisms can not explain the entire inter-individual variability in warfarin dose response. In addition, CYP2C9*2,*3 allele frequencies in various world populations were not entirely matching to previous epidemiological findings of ethnic differences in warfarin dose requirements, suggesting that individuals of Asian origin are relatively low dose requirers and individuals of African origin are high dose requirers compared to Caucasians (Absher et al., 2002; Dang et al., 2005). Conversely, CYP2C9*2 and *3 were found prevalent in Caucasians (12% and 8% respectively), but were hardly present in African or Asian populations (Moyer et al., 2009; Stehle et al., 2008).

Recent studied suggested implication of yet another cytochrome P450 in warfarin dose, CYP4F2, showing that coding and exceptionally common Val433Met polymorphism (up to 30% allele frequency in white populations) is associated with 4-12% increase in warfarin dose requirements (Borgiani et al., 2009; Caldwell et al., 2008). Contribution of this factor was further supported in recent GWAS showing that when CYP2C9 and VKORC1 effects were removed through multiple regression adjustments, an additional signal for CYP4F2 was observed (Takeuchi et al., 2009). Although the effect of this CYP4F2 polymorphism is probably small (about 1.1% variability explained), the suggested molecular explanation of this effect is interesting. CYP4F2 was shown to catalyze vitamin K oxidation, while the presence of 433Met variation reduced its catalytic ability, potentially leading to accumulation of the VKORC1 substrate - vitamin K epoxide and larger warfarin doses required for inhibition of this pathway (McDonald et al., 2009). CYP4F2 Val433Met was also associated with acenocoumarol dose requirements with similar modest effect (1.2-1.3%) (Perez-Andreu et al., 2009; Teichert et al., 2009).

A major step forward has been taken with discovery of an enzyme responsible for warfarin pharmacodynamics and direct warfarin target, the vitamin K epoxide reductase (VKOR). When VKOR is blocked by warfarin, vitamin K epoxide cannot be reduced to replenish the active form of vitamin K, which is necessary for activation of coagulation factors by γ-carboxylation (Figure 1). Therefore, lack of active vitamin K eventually results in less activated coagulation factors and decreased coagulation activity. After more than 50 years of search for the warfarin target, the gene encoding the VKOR catalytic subunit (VKORC1) was identified in parallel by two independent groups (Li et al., 2004; Rost et al., 2004), the latter also provided first evidence of rare VKORC1 mutations in patients with exceptionally high warfarin dose requirements (i.e. warfarin resistance). Shortly after, several studies reported that VKORC1 polymorphisms affect warfarin dose response (Bodin et al., 2005; D'Andrea et al., 2005; Sconce et al., 2005) and studies considering both CYP2C9 and VKORC1 polymorphisms suggested that they provide relatively good explanation of low dose requirements conditional on enzymes insufficiencies and a total of about 50% variability explained (Bodin et al., 2005; Sconce et al., 2005). A landmark study (Rieder et al., 2005) revealed a series of VKORC1 polymorphisms (10 SNPs including previously reported) that construct high-linkage disequilibrium haplotype structure with distinct frequencies among human populations. Specifically, haplotypes H1 and H2 containing promoter -1639G>A (also 3673G>A), and intragenic 1173C>T (also 6486C>T), 6853G>C and 7566C>T variations were associated with reduced VKORC1 transcription and lower warfarin doses, consistent with the notion that lower target enzyme production leads to lower requirement of its specific inhibitor. Since then, numerous studies have supported the notion that H1 and H2 haplotype variants (also VKORC1*2 (Geisen et al., 2005) are associated with warfarin sensitivity. Studies examining VKORC1 haplotype frequencies in various world populations confirmed that VKORC1 alleles/haplotypes are important genetic factors in determining individual as well as populational warfarin dose response variability, particularly the occurrence of warfarin sensitivity (Mushiroda et al., 2006; Takahashi et al., 2006; Veenstra et al., 2005). A paramount analysis of VKORC1 alleles/haplotypes in 8,750 patients from 11 countries partaking in the International Warfarin Pharmacogenetics Consortium (IWPC) , the largest cohort representing three racial groups (Asians, whites and blacks) (Limdi et al., 2010), showed that the -1639G>A marker is sufficient to explain the variance across all three racial groups. In fact, the -1639G>A marker has been incorporated into all warfarin genetic testing kits approved by the FDA. However this study acknowledged that the contribution of VKORC1 to dose requirements is higher in whites than in non-whites. The most compelling evidence for VKORC1 contribution to warfarin sensitivity were provided by the IWPC study of over 5,000 patients (Klein et al., 2009), showing that patients with -1639 GG,

GA, and AA genotypes had mean warfarin weekly doses of 42.6mg [41.5-43.7], 30.7mg [29.9-31.5] and 20.3mg [19.8-20.8], respectively, corresponding to approximately 25% dose reduction per A allele. Moreover, the -1639A allele was associated with other clinical outcomes indicative of increased warfarin sensitivity, specifically with higher INR values and shorter time spent within the therapeutic range, but not with bleeding complications (Limdi et al, 2008; Schwarz et al, 2008; Wadelius et al, 2009), as previously mentioned, evaluation of bleeding risks may require larger studies. VKORC1 alleles/haplotypes were shown to have similar effects on increased sensitivity to acenocoumarol (Stehle et al., 2008).

Thus, added genetic data on CYP2C9 and VKORC1 provided sufficiently good resolution of warfarin sensitivity but not of warfarin resistance, showing by default that patients of African origin (African-Americans), in which warfarin resistance is common, are essentially lacking markers of warfarin sensitivity. In addition, use of correlation analyses and more complex models accounting for other genetic and non genetic factors in African-American patients, did not reach the values achieved in Caucasian and Asian patients (Momary et al., 2007; Schelleman et al., 2007). Rare VKORC1 mutations identified in singular families with multiple coagulation factor deficiency (Rost et al., 2004) and rare patients with severe warfarin resistance (Harrington et al., 2005) also could not explain the relatively common occurrence of warfarin resistance in patients of African origin. Other gene variants, such as polymorphisms in the microsomal epoxide hydrolase (EPHX1) and calumenin (CALU), were shown to have only marginal contribution to higher warfarin doses (Loebstein et al., 2005; Wadelius et al., 2007). This gap of knowledge was resolved by two studies reporting a common warfarin resistance marker, the VKORC1 Asp36Tyr mutation, with significant contribution to high warfarin doses (>70 mg/week) and dominant effect over warfarin sensitivity markers in the same individual (Loebstein et al., 2007; Scott et al., 2008). Initially described in the Jewish Ashkenazi (4% allele frequency), Asp36Tyr was further found surprisingly prevalent in individuals from Ethiopia (15%) (Aklillu et al., 2008). Most recent study specifically focusing on high-dose coumarins requirers reported that Asp36Tyr is the most common VKORC1 mutation also among European warfarin resistant patients and appears to affect phenprocoumon therapeutic in the same way (Watzka et al., 2011).

5. Implementation of warfarin pharmacogenetics

Prior to the genetic era, warfarin dose prediction at the initiation of therapy used a clinical algorithm, including variables such as age, weight or height, race, concomitant medication and dietary vitamin K consumption, all together accounting for 20-30% of warfarin dose variability (Gage et al., 2008). Taken together, CYP2C9 and VKORC1 genotypes could explain additional 20-30% of warfarin dose variability (Wu, 2007) and by other estimates even 30-40% (Manolopoulos et al., 2010), again showing an overriding effect of genetic factors. These observations raised the possibility that genetic testing of patients prior to therapy initiation might provide information that could enhance the clinical algorithm. Several prospective studies examined potential clinical utility of the pharmacogenetic algorithm including genetic and clinical data. The first prospective randomized study comparing between the pharmacogenetically-guided and standard dosing algorithms for 206 patients initiating warfarin therapy (Anderson et al., 2007b) failed to show significant differences between groups for the primary endpoint, i.e. the number of out-of-range INR standardized by the number of INRs obtained (30.7%±22.9 in pharmacogenetic-guided *versus* 33.1%±22.9 in standard dosing group). However, the investigators succeeded to show that the pharmacogenetic algorithm slightly, but significantly, decreased the number of dose adjustments from 3.6 to 3.0 per patient (mean decrease of 0.62 adjustments [0.04–1.19], p=0.035). While it was clear that a patient's genetics influences warfarin dosing, it was still unclear how this data could be utilized in the clinic. Several groups suggested other pharmacogenetic algorithms, using genetic and clinical factors (Gage et al., 2008; Limdi et al., 2008; Takahashi et al., 2006). The IWPC pharmacogenetic algorithm was constructed on the basis of analysis of 4000 patients of various ethnicities, accounting for patients' genetic (VKORC1 and CYP2C9) and clinical data (age, weight and early INR values) (Klein et al., 2009). The predictive value of this pharmacogenetic algorithm was then validated in a cohort of 1000 patients, calculating the percentage of patients whose predicted dose was within 20% of the actual stable therapeutic dose. The investigators found that the pharmacogenetically-guided dosing was more accurate compared to the traditional approach. The greatest predictive value of the pharmacogenetic algorithm was seen in patients receiving weekly doses of 21mg or less, and 49mg or more to achieve the target INR, 49.4% in pharmacogenetically-guided *versus* 33.3% in traditional among patients requiring ≤ 21mg and 24.8% *versus* 7.2% among patients requiring ≥ 49mg (p<0.001 for both comparisons). Thus, the conclusion was that the addition of genotype information enhanced outcomes, especially for patients who required unusually high or low warfarin doses (outliers). CYP4F2 was not included in this algorithm but has been included in several algorithms developed later (Sagreiya et al., 2010; Zambon et al., 2011). Probably the most direct evidence for benefits of the pharmacogenetically-guided approach were provided in the latest study comparing nearly 900 patients for whom genetic information on CYP2C9 and VKORC1 was made available to prescribing physicians with matched 2,690 patients control group who started warfarin therapy without genetic information (Epstein et al., 2010). Six months after warfarin initiation, the genotyped cohort had 31% fewer hospitalizations overall (HR=0.69 [0.58-0.82], p< 0.001) and 28% fewer hospitalizations for bleeding or thromboembolism (HR=0.72 [0.53-0.97], p=0.029)

In February 2010, the FDA revised warfarin label providing genotype-specific ranges of doses and recommending, but not requiring, that genotypes be taken into consideration when the drug is prescribed. The wide availability of CYP2C9 and VKORC1 genotyping and the release of both Web-based and personal decision-support tools have facilitated clinical use of this information. Nevertheless, clinical adoption of genotype-guided administration of warfarin has been slow (Ansell et al., 2008). Several prospective clinical trials are currently ongoing to fill the need for prospective assessment of the value of genetic information in warfarin therapy (Ginsburg & Voora, 2010). Alternative anticoagulant therapies are also being developed that might replace warfarin, perhaps in patients with genotypes associated with extreme warfarin dose response (Kanagasabapathy et al., 2010).

6. Antiplatelet therapies

Platelets play a central role in cardiovascular arterial thrombosis caused by endothelial damage due to a ruptured atherosclerotic plaque, they adhere to the damaged sub-endothelial matrix and aggregate with each other to form a prothrombotic surface that promotes clot formation and subsequently vascular occlusion. Treatment of cardiovascular arterial disease has been using drugs targeting key pathways of platelet activation, including thromboxane A_2 synthesis and ADP-mediated and integrin $\alpha_{IIb}\beta_3$ signaling pathways. The most common antiplatelet agents include aspirin, clopidogrel and integrin $\alpha_{IIb}\beta_3$ antagonists (Figure 2). Numerous clinical trials have accumulated substantial evidence for efficacy of aspirin and clopidogrel, or both, in the primary and secondary prevention of MI, stroke and cardiovascular death (Wang et al., 2006). However, these trials have also demonstrated subsets of patients in which failure of antiplatelet therapy increased risks of vascular event and death. It has been estimated that 10-15% of the population is resistant to aspirin and close to 30% to clopidogrel, while resistance to both aspirin and clopidogrel occurs in 9% (Dupont et al., 2009). A lot of focus has been drawn to defining antiplatelet drug resistance and understanding how it develops. The term 'resistance' has been coined for lack of ability to attain the expected pharmacologic effect in the laboratory *in vitro* tests of platelet function (Barragan et al., 2003; Mehta et al., 1978; Muller et al., 2003). However, lack of agreement on a standardized definition for antiplatelet resistance contributed to the disparity in its incidence among different studies. Multiple assays for platelet function have been developed, among them the test considered the gold standard for aspirin response - light transmittance aggregometry (LTA), the point-of-care platelet function analyzer PFA-100 device and the newly introduced 'VeryfyNow' assays for aspirin and clopidogrel. One problem is the extent to which these laboratory methods correlate with one another, recent study using six different platelet function test has demonstrated that their results are weakly comparable regarding aspirin response (Lordkipanidze et al., 2007). The other problem is that the phenomenon of resistance is not well understood and, apart from genetic factors, is highly dependent on drug-drug interactions, diet and clinical conditions associated with high platelet turnover, such as inflammation, chronic infection and other disorders (Musallam et al., 2011). Therefore, a more subtle term, i.e. "non-responsiveness", have been suggested (Hennekens et al., 2004) until the reasons for antiplatelet treatment failure are better recognized.

7. Aspirin

For over 50 years, aspirin has been the foundation of antiplatelet therapy. Aspirin (acetylsaliylic acid) irreversibly acetylates the platelet cyclooxygenase-1 (COX1) at serine 529, which reduces the production of thromboxane A2, a potent platelet activator (Figure 2). Oral aspirin is rapidly absorbed from the stomach and small intestine, reaching peak plasma levels in 1-4 hours, its plasma half-life is only 15–20 minutes, but the platelet inhibitory effect lasts for platelets lifespan because of the irreversible inactivation of COX1 (Patrono et al., 2008). In high-risk patients, aspirin reduces vascular death by approximately 15% and non-fatal vascular events by 30% (Patrono et al., 2008). Aspirin may also be of benefit in the primary prevention of cardiovascular events, but the effect is more modest (Patrono et al., 2008). Consensus guidelines on the role of laboratory testing for aspirin response remain lacking, as evaluation of platelet function for aspirin is highly test specific. The very low cost of the drug is a major advantage.

Potential contribution of genetic factors to aspirin resistance has been investigated in numerous studies, but has not been entirely resolved. Early studies suggested that polymorphisms in the COX1 gene could be responsible for partial resistance to low dose aspirin (Eikelboom et al., 2002; M.K. Halushka & P.V.Halushka, 2002). Further study of 144 CVD patients on aspirin using LTA for platelet activity studies (Maree et al., 2005) confirmed that polymorphisms in COX1 significantly affect arachidonic acid (AA)-induced platelet aggregation and serum thromboxane A_2 levels (p=0.004). However, more recent systematic review has not supported the association between COX1 polymorphisms and aspirin resistance (Goodman et al., 2008). Candidate polymorphisms in platelet glycoprotein receptors (GPIa/IIa, GP Ibα and GPIIIa) have been also considered as potential contributors to variability in aspirin response. An original study of 100 patients on low dose aspirin using PFA-100 method for measuring platelet-induced hemostasis *in vitro* (Macchi et al., 2003) reported that patients with poor platelet response to aspirin therapy had significantly more often GPIIIa A1/A1 genotype (86.2%) than good responsers (59.4%; p = 0.01). No relation was found between aspirin resistance and other GP genotypes. Association between homozygosity for the GPIIIa A1 allele and resistance to aspirin inhibition was furhter supported by several studies (Dropinski et al., 2007; Feher et al., 2009; Papp et al., 2005), but refuted by others (Lev et al., 2007). Another interesting study re-assessing the effects of various polymorphisms in COX1 or platelet glycoprotein receptors on variable response to aspirin, used both PFA-100 and LTA platelet activity assays (Lepantalo et al., 2006). This study emphasized the effect that the two methods may have on association findings, in addition, the authors suggested that the poor response to aspirin was also associated with female gender (p=0.019). Several studies using female platelets have shown increased platelet reactivity at baseline and a less effective inhibition of platelet aggregation by aspirin (Zuern et al., 2009). The mechanisms underlying these differences are still to be elucidated, but influences of female sex hormones may play an important role. As a consequence, inhibition of platelet aggregation in women treated with aspirin may be insufficient, and female patients might benefit from higher maintenance dosages or the use of alternative antiplatelet medications.

Thus, the potential causes, incidence and clinical impact of aspirin resistance are still obscure. Measured variability in response to aspirin is most probably multifactorial, with genetics playing what appears to be a small, undefined role. Others suggest that the actual incidence of true clinical aspirin resistance is very low, and that aspirin failure has little to do with ex vivo-determined responsiveness (Cuisset et al., 2009). Alternate pathways for platelets activation that are not inhibited by aspirin, such as erythrocyte induced platelet activation (Santos et al., 1991), may be responsible for aspirin resistance. Based on these notions and the mixed results shown in the above studies, there is currently no defined role for pharmacogenetic testing to dose aspirin.

8. Clopidogrel high-risk pharmacokinetics

Thienopyridines, such as clopidogrel and prasugrel, irreversibly bind to the purinoceptor $P2Y_{12}$ receptor resulting in inhibition of platelets activation in response to adenosine diphosphate (ADP) and inhibition of platelet aggregation (Figure 2). Clopidogrel is given orally in a daily universal dose, it has substantial benefits in patients after PCI and stent implantation (Anderson et al., 2007a). Dual antiplatelet therapy (aspirin plus clopidogrel) is the standard of care for patients with acute coronary syndrome managed medically after coronary stenting or by PCI (Anderson et al., 2007a). However, major adverse cardiovascular events including stent thrombosis can occur despite antiplatelet therapy, recent meta-analysis showed that persistent platelet reactivity on clopidogrel treatment confers a five-fold increased risk of major adverse cardiovascular events (Sofi et al.,2010). All thienopyridines are pro-drugs requiring activation by the hepatic cytochrome P450 enzyme system. Clopidogrel is metabolized to its active metabolite through a two-step process mediated by various CYPs, among which CYP2C9 and CYP2C19 play a major role (Brandt et al., 2007), the activation of prasugrel, in contrast, is mediated by esterases and by CYP3As with lesser contribution of CYP2C9 and CYP2C19 (Jakubowski et al., 2007). Inter-patient response variability to clopidogrel became evident from platelet function assays *in vitro* (Barragan et al., 2003; Muller et al., 2003) and from associations of poor clopidogrel response *in vitro* (clopidogrel resistance or none-responsiveness) to poor clinical response evidenced by major adverse events (Snoep et al., 2007).

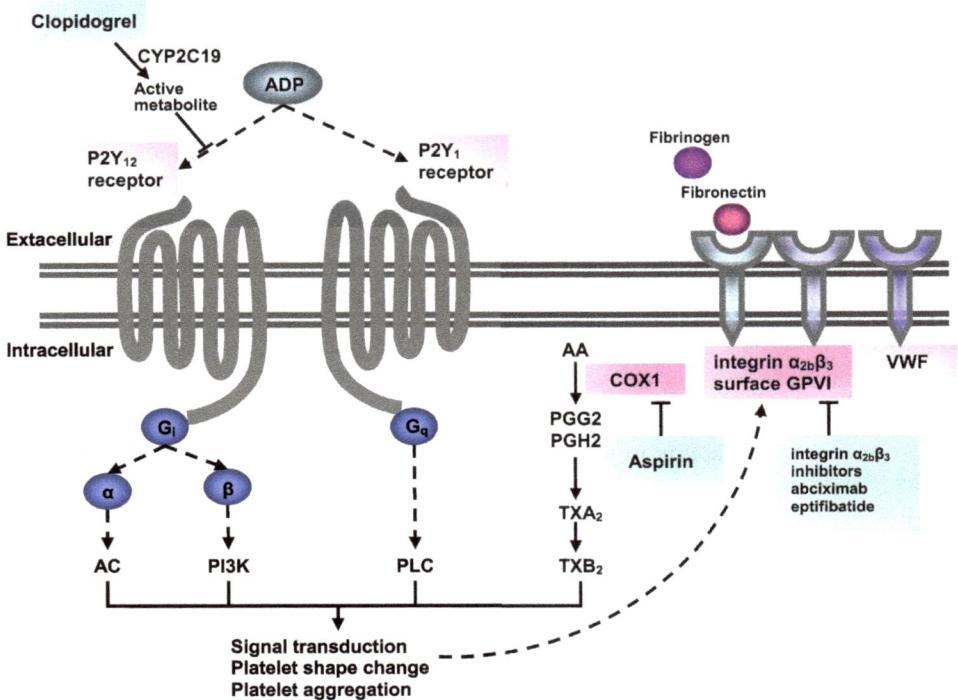

Abbreviations: CYP2C19 cytochrome P450 enzyme; ADP adenosine diphosphate; P2Y$_{12}$ and P2Y$_1$ purinoceptor receptors; coupled G$_i$ and G$_q$ proteins; G$_i$ protein α and β subunits; AC adenyl cyclase; PI3K phosphatidylinositol 3-kinase; PLC phospholipase C; AA arachidonic acid; PGG2 and PGH2 endoperoxides; TXA$_2$ TXB$_2$ thromboxanes; COX1 cyclooxygenase 1; surface GPVI glycoprotein VI and integrin $\alpha_{2b}\beta_1$; VWF von Willebrand factor; arrows indicate activation and blocked lines inhibition.

Fig. 2. Targets of several antiplatelet agents, clopidogrel, aspirin and integrin $\alpha_{2b}\beta_3$ inhibitors

Multiple factor have been implicated in high-on clopidogrel platelet reactivity, including drug compliance, drug-drug interactions, age, diabetes, body-mass index, left ventricle ejection function and inflammation (Giusti et al., 2010). Several studies have demonstrated that common and functional polymorphisms in CYPs responsible for clopidogrel pharmacokinetics can affect clopidogrel responsiveness. In a key study (Brandt et al., 2007), the investigators hypothesized that polymorphisms inducing loss-of-function of CYP2C19, CYP2C9, and CYP3A5 could contribute to decreased formation of the active clopidogrel metabolite and thereby affect inhibition of platelet activation. They examined the effect of loading doses of clopidogrel and prasugrel on platelet function *in vitro*, showing significant association between the CYP2C19*2 allele encoding a truncated protein product with little enzymatic activity and poor response to clopidogrel, but not to prasugrel. CYP2C9*2 and *3 showed similar tendencies. Carriers of CYP2C19*2 were more frequency poor responders compared to patients without the allele (72% *versus* 41% respectively, p=0.030). A similar trend was observed among CYP2C9*2,*3 homozygotes compared to patients with the wild type genotype (75% *versus* 41.4%, p=0.024). Overall, the presence of either CYP2C19*2 or CYP2C9 (*2/*2 or *3) was strongly associated with poor clopidogrel response (p<0.001). No association was found between CYP3A5 polymorphisms and clopidogrel response. In addition, the presence of these or any other CYP polymorphisms had no effect on response to prasugrel. The effect CYP3A5 polymorphisms on clopidogrel response is still elusive, a follow up study of 348 patients treated with clopidogrel after stent placement (Suh et al., 2006) suggested that the CYP3A5*3 'non-expressor' allele contributed to significantly increased risk of atherothrombotic events, however these findings could not be reproduced by others (Simon et al., 2009). Since CYP3A5 and A4 have an overlapping substrate specificity (Lamba et al., 2002), variability in CYP3A4 activity was also associated with clopidogrel response (Lau et al., 2004). As a result, other drugs that are metabolized by CYP3A4, e.g. certain statins commonly used in patients with athrosclerosis, could interfere with clopidogrel activation.

The concept of high-risk pharmacokinetics in response to clopidogrel and specifically the role of CYP2C19*2 became increasingly recognized owing to several recent studies. Sub-group analysis of the EXCELSIOR study examined whether the loss-of-function CYP2C19*2 allele is associated with increased platelet reactivity despite clopidogrel treatment in patients undergoing elective PCI with stent placement (Trenk et al., 2008). CYP2C19*2 was significantly associated with residual platelet aggregation (RPA>14%) before hospital discharge. Patients with RPA>14% had significantly increased risk of death or MI (HR=3.0 [1.4–6.8], p=0.004) 1-year post-procedure. The authors concluded that patients carrying at least one CYP2C19*2 allele are more prone to high-on clopidogrel platelet reactivity, although this study was not adequately powered to determine the effect of variant alleles on clinical outcomes. A consecutive study (Shuldiner et al., 2009) clarified the association between CYP2C19*2 and clinical outcomes, by doing GWAS and CYP2C19*2 genotyping in conjunction with platelet function assays in 429 healthy Amish volunteers on clopidogrel from the Amish Pharmacogenomics of Antiplatelet Intervention (PAPI) study, and then re-examining PAPI findings in relation to cardiovascular outcomes in an independent cohort of 227 clopidogrel-treated patients after PCI. The investigators established that CYP2C19*2 was associated with reduced clopidogrel response in PAPI study accounting for 12% of the variability in ADP-induced platelet aggregation (p=4.3×10^{-11}). The relation between CYP2C19*2 genotype and platelet aggregation was replicated in the patients cohort (p=0.02). Moreover, patients with the CYP2C19*2 variant were more likely (20.9% *versus* 10.0%) to have cardiovascular ischemic events or death during the 1-year follow-up period (HR=2.42 [1.18-4.99], p=0.02) (Shuldiner et al., 2009). In patients no longer taking clopidogrel after 1-year, no increase was observed between carriers and non-carriers of CYP2C19*2 (Mega et al.,

2009a). Apart from the CYP2C19*2 contribution (12%), age, body mass, and lipid levels accounted for additional 10% of clopidogrel response. Essential confirmation of CYP2C19*2 as an important determinant of clopidogrel response was provided by a sub-analysis of the randomized TRITON-TIMI 38 trial of clopidogrel and prasugrel outcomes using similar two-phase approach (Mega et al., 2009a). This study tested associations between CYP2C19 reduced-function alleles (five alleles were tested) and measurements of active drug metabolite in plasma and platelet aggregation in response to clopidogrel in healthy individuals (n=162), and then re-evaluated these associations in a separate cohort of patients with acute coronary syndrome (n=1477) considering cardiovascular outcomes. In healthy individuals, carriers of at least one CYP2C19 reduced-function allele (approximately 30% of the population) had 32.4% reduction in plasma exposure to the active drug metabolite and reduction in maximal platelet aggregation in response to clopidogrel, as compared to non-carriers (both p<0.001). Among TRITON–TIMI 38 patients, carriers of the CYP2C19 reduced-function allele had 53% increase in the risk of death from cardiovascular causes, MI or stroke compared to non-carriers (12.1% *versus* 8.0%, HR=1.53 for carriers [1.07-2.19], p=0.01) and increase in the risk of stent thrombosis (2.6% *versus* 0.8%, HR=3.09 [1.19-8.00], p=0.02). These findings imply that in patients receiving clopidogrel reduced-function CYP2C19 alleles can lead to reduced exposure to the active metabolite, less platelet inhibition and reduced protection from ischemic events, including stent thrombosis. Interestingly, no associations were found with any of these CYP variants among patients randomized to prasugrel therapy in the TRITON trial (Mega et al., 2009b). One drawback raised in a parallel study of the French FAST-MI registry including 2,208 patients (Simon et al., 2009), suggested that only carriers of two loss-of-function alleles CYP2C19*2, *3, *4, or *5 (i.e. homozygotes or compound heterozygotes) have increased risk of death, nonfatal MI or stroke during 1-year period (21.5% *versus* 13.3%, HR=1.98 [1.10–3.58]). This risk was increased even further in PCI (HR=3.58 [1.71–7.51]). This question has been resolved in the a meta-analysis including 9,685 patients with acute coronary syndrome or PCI (Mega et al., 2010b), showing that carriers of even one reduced-function CYP2C19 allele may have significantly increased risks of major adverse cardiovascular events, particularly stent thrombosis.

Platelet response to clopidogrel is not fully explained by the CYP2C19 loss-of-function alleles. Other pharmacokinetic sources of inter-patient variability have been suggested, specifically the effect of the 3435C>T polymorphism in the p-glycoprotein ABCB1 on clopidogrel absorption and metabolism (Hoffmeyer et al., 2000; Owen et al., 2005; Taubert et al., 2006). However, this issue remains controversial in the recent sub-analysis of TRITON–TIMI 38 and PLATO trials considering ABCB1 genotypes and clinical outcomes of patients on clopidogrel (Mega et al., 2010a; Wallentin et al., 2010a). Most recently, a novel determinant of clopidogrel efficacy was proposed (Bouman et al., 2011), namely the estrase PON1, a key enzyme in the rate limiting step of clopidogrel bioactivation and that a coding Q192R PON1 polymorphism can affect plasma concentrations of active metabolite, clopidogrel inhibition and risk of stent thrombosis,. Large randomized replication studies are needed to confirm these interesting and new observations. In addition, few contrasting data are available on pharmacodynamic factors, particularly polymorphisms in genes encoding platelet glycoproteins involved in thienopyridines intestinal absorption and platelet receptors that serve as thienopyridines targets. Effects of polymorphisms in glycoprotein GPIIIa, and platelet receptors P2Y12 and P2Y1 related to aspirin and clopidogrel response were evaluated in a preliminary study (Lev et al., 2007), finding no definitive associations between various polymorphisms and clopidogrel response assessed by platelet aggregation studies. Another study (Shuldiner et al., 2009) relating to clinical outcomes also did not find an association between the P2Y12 polymorphism and the risk of death, non-fatal MI, or stroke in patients treated with clopidogrel.

9. Implementation of clopidogrel pharmacogenetics

Early in 2010, the FDA added a boxed warning to prescribing information for clopidogrel, stating that persons with the low-rate metabolizing *CYP2C19* variant might require dose adjustment or the use of another drug. After this FDA action, the American Heart Association and the American College of Cardiology issued a joint endorsement of *CYP2C19* genotyping for patients at moderate or high risk for cardiovascular events who are treated with clopidogrel (Holmes et al., 2010), this genetic test is now widely available in the US. Despite that, there are studies that challenge the clinical impact of polymorphisms on the effectiveness of clopidogrel. Most recently, the CHARISMA genomic sub-study reported at the TCT 2009 meeting http://www.theheart.org/article/1008623.do that while patients homozygous for the loss-of-function CYP2C19 allele appeared to have an increased risk of ischemia when compared with patients with the wild-type allele, they also had fewer bleeding events. Conflicting results of many different studies exemplify many unanswered questions regarding clinical significance of pharmacogenetics in antiplatelet drugs. Being able to predict the specific response of an individual patient based on his or her genetic code has yet to be defined, especially for clopidogrel. Despite the lack of clear guidance regarding how clinicians could utilize the pharmacogenetic information on clopidogrel, some clinical laboratories, especially in the US, now offer genetic screening for markers associated with response to antithrombotics including clopidogrel.

10. New generation antithrombotic drugs

Novel orally active antiplatelet agents are now available. Prasugrel, the third-generation thienopyridine, has been associated with greater active metabolite generation, superior inhibition of platelet aggregation and less response variability than clopidogrel (Gurbel & Tantry, 2008). In the TRITON-TIMI 38 trial of patients with acute coronary syndrome undergoing PCI, the prevalence of cardiovascular death, non-fatal MI or stroke was lower with prasugrel than with clopidogrel, although rates of bleeding were higher in the prasugrel group (Wiviott et al., 2007). A novel selective inhibitor of P2Y12-receptor, ticagrelor has been also evaluated against clopidogrel in patients with acute coronary syndrome in the PLATO trial (Wallentin et al., 2009). Ticagrelor was associated with significant reduction in cardiovascular death, MI and stroke, without any difference in the overall incidence of major bleeding, but with increase in major bleeding related to noncoronary-artery bypass graft.

In October 2010, the FDA approved the oral anticoagulant dabigatran (Pradaxa; Boehringer Ingelheim), a direct thrombin inhibitor (DTI), for stroke prevention in patients with AF (SPAF). The clinical community is excited at the prospect of having an alternative for warfarin therapy, the current gold standard therapy for stroke prevention, a challenge that has taken more than 50 years. SPAF is not the only indication for dabigatran and other new DTIs, ongoing trials are evaluating DTIs for the treatment of acute coronary syndromes and VTE after major orthopaedic surgery (Hughes, 2010). Initially, dabigatran will probably substitute warfarin in patients who have problems with INR management, investigators of the Phase III RE-LY trial comparing between dabigatran and warfarin effects in 18,113 patients suggest that the rates of adverse events were similar for dabigatran and warfarin in patients with good INR control, whereas dabigatran was always superior to warfarin in patients with poor INR control (Wallentin et al., 2010b). Thus, successful entry of dabigatran may benefit from identification of warfarin dose outliers by genetic testing for CYP2C9 and VKORC1 markers and in the same way, the next generation DTIs, rivaroxaban and apixaban that are currently tested in the Phase III ROCKET-AF and ARISTOTLE trials, respectively (http://clinicaltrials.gov/).

11. Conclusions

Pharmacogenetics is one of the major components of personalized therapy. However, even though the conceptual basis for pharmacogenetics has existed for over half century and recent scientific and technological advancements in the field, and the FDA awareness of the necessity to integrate genomic data into regulatory review, the translation of pharmacogenetics into the clinic has been slow. The cardiovascular field and particularly the antithrombotic drug therapy have provided some excellent examples of clinical utility of pharmacogenetic approaches. The impact of VKORC1 and CYP2C9 variants on warfarin response, established the value of genetic variability to predict the appropriate warfarin dose for improving and easing the transition to a therapeutic INR level. In fact, the labeling for warfarin now includes recommendations for genetic testing. Nevertheless, the clinical application of this information has yet to become universal, in part due to ethical and confidentiality issues regarding genetic information, logistic issues with obtaining timely genotyping, and resolution of appropriate genetically-guided dosing algorithms for warfarin in various populations. Specifically to this last point, the validity of the existing genetically-guided dosing algorithms in ethnically heterogonous populations, such as in the US, has been seriously compromised by ethnic stratification of certain genetic warfarin dosing markers and inability to predict with equivalent degree of confidence in individual dose response. In addition, as warfarin pharmacogenetics is extensively affected by environmental interactions, differences in lifestyle, nutrition and traditional medical routines may have significant impact on how warfarin genetic testing is translated to clinical decision making in various population. Once again, large-scale prospective studies are needed to confirm the usefulness and pharmacoeconomic benefits of personalized genetically-guided treatment for warfarin on a population basis.

Similar to the evolution of personalized medicine for the anticoagulant warfarin, the antiplatelet drug clopidogrel has also demonstrated strong potential for improving therapy by pharmacogenetic approach. For now, however, clopidogrel pharmacogenetics is even farther from obtaining widespread application than warfarin. There is a much smaller percentage of variability explained by the current paradigm and fewer prospective studies confirming the worthiness of genetic information for improving clinical outcomes. Likewise, any potential economic savings of this strategy have not been demonstrated. Most importantly, it is unclear how the genetic information on CYP2C19 can be utilized for adjustment of the treatment regime, for example by increasing the dosing of clopidogrel or by substituting clopidogrel for the recently approved prasugrel or for the potentially soon to be available ticagrelor. The appropriate use of these strategies is difficult to assess in the absence of genetic information on clopidogrel alternatives, and incomplete understanding about other potential predictors, i.e. genetic, epigenetic and environmental modulators of response to antiplatelet agents. This problem is moreover accentuated by lack of reliable and validated assays for measuring platelet function with sensitivity, consistency, standardization and correlation with clinical outcomes, in order to tailor with confidence personalized antiplatelet therapy.

There has been significant discussion in the scientific press (Collins, 2010; Varmus, 2010; Venter, 2010; Woodcock, 2010) about the slow pace of the application of genomics to clinical practice. All parties point to the need for increasingly large and complex studies to test pharmacogenomic paradigms in the clinical setting; economic disincentives for pharmaceutical industry to accept the implications of individualized drug response; and the slow pace of the incorporation of pharmacogenomics into the drug evaluation process. In line with this critique, the FDA has recently released several regulatory guidelines (Guidance for Industry: Pharmacogenomic Data Submission 2005 and Companion Guidance 2007) on integration of genomic data in the evaluation process of new drug applications. Finally, there is a need for concerted effort directed at the education of healthcare professionals as well as patients to understand, accept and utilize genomic information

As time progresses, technology will continue to decrease the cost of whole-genome scans and other genetic tools, allowing more efficient and secure transfer of genetic information. Challenges that are associated with replication of study findings and evaluation of the clinical significance of genetic variants, underscore the importance of functional experiments to test their biological implications and to extend our understanding of drug mechanisms. These advances, along with development of logistical platforms for universal application of genetic information will allow realization of personalized medicine across all therapeutic areas, antithrombotic drug therapy. Finally, additional scientific, regulatory, and psychological factors must be addressed before pharmacogenomic tests will become a routine part of medicine. The FDA-mandated incorporation of pharmacogenomic information in drug labeling will remain an important step in the acceptance of pharmacogenomics in clinical practice. Perhaps equally important will be the willingness of physicians to reexamine suboptimal pharmacologic management programs.

12. References

Absher RK, Moore ME, Parker MH. 2002. Patient-specific factors predictive of warfarin dosage requirements. Ann Pharmacother 36(10):1512-7.

Aithal GP, Day CP, Kesteven PJ, Daly AK. 1999. Association of polymorphisms in the cytochrome P450 CYP2C9 with warfarin dose requirement and risk of bleeding complications. Lancet 353(9154):717-9.

Aklillu E, Leong C, Loebstein R, Halkin H, Gak E. 2008. VKORC1 Asp36Tyr warfarin resistance marker is common in Ethiopian individuals. Blood 111(7):3903-4.

Anderson JL, Adams CD, Antman EM, Bridges CR, Califf RM, Casey DE, Jr., Chavey WE, 2nd, Fesmire FM, Hochman JS, Levin TN and others. 2007a. ACC/AHA 2007 guidelines for the management of patients with unstable angina/non ST-elevation myocardial infarction: a report of the American College of Cardiology/American Heart Association Task Force on Practice Guidelines (Writing Committee to Revise the 2002 Guidelines for the Management of Patients With Unstable Angina/Non ST-Elevation Myocardial Infarction): developed in collaboration with the American College of Emergency Physicians, the Society for Cardiovascular Angiography and Interventions, and the Society of Thoracic Surgeons: endorsed by the American Association of Cardiovascular and Pulmonary Rehabilitation and the Society for Academic Emergency Medicine. Circulation 116(7):e148-304.

Anderson JL, Horne BD, Stevens SM, Grove AS, Barton S, Nicholas ZP, Kahn SF, May HT, Samuelson KM, Muhlestein JB and others. 2007b. Randomized trial of genotype-guided versus standard warfarin dosing in patients initiating oral anticoagulation. Circulation 116(22):2563-70.

Ansell J, Hirsh J, Hylek E, Jacobson A, Crowther M, Palareti G. 2008. Pharmacology and management of the vitamin K antagonists: American College of Chest Physicians Evidence-Based Clinical Practice Guidelines (8th Edition). Chest 133(6 Suppl):160S-198S.

Aspinall MG, Hamermesh RG. 2007. Realizing the promise of personalized medicine. Harv Bus Rev 85(10):108-17, 165.

Barragan P, Bouvier JL, Roquebert PO, Macaluso G, Commeau P, Comet B, Lafont A, Camoin L, Walter U, Eigenthaler M. 2003. Resistance to thienopyridines: clinical detection of coronary stent thrombosis by monitoring of vasodilator-stimulated phosphoprotein phosphorylation. Catheter Cardiovasc Interv 59(3):295-302.

Bodin L, Verstuyft C, Tregouet DA, Robert A, Dubert L, Funck-Brentano C, Jaillon P, Beaune P, Laurent-Puig P, Becquemont L and others. 2005. Cytochrome P450 2C9 (CYP2C9) and vitamin K epoxide reductase (VKORC1) genotypes as determinants of acenocoumarol sensitivity. Blood 106(1):135-40.

Bonello L, Camoin-Jau L, Arques S, Boyer C, Panagides D, Wittenberg O, Simeoni MC, Barragan P, Dignat-George F, Paganelli F. 2008. Adjusted clopidogrel loading doses according to vasodilator-stimulated phosphoprotein phosphorylation index decrease rate of major adverse cardiovascular events in patients with clopidogrel resistance: a multicenter randomized prospective study. J Am Coll Cardiol 51(14):1404-11.

Borgiani P, Ciccacci C, Forte V, Sirianni E, Novelli L, Bramanti P, Novelli G. 2009. CYP4F2 genetic variant (rs2108622) significantly contributes to warfarin dosing variability in the Italian population. Pharmacogenomics 10(2):261-6.

Bouman HJ, Schomig E, van Werkum JW, Velder J, Hackeng CM, Hirschhauser C, Waldmann C, Schmalz HG, ten Berg JM, Taubert D. 2011. Paraoxonase-1 is a major determinant of clopidogrel efficacy. Nat Med 17(1):110-6.

Brandt JT, Close SL, Iturria SJ, Payne CD, Farid NA, Ernest CS, 2nd, Lachno DR, Salazar D, Winters KJ. 2007. Common polymorphisms of CYP2C19 and CYP2C9 affect the pharmacokinetic and pharmacodynamic response to clopidogrel but not prasugrel. J Thromb Haemost 5(12):2429-36.

Budnitz DS, Shehab N, Kegler SR, Richards CL. 2007. Medication use leading to emergency department visits for adverse drug events in older adults. Ann Intern Med 147(11):755-65.

Caldwell MD, Awad T, Johnson JA, Gage BF, Falkowski M, Gardina P, Hubbard J, Turpaz Y, Langaee TY, Eby C and others. 2008. CYP4F2 genetic variant alters required warfarin dose. Blood 111(8):4106-12.

Collins F. 2010. Has the revolution arrived? Nature 464(7289):674-5.

Cuisset T, Frere C, Quilici J, Gaborit B, Bali L, Poyet R, Faille D, Morange PE, Alessi MC, Bonnet JL. 2009. Aspirin noncompliance is the major cause of "aspirin resistance" in patients undergoing coronary stenting. Am Heart J 157(5):889-93.

Cushman M. 2007. Epidemiology and risk factors for venous thrombosis. Semin Hematol 44(2):62-9.

D'Andrea G, D'Ambrosio RL, Di Perna P, Chetta M, Santacroce R, Brancaccio V, Grandone E, Margaglione M. 2005. A polymorphism in the VKORC1 gene is associated with an interindividual variability in the dose-anticoagulant effect of warfarin. Blood 105(2):645-9.

Daly AK, King BP. 2003. Pharmacogenetics of oral anticoagulants. Pharmacogenetics 13(5):247-52.

Dang MT, Hambleton J, Kayser SR. 2005. The influence of ethnicity on warfarin dosage requirement. Ann Pharmacother 39(6):1008-12.

Dobrzanski S, Duncan SE, Harkiss A, Wardlaw A. 1983. Age and weight as determinants of warfarin requirements. J Clin Hosp Pharm 8(1):75-7.

Dropinski J, Musial J, Sanak M, Wegrzyn W, Nizankowski R, Szczeklik A. 2007. Antithrombotic effects of aspirin based on PLA1/A2 glycoprotein IIIa polymorphism in patients with coronary artery disease. Thromb Res 119(3):301-3.

Dupont AG, Gabriel DA, Cohen MG. 2009. Antiplatelet therapies and the role of antiplatelet resistance in acute coronary syndrome. Thromb Res 124(1):6-13.

Eikelboom JW, Hirsh J, Weitz JI, Johnston M, Yi Q, Yusuf S. 2002. Aspirin-resistant thromboxane biosynthesis and the risk of myocardial infarction, stroke, or cardiovascular death in patients at high risk for cardiovascular events. Circulation 105(14):1650-5.

Epstein RS, Moyer TP, Aubert RE, DJ OK, Xia F, Verbrugge RR, Gage BF, Teagarden JR. 2010. Warfarin genotyping reduces hospitalization rates results from the MM-WES (Medco-Mayo Warfarin Effectiveness study). J Am Coll Cardiol 55(25):2804-12.

Feero WG, Guttmacher AE, Collins FS. 2010. Genomic medicine--an updated primer. N Engl J Med 362(21):2001-11.

Feher G, Feher A, Pusch G, Lupkovics G, Szapary L, Papp E. 2009. The genetics of antiplatelet drug resistance. Clin Genet 75(1):1-18.

Fuster V, Ryden LE, Cannom DS, Crijns HJ, Curtis AB, Ellenbogen KA, Halperin JL, Le Heuzey JY, Kay GN, Lowe JE and others. 2006. ACC/AHA/ESC 2006 Guidelines for the Management of Patients with Atrial Fibrillation: a report of the American

College of Cardiology/American Heart Association Task Force on Practice Guidelines and the European Society of Cardiology Committee for Practice Guidelines (Writing Committee to Revise the 2001 Guidelines for the Management of Patients With Atrial Fibrillation): developed in collaboration with the European Heart Rhythm Association and the Heart Rhythm Society. Circulation 114(7):e257-354.

Fuster V, Sweeny JM. 2010. Clopidogrel and the reduced-function CYP2C19 genetic variant: a limited piece of the overall therapeutic puzzle. Jama 304(16):1839-40.

Gage BF, Eby C, Johnson JA, Deych E, Rieder MJ, Ridker PM, Milligan PE, Grice G, Lenzini P, Rettie AE and others. 2008. Use of pharmacogenetic and clinical factors to predict the therapeutic dose of warfarin. Clin Pharmacol Ther 84(3):326-31.

Galanis T, Thomson L, Palladino M, Merli GJ. 2011. New oral anticoagulants. J Thromb Thrombolysis 31(3):310-20.

Geisen C, Watzka M, Sittinger K, Steffens M, Daugela L, Seifried E, Muller CR, Wienker TF, Oldenburg J. 2005. VKORC1 haplotypes and their impact on the inter-individual and inter-ethnical variability of oral anticoagulation. Thromb Haemost 94(4):773-9.

Ginsburg GS, Donahue MP, Newby LK. 2005. Prospects for personalized cardiovascular medicine: the impact of genomics. J Am Coll Cardiol 46(9):1615-27.

Ginsburg GS, Voora D. 2010. The long and winding road to warfarin pharmacogenetic testing. J Am Coll Cardiol 55(25):2813-5.

Giorgi MA, Cohen Arazi H, Gonzalez CD, Di Girolamo G. 2011. Beyond efficacy: pharmacokinetic differences between clopidogrel, prasugrel and ticagrelor. Expert Opin Pharmacother 12(8):1285-95.

Giusti B, Gori AM, Marcucci R, Abbate R. 2010. Relation of CYP2C19 loss-of-function polymorphism to the occurrence of stent thrombosis. Expert Opin Drug Metab Toxicol 6(4):393-407.

Goodman T, Ferro A, Sharma P. 2008. Pharmacogenetics of aspirin resistance: a comprehensive systematic review. Br J Clin Pharmacol 66(2):222-32.

Greenblatt DJ, von Moltke LL. 2005. Interaction of warfarin with drugs, natural substances, and foods. J Clin Pharmacol 45(2):127-32.

Gurbel PA, Tantry US. 2008. Prasugrel, a third generation thienopyridine and potent platelet inhibitor. Curr Opin Investig Drugs 9(3):324-36.

Halushka MK, Halushka PV. 2002. Why are some individuals resistant to the cardioprotective effects of aspirin? Could it be thromboxane A2? Circulation 105(14):1620-2.

Harrington DJ, Underwood S, Morse C, Shearer MJ, Tuddenham EG, Mumford AD. 2005. Pharmacodynamic resistance to warfarin associated with a Val66Met substitution in vitamin K epoxide reductase complex subunit 1. Thromb Haemost 93(1):23-6.

Heit JA. 2005. Venous thromboembolism: disease burden, outcomes and risk factors. J Thromb Haemost 3(8):1611-7.

Hennekens CH, Schror K, Weisman S, FitzGerald GA. 2004. Terms and conditions: semantic complexity and aspirin resistance. Circulation 110(12):1706-8.

Higashi MK, Veenstra DL, Kondo LM, Wittkowsky AK, Srinouanprachanh SL, Farin FM, Rettie AE. 2002. Association between CYP2C9 genetic variants and anticoagulation-related outcomes during warfarin therapy. Jama 287(13):1690-8.

Hirsch AT, Haskal ZJ, Hertzer NR, Bakal CW, Creager MA, Halperin JL, Hiratzka LF, Murphy WR, Olin JW, Puschett JB and others. 2006. ACC/AHA 2005 Practice Guidelines for the management of patients with peripheral arterial disease (lower extremity, renal, mesenteric, and abdominal aortic): a collaborative report from the American Association for Vascular Surgery/Society for Vascular Surgery, Society for Cardiovascular Angiography and Interventions, Society for Vascular Medicine and Biology, Society of Interventional Radiology, and the ACC/AHA Task Force on Practice Guidelines (Writing Committee to Develop Guidelines for the Management of Patients With Peripheral Arterial Disease): endorsed by the American Association of Cardiovascular and Pulmonary Rehabilitation; National Heart, Lung, and Blood Institute; Society for Vascular Nursing; TransAtlantic Inter-Society Consensus; and Vascular Disease Foundation. Circulation 113(11):e463-654.

Hirsh J, Guyatt G, Albers GW, Harrington R, Schunemann HJ. 2008. Executive summary: American College of Chest Physicians Evidence-Based Clinical Practice Guidelines (8th Edition). Chest 133(6 Suppl):71S-109S.

Hoffmeyer S, Burk O, von Richter O, Arnold HP, Brockmoller J, Johne A, Cascorbi I, Gerloff T, Roots I, Eichelbaum M and others. 2000. Functional polymorphisms of the human multidrug-resistance gene: multiple sequence variations and correlation of one allele with P-glycoprotein expression and activity in vivo. Proc Natl Acad Sci U S A 97(7):3473-8.

Holbrook AM, Pereira JA, Labiris R, McDonald H, Douketis JD, Crowther M, Wells PS. 2005. Systematic overview of warfarin and its drug and food interactions. Arch Intern Med 165(10):1095-106.

Holmes DR, Jr., Dehmer GJ, Kaul S, Leifer D, O'Gara PT, Stein CM. 2010. ACCF/AHA clopidogrel clinical alert: approaches to the FDA "boxed warning": a report of the American College of Cardiology Foundation Task Force on clinical expert consensus documents and the American Heart Association endorsed by the Society for Cardiovascular Angiography and Interventions and the Society of Thoracic Surgeons. J Am Coll Cardiol 56(4):321-41.

Huang E, Ishida S, Pittman J, Dressman H, Bild A, Kloos M, D'Amico M, Pestell RG, West M, Nevins JR. 2003. Gene expression phenotypic models that predict the activity of oncogenic pathways. Nat Genet 34(2):226-30.

Hughes B. 2010.First oral warfarin alternative approved in the US. Nat Rev Drug Discov 9(12):903-6.

Jakubowski JA, Winters KJ, Naganuma H, Wallentin L. 2007. Prasugrel: a novel thienopyridine antiplatelet agent. A review of preclinical and clinical studies and the mechanistic basis for its distinct antiplatelet profile. Cardiovasc Drug Rev 25(4):357-74.

Kamali F, Wynne H. 2010. Pharmacogenetics of warfarin. Annu Rev Med 61:63-75.

Kaminsky LS, Zhang ZY. 1997. Human P450 metabolism of warfarin. Pharmacol Ther 73(1):67-74.

Kanagasabapathy P, Chowdary P, Gatt A. 2010. Alternatives to Warfarin-The Next Generation of Anticoagulants. Cardiovasc Ther.

Klein TE, Altman RB, Eriksson N, Gage BF, Kimmel SE, Lee MT, Limdi NA, Page D, Roden DM, Wagner MJ and others. 2009. Estimation of the warfarin dose with clinical and pharmacogenetic data. N Engl J Med 360(8):753-64.

Kroese M, Zimmern RL, Pinder SE. 2007. HER2 status in breast cancer--an example of pharmacogenetic testing. J R Soc Med 100(7):326-9.

Lamba JK, Lin YS, Schuetz EG, Thummel KE. 2002. Genetic contribution to variable human CYP3A-mediated metabolism. Adv Drug Deliv Rev 54(10):1271-94.

Lau WC, Gurbel PA, Watkins PB, Neer CJ, Hopp AS, Carville DG, Guyer KE, Tait AR, Bates ER. 2004. Contribution of hepatic cytochrome P450 3A4 metabolic activity to the phenomenon of clopidogrel resistance. Circulation 109(2):166-71.

Lepantalo A, Mikkelsson J, Resendiz JC, Viiri L, Backman JT, Kankuri E, Karhunen PJ, Lassila R. 2006. Polymorphisms of COX-1 and GPVI associate with the antiplatelet effect of aspirin in coronary artery disease patients. Thromb Haemost 95(2):253-9.

Lev EI, Patel RT, Guthikonda S, Lopez D, Bray PF, Kleiman NS. 2007. Genetic polymorphisms of the platelet receptors P2Y(12), P2Y(1) and GP IIIa and response to aspirin and clopidogrel. Thromb Res 119(3):355-60.

Li T, Chang CY, Jin DY, Lin PJ, Khvorova A, Stafford DW. 2004. Identification of the gene for vitamin K epoxide reductase. Nature 427(6974):541-4.

Limdi NA, Arnett DK, Goldstein JA, Beasley TM, McGwin G, Adler BK, Acton RT. 2008. Influence of CYP2C9 and VKORC1 on warfarin dose, anticoagulation attainment and maintenance among European-Americans and African-Americans. Pharmacogenomics 9(5):511-26.

Limdi NA, Wadelius M, Cavallari L, Eriksson N, Crawford DC, Lee MT, Chen CH, Motsinger-Reif A, Sagreiya H, Liu N and others. 2010. Warfarin pharmacogenetics: a single VKORC1 polymorphism is predictive of dose across 3 racial groups. Blood 115(18):3827-34.

Lindh JD, Holm L, Andersson ML, Rane A. 2009. Influence of CYP2C9 genotype on warfarin dose requirements--a systematic review and meta-analysis. Eur J Clin Pharmacol 65(4):365-75.

Lloyd-Jones D, Adams R, Carnethon M, De Simone G, Ferguson TB, Flegal K, Ford E, Furie K, Go A, Greenlund K and others. 2009. Heart disease and stroke statistics--2009 update: a report from the American Heart Association Statistics Committee and Stroke Statistics Subcommittee. Circulation 119(3):e21-181.

Loebstein R, Dvoskin I, Halkin H, Vecsler M, Lubetsky A, Rechavi G, Amariglio N, Cohen Y, Ken-Dror G, Almog S and others. 2007. A coding VKORC1 Asp36Tyr polymorphism predisposes to warfarin resistance. Blood 109(6):2477-80.

Loebstein R, Vecsler M, Kurnik D, Austerweil N, Gak E, Halkin H, Almog S. 2005. Common genetic variants of microsomal epoxide hydrolase affect warfarin dose requirements beyond the effect of cytochrome P450 2C9. Clin Pharmacol Ther 77(5):365-72.

Lordkipanidze M, Pharand C, Schampaert E, Turgeon J, Palisaitis DA, Diodati JG. 2007. A comparison of six major platelet function tests to determine the prevalence of aspirin resistance in patients with stable coronary artery disease. Eur Heart J 28(14):1702-8.

Macchi L, Christiaens L, Brabant S, Sorel N, Ragot S, Allal J, Mauco G, Brizard A. 2003. Resistance in vitro to low-dose aspirin is associated with platelet PlA1 (GP IIIa) polymorphism but not with C807T(GP Ia/IIa) and C-5T Kozak (GP Ibalpha) polymorphisms. J Am Coll Cardiol 42(6):1115-9.

Mackman N. 2008. Triggers, targets and treatments for thrombosis. Nature 451(7181):914-8.

Manolio TA. 2010. Genomewide association studies and assessment of the risk of disease. N Engl J Med 363(2):166-76.

Manolopoulos VG, Ragia G, Tavridou A. 2010. Pharmacogenetics of coumarinic oral anticoagulants. Pharmacogenomics 11(4):493-6.

Maree AO, Curtin RJ, Chubb A, Dolan C, Cox D, O'Brien J, Crean P, Shields DC, Fitzgerald DJ. 2005. Cyclooxygenase-1 haplotype modulates platelet response to aspirin. J Thromb Haemost 3(10):2340-5.

McDonald MG, Rieder MJ, Nakano M, Hsia CK, Rettie AE. 2009. CYP4F2 is a vitamin K1 oxidase: An explanation for altered warfarin dose in carriers of the V433M variant. Mol Pharmacol 75(6):1337-46.

Mega JL, Close SL, Wiviott SD, Shen L, Hockett RD, Brandt JT, Walker JR, Antman EM, Macias W, Braunwald E and others. 2009a. Cytochrome p-450 polymorphisms and response to clopidogrel. N Engl J Med 360(4):354-62.

Mega JL, Close SL, Wiviott SD, Shen L, Hockett RD, Brandt JT, Walker JR, Antman EM, Macias WL, Braunwald E and others. 2009b. Cytochrome P450 genetic polymorphisms and the response to prasugrel: relationship to pharmacokinetic, pharmacodynamic, and clinical outcomes. Circulation 119(19):2553-60.

Mega JL, Close SL, Wiviott SD, Shen L, Walker JR, Simon T, Antman EM, Braunwald E, Sabatine MS. 2010a. Genetic variants in ABCB1 and CYP2C19 and cardiovascular outcomes after treatment with clopidogrel and prasugrel in the TRITON-TIMI 38 trial: a pharmacogenetic analysis. Lancet 376(9749):1312-9.

Mega JL, Simon T, Collet JP, Anderson JL, Antman EM, Bliden K, Cannon CP, Danchin N, Giusti B, Gurbel P and others. 2010b. Reduced-function CYP2C19 genotype and risk of adverse clinical outcomes among patients treated with clopidogrel predominantly for PCI: a meta-analysis. Jama 304(16):1821-30.

Mehta J, Mehta P, Burger C, Pepine CJ. 1978. Platelet aggregation studies in coronary artery disease. Past 4. Effect of aspirin. Atherosclerosis 31(2):169-75.

Melnikova I. 2009. The anticoagulants market. Nat Rev Drug Discov 8(5):353-4.

Michelson AD. 2010. Antiplatelet therapies for the treatment of cardiovascular disease. Nat Rev Drug Discov 9(2):154-69.

Momary KM, Shapiro NL, Viana MA, Nutescu EA, Helgason CM, Cavallari LH. 2007. Factors influencing warfarin dose requirements in African-Americans. Pharmacogenomics 8(11):1535-44.

Motulsky AG. 1965. The Genetics of Abnormal Drug Responses. Ann N Y Acad Sci 123:167-77.

Moyer TP, O'Kane DJ, Baudhuin LM, Wiley CL, Fortini A, Fisher PK, Dupras DM, Chaudhry R, Thapa P, Zinsmeister AR and others. 2009. Warfarin sensitivity genotyping: a review of the literature and summary of patient experience. Mayo Clin Proc 84(12):1079-94.

Muller I, Besta F, Schulz C, Massberg S, Schonig A, Gawaz M. 2003. Prevalence of clopidogrel non-responders among patients with stable angina pectoris scheduled for elective coronary stent placement. Thromb Haemost 89(5):783-7.

Musallam KM, Charafeddine K, Bitar A, Khoury M, Assaad S, Beresian J, Alam S, Taher AT. 2011. Resistance to aspirin and clopidogrel therapy. Int J Lab Hematol 33(1):1-18.

Mushiroda T, Ohnishi Y, Saito S, Takahashi A, Kikuchi Y, Saito S, Shimomura H, Wanibuchi Y, Suzuki T, Kamatani N and others. 2006. Association of VKORC1 and CYP2C9 polymorphisms with warfarin dose requirements in Japanese patients. J Hum Genet 51(3):249-53.

Owen A, Goldring C, Morgan P, Chadwick D, Park BK, Pirmohamed M. 2005. Relationship between the C3435T and G2677T(A) polymorphisms in the ABCB1 gene and P-glycoprotein expression in human liver. Br J Clin Pharmacol 59(3):365-70.

Papp E, Havasi V, Bene J, Komlosi K, Czopf L, Magyar E, Feher C, Feher G, Horvath B, Marton Z and others. 2005. Glycoprotein IIIA gene (PlA) polymorphism and aspirin resistance: is there any correlation? Ann Pharmacother 39(6):1013-8.

Pare G, Mehta SR, Yusuf S, Anand SS, Connolly SJ, Hirsh J, Simonsen K, Bhatt DL, Fox KA, Eikelboom JW. 2010. Effects of CYP2C19 genotype on outcomes of clopidogrel treatment. N Engl J Med 363(18):1704-14.

Patrono C, Baigent C, Hirsh J, Roth G. 2008. Antiplatelet drugs: American College of Chest Physicians Evidence-Based Clinical Practice Guidelines (8th Edition). Chest 133(6 Suppl):199S-233S.

Perez-Andreu V, Roldan V, Anton AI, Garcia-Barbera N, Corral J, Vicente V, Gonzalez-Conejero R. 2009. Pharmacogenetic relevance of CYP4F2 V433M polymorphism on acenocoumarol therapy. Blood 113(20):4977-9.

Rettie AE, Wienkers LC, Gonzalez FJ, Trager WF, Korzekwa KR. 1994. Impaired (S)-warfarin metabolism catalysed by the R144C allelic variant of CYP2C9. Pharmacogenetics 4(1):39-42.

Rieder MJ, Reiner AP, Gage BF, Nickerson DA, Eby CS, McLeod HL, Blough DK, Thummel KE, Veenstra DL, Rettie AE. 2005. Effect of VKORC1 haplotypes on transcriptional regulation and warfarin dose. N Engl J Med 352(22):2285-93.

Rost S, Fregin A, Ivaskevicius V, Conzelmann E, Hortnagel K, Pelz HJ, Lappegard K, Seifried E, Scharrer I, Tuddenham EG and others. 2004. Mutations in VKORC1 cause warfarin resistance and multiple coagulation factor deficiency type 2. Nature 427(6974):537-41.

Sacco RL, Adams R, Albers G, Alberts MJ, Benavente O, Furie K, Goldstein LB, Gorelick P, Halperin J, Harbaugh R and others. 2006. Guidelines for prevention of stroke in patients with ischemic stroke or transient ischemic attack: a statement for healthcare professionals from the American Heart Association/American Stroke Association Council on Stroke: co-sponsored by the Council on Cardiovascular

Radiology and Intervention: the American Academy of Neurology affirms the value of this guideline. Circulation 113(10):e409-49.

Sadee W, Dai Z. 2005. Pharmacogenetics/genomics and personalized medicine. Hum Mol Genet 14 Spec No. 2:R207-14.

Sagreiya H, Berube C, Wen A, Ramakrishnan R, Mir A, Hamilton A, Altman RB. 2010. Extending and evaluating a warfarin dosing algorithm that includes CYP4F2 and pooled rare variants of CYP2C9. Pharmacogenet Genomics 20(7):407-13.

Sanderson S, Emery J, Higgins J. 2005. CYP2C9 gene variants, drug dose, and bleeding risk in warfarin-treated patients: a HuGEnet systematic review and meta-analysis. Genet Med 7(2):97-104.

Santos MT, Valles J, Marcus AJ, Safier LB, Broekman MJ, Islam N, Ullman HL, Eiroa AM, Aznar J. 1991. Enhancement of platelet reactivity and modulation of eicosanoid production by intact erythrocytes. A new approach to platelet activation and recruitment. J Clin Invest 87(2):571-80.

Schelleman H, Chen Z, Kealey C, Whitehead AS, Christie J, Price M, Brensinger CM, Newcomb CW, Thorn CF, Samaha FF and others. 2007. Warfarin response and vitamin K epoxide reductase complex 1 in African Americans and Caucasians. Clin Pharmacol Ther 81(5):742-7.

Sconce EA, Khan TI, Wynne HA, Avery P, Monkhouse L, King BP, Wood P, Kesteven P, Daly AK, Kamali F. 2005. The impact of CYP2C9 and VKORC1 genetic polymorphism and patient characteristics upon warfarin dose requirements: proposal for a new dosing regimen. Blood 106(7):2329-33.

Scott SA, Edelmann L, Kornreich R, Desnick RJ. 2008. Warfarin pharmacogenetics: CYP2C9 and VKORC1 genotypes predict different sensitivity and resistance frequencies in the Ashkenazi and Sephardi Jewish populations. Am J Hum Genet 82(2):495-500.

Shuldiner AR, O'Connell JR, Bliden KP, Gandhi A, Ryan K, Horenstein RB, Damcott CM, Pakyz R, Tantry US, Gibson Q and others. 2009. Association of cytochrome P450 2C19 genotype with the antiplatelet effect and clinical efficacy of clopidogrel therapy. Jama 302(8):849-57.

Simon T, Verstuyft C, Mary-Krause M, Quteineh L, Drouet E, Meneveau N, Steg PG, Ferrieres J, Danchin N, Becquemont L. 2009. Genetic determinants of response to clopidogrel and cardiovascular events. N Engl J Med 360(4):363-75.

Snoep JD, Hovens MM, Eikenboom JC, van der Bom JG, Huisman MV. 2007. Association of laboratory-defined aspirin resistance with a higher risk of recurrent cardiovascular events: a systematic review and meta-analysis. Arch Intern Med 167(15):1593-9.

Sofi F, Marcucci R, Gori AM, Giusti B, Abbate R, Gensini GF. 2010. Clopidogrel non-responsiveness and risk of cardiovascular morbidity. An updated meta-analysis. Thromb Haemost 103(4):841-8.

Stehle S, Kirchheiner J, Lazar A, Fuhr U. 2008. Pharmacogenetics of oral anticoagulants: a basis for dose individualization. Clin Pharmacokinet 47(9):565-94.

Steinhubl SR, Berger PB, Mann JT, 3rd, Fry ET, DeLago A, Wilmer C, Topol EJ. 2002. Early and sustained dual oral antiplatelet therapy following percutaneous coronary intervention: a randomized controlled trial. Jama 288(19):2411-20.

Suh JW, Koo BK, Zhang SY, Park KW, Cho JY, Jang IJ, Lee DS, Sohn DW, Lee MM, Kim HS. 2006. Increased risk of atherothrombotic events associated with cytochrome P450 3A5 polymorphism in patients taking clopidogrel. Cmaj 174(12):1715-22.

Takahashi H, Kashima T, Nomoto S, Iwade K, Tainaka H, Shimizu T, Nomizo Y, Muramoto N, Kimura S, Echizen H. 1998. Comparisons between in-vitro and in-vivo metabolism of (S)-warfarin: catalytic activities of cDNA-expressed CYP2C9, its Leu359 variant and their mixture versus unbound clearance in patients with the corresponding CYP2C9 genotypes. Pharmacogenetics 8(5):365-73.

Takahashi H, Wilkinson GR, Nutescu EA, Morita T, Ritchie MD, Scordo MG, Pengo V, Barban M, Padrini R, Ieiri I and others. 2006. Different contributions of polymorphisms in VKORC1 and CYP2C9 to intra- and inter-population differences in maintenance dose of warfarin in Japanese, Caucasians and African-Americans. Pharmacogenet Genomics 16(2):101-10.

Takeuchi F, McGinnis R, Bourgeois S, Barnes C, Eriksson N, Soranzo N, Whittaker P, Ranganath V, Kumanduri V, McLaren W and others. 2009. A genome-wide association study confirms VKORC1, CYP2C9, and CYP4F2 as principal genetic determinants of warfarin dose. PLoS Genet 5(3):e1000433.

Taubert D, von Beckerath N, Grimberg G, Lazar A, Jung N, Goeser T, Kastrati A, Schomig A, Schomig E. 2006. Impact of P-glycoprotein on clopidogrel absorption. Clin Pharmacol Ther 80(5):486-501.

Teichert M, van Schaik RH, Hofman A, Uitterlinden AG, de Smet PA, Stricker BH, Visser LE. 2009. Genotypes associated with reduced activity of VKORC1 and CYP2C9 and their modification of acenocoumarol anticoagulation during the initial treatment period. Clin Pharmacol Ther 85(4):379-86.

Trenk D, Hochholzer W, Fromm MF, Chialda LE, Pahl A, Valina CM, Stratz C, Schmiebusch P, Bestehorn HP, Buttner HJ and others. 2008. Cytochrome P450 2C19 681G>A polymorphism and high on-clopidogrel platelet reactivity associated with adverse 1-year clinical outcome of elective percutaneous coronary intervention with drug-eluting or bare-metal stents. J Am Coll Cardiol 51(20):1925-34.

Varmus H. 2010. Ten years on--the human genome and medicine. N Engl J Med 362(21):2028-9.

Veenstra DL, You JH, Rieder MJ, Farin FM, Wilkerson HW, Blough DK, Cheng G, Rettie AE. 2005. Association of Vitamin K epoxide reductase complex 1 (VKORC1) variants with warfarin dose in a Hong Kong Chinese patient population. Pharmacogenet Genomics 15(10):687-91.

Venter JC. 2010. Multiple personal genomes await. Nature 464(7289):676-7.

Wadelius M, Chen LY, Eriksson N, Bumpstead S, Ghori J, Wadelius C, Bentley D, McGinnis R, Deloukas P. 2007. Association of warfarin dose with genes involved in its action and metabolism. Hum Genet 121(1):23-34.

Wadelius M, Chen LY, Lindh JD, Eriksson N, Ghori MJ, Bumpstead S, Holm L, McGinnis R, Rane A, Deloukas P. 2009. The largest prospective warfarin-treated cohort supports genetic forecasting. Blood 113(4):784-92.

Wallentin L, Becker RC, Budaj A, Cannon CP, Emanuelsson H, Held C, Horrow J, Husted S, James S, Katus H and others. 2009. Ticagrelor versus clopidogrel in patients with acute coronary syndromes. N Engl J Med 361(11):1045-57.

Wallentin L, James S, Storey RF, Armstrong M, Barratt BJ, Horrow J, Husted S, Katus H, Steg PG, Shah SH and others. 2010a. Effect of CYP2C19 and ABCB1 single nucleotide polymorphisms on outcomes of treatment with ticagrelor versus clopidogrel for acute coronary syndromes: a genetic substudy of the PLATO trial. Lancet 376(9749):1320-8.

Wallentin L, Yusuf S, Ezekowitz MD, Alings M, Flather M, Franzosi MG, Pais P, Dans A, Eikelboom J, Oldgren J and others. 2010b. Efficacy and safety of dabigatran compared with warfarin at different levels of international normalised ratio control for stroke prevention in atrial fibrillation: an analysis of the RE-LY trial. Lancet 376(9745):975-83.

Wang L, McLeod HL, Weinshilboum RM. 2011. Genomics and drug response. N Engl J Med 364(12):1144-53.

Wang TH, Bhatt DL, Topol EJ. 2006. Aspirin and clopidogrel resistance: an emerging clinical entity. Eur Heart J 27(6):647-54.

Watzka M, Geisen C, Bevans CG, Sittinger K, Spohn G, Rost S, Seifried E, Muller CR, Oldenburg J. 2011. Thirteen novel VKORC1 mutations associated with oral anticoagulant resistance: insights into improved patient diagnosis and treatment. J Thromb Haemost 9(1):109-18.

Weinshilboum RM, Wang L. 2006. Pharmacogenetics and pharmacogenomics: development, science, and translation. Annu Rev Genomics Hum Genet 7:223-45.

Wiviott SD, Braunwald E, McCabe CH, Montalescot G, Ruzyllo W, Gottlieb S, Neumann FJ, Ardissino D, De Servi S, Murphy SA and others. 2007. Prasugrel versus clopidogrel in patients with acute coronary syndromes. N Engl J Med 357(20):2001-15.

Woodcock J. 2010. Assessing the clinical utility of diagnostics used in drug therapy. Clin Pharmacol Ther 88(6):765-73.

Wu AH. 2007. Use of genetic and nongenetic factors in warfarin dosing algorithms. Pharmacogenomics 8(7):851-61.

Wynne H, Cope L, Kelly P, Whittingham T, Edwards C, Kamali F. 1995. The influence of age, liver size and enantiomer concentrations on warfarin requirements. Br J Clin Pharmacol 40(3):203-7.

Wysowski DK, Nourjah P, Swartz L. 2007. Bleeding complications with warfarin use: a prevalent adverse effect resulting in regulatory action. Arch Intern Med 167(13):1414-9.

Yusuf S, Zhao F, Mehta SR, Chrolavicius S, Tognoni G, Fox KK. 2001. Effects of clopidogrel in addition to aspirin in patients with acute coronary syndromes without ST-segment elevation. N Engl J Med 345(7):494-502.

Zambon CF, Pengo V, Padrini R, Basso D, Schiavon S, Fogar P, Nisi A, Frigo AC, Moz S, Pelloso M and others. 2011.VKORC1, CYP2C9 and CYP4F2 genetic-based algorithm for warfarin dosing: an Italian retrospective study. Pharmacogenomics 12(1):15-25.

Zhang W, Huang RS, Dolan ME. 2008. Integrating Epigenomics into Pharmacogenomic
    Studies. Pharmgenomics Pers Med 2008(1):7-14.
Zuern CS, Lindemann S, Gawaz M. 2009. Platelet function and response to aspirin: gender-
    specific features and implications for female thrombotic risk and management.
    Semin Thromb Hemost. 35(3):295-306.

Part 4

Emerging Role of
Pharmacogenetics in Other Disciplines

8

Neuropharmacogenetics of Major Depression: Has the Time Come to Take both Sexes into Account?

Pothitos M. Pitychoutis, Despina Sanoudou,
Christina Dalla and Zeta Papadopoulou-Daifoti
Department of Pharmacology, Medical School,
National and Kapodistrian University of Athens
Greece

1. Introduction

According to the *World Health Organization* (WHO), by 2020 depression is expected to rise to the number two contributor to global burden of disease (WHO, 2005). However according to recent reports, depression comprises the most costly brain disorder in Europe, accounting for 33% of the total cost that corresponds to about 1% of the European gross domestic product (GDP) (Sobocki et al., 2006). Despite the fact that our knowledge regarding the pathophysiology and the neurobiological substrate of depression has grown exponentially over the last decades, there is still a significant percentage of patients who respond poorly or do not tolerate current antidepressant pharmacotherapies (Rush, 2007). Most likely, the latter reflects the fact that the term "depression" encompasses a group of disorders, with each being characterized by a unique *endophenotype* that deserves tailor-made treatment strategies (Hasler et al., 2004; Antonijevic, 2006).

Major depression is a leading cause of disability among women 15-44 years and twice as many women as men suffer from this debilitating condition annually (Kessler et al., 1994; Young et al., 2009). Paradoxically, research regarding the neurobiological substrate of depressive disorders, as well as response to antidepressant medications has focused almost exclusively on the male sex. However, as noted in a recent review, evidence exist that genetic variations in *loci* related to central neurotransmitter and neuromodulatory systems, may be implicated in the sex-differentiated manifestation of depressive symptomatology and differential responsiveness to various antidepressant drugs (Pitychoutis et al., 2010a).

The selective serotonin (5-hydroxytryptamine; 5-HT) reuptake inhibitors (SSRIs) comprise the most widely prescribed class of antidepressants worldwide. However, they present with variable therapeutic efficacy, which is often accompanied by numerous side-effects. Most importantly, the protracted period of time (3-4 weeks) in order for these agents to induce a clinically meaningful improvement in depressive symptomatology has been associated with increased drop-out rates. Not surprisingly, only 60-65% of adult depressed patients respond to the first course of therapy and among responders less than half either reach remission or become free of symptoms (Rosenzweig-Lipson *et al.*, 2007). Thus, the need for more effective pharmacotherapies to combat depression is an ever-growing concern due to the enormous societal and financial ramifications of these disorders.

The present chapter focuses on current advances in the field of pharmacogenetics of major depression under the prism of sex differences. In order to treat depression, a personalized approach including better-targeted therapies may be needed. Understanding sex differences in response to antidepressant medications is a major step towards this direction.

2. Sex differences in major depression

Major depression occurs more frequently in women than in men. Despite the fact that the aetiology behind this sex difference is still elusive, scientists agree that it possibly reflects a complex genetic, hormonal, biochemical and social interplay. Prior to puberty, no significant differences are detected regarding the precipitation of depressive symptomatology between the male and the female sex (Kuehner, 2003), whereas during the reproductive period women appear to experience major depression at roughly twice the rate of men (Marcus *et al.*, 2005; Grigoriadis & Robinson, 2007; Pitychoutis & Papadopoulou-Daifoti, 2010). Of note, an increasing amount of data suggests that associations between stressful interpersonal events and depression are stronger in women than in men (Oldehinkel & Bouma, 2011).

Interestingly, in depression, a sex-specific symptom pattern may occur. According to some reports men seem to lose more weight while women tend to report more appetite and weight increase, accompanied by hypochondriasis and somatic concerns (Young *et al.*, 1990; Kornstein *et al.*, 2000b). More recently, Marcus *et al.* (2005) analyzed data from the STAR*D (Sequenced Treatment Alternatives to Relieve Depression) multicenter trial; in this sample women reported an earlier onset of the first major depressive episode, as well as a trend towards a greater length of the current episode. In the same study, alcohol and drug dependence were more common in men. Importantly, even though women reported greater likelihood of having attempted a suicide in the past, men were characterized by greater psychomotor agitation and suicidal ideation (Marcus *et al.*, 2005).

Even though these statistics have been partly attributed to the fact that women are more likely to seek psychiatric assistance in view of a negative affective *status* and to be over-diagnosed with major depression compared to men (Grigoriadis & Robinson, 2007), nowadays there is enough evidence for sex-differentiated biological pathways in affective disorders. Notably, a variety of serotonergic sexual dimorphisms have been hypothesized to confer increased vulnerability of females to depression. In this context, whole brain 5-HT synthesis and 5-HT$_2$ receptor binding have been reported to be lower in several regions of the female brain (for review see Rubinow *et al.*, 1998).

3. Sex differences in antidepressant response: Insights from the clinic and from animal models of depression

Converging albeit inconclusive evidence support the existence of a sex-differentiated responsiveness to antidepressant drugs (Dalla *et al.*, 2011; Sloan & Kornstein, 2003; Marcus *et* *al.*, 2005). Indeed, earlier studies reported that women presented a slower response to tricyclic antidepressants (TCAs) (Prange *et al.*, 1969), while also being less likely to achieve remission (Glassman *et al.*, 1977). In an intriguing study conducted in a sample of 235 male and 400 female depressed outpatients, women were more likely to show a favourable response to the SSRI sertraline than to the TCA imipramine, while the opposite association seemed to hold true for men (Kornstein *et al.*, 2000a). This sex-differentiated interplay was also accompanied by a sex-based adverse effect profile; while depressed men treated with imipramine reported sexual dysfunction, urinary frequency and dyspepsia at a higher percentage, depressed women treated with sertraline complained more frequently about nausea and dizziness (Kornstein *et al.*, 2000a). The STAR*D is the largest study of major depression ever conducted in the US and the largest to address sex differences in prospective treatment using a representative sample of 2,876 treatment-seeking depressed patients (Rush *et al.*, 2004; Young *et al.*, 2009). Using data from this study, Young *et al.* (2009) reported that women that received the SSRI citalopram for 12-14 weeks presented 33% greater likelihood of remission as compared to male depressed patients (Young *et al.*, 2009). Importantly, this sex difference was attributed to sex-specific biological differences in the serotonergic system (Young *et al.*, 2009). However, it should be noted that other studies have not detected sex-related effects of antidepressants in humans. For instance, Quitkin *et al.* (2002) found no significant difference in response to the SSRI fluoxetine in a sample of 840 outpatients. In another study, Thiels *et al.* (2005) did not report a significant difference in response to 6-month treatment with the SSRI sertraline. Therefore, the clinical significance of these findings still remains controversial (Quitkin *et al.*, 2002; Hildebrandt *et al.*, 2003; Thiels *et al.*, 2005).

Sex differences in response to antidepressant pharmacotherapy have been largely attributed to the sex-differentiated pharmacokinetic disposition of psychotropic agents. Studies in humans and in laboratory animals have shown that females are characterized by increased levels of hepatic cytochrome P450 (CYP) 3A. Thus, it has been suggested that over-expression of CYP3A, may modulate the effectiveness of drugs in women (Paine *et al.*, 2005; Waxman & Holloway, 2009). Moreover, the estrogen-altering oral contraceptives and hormonal replacement therapies may ultimately influence the pharmacokinetic disposition of antidepressants (Yonkers *et al.*, 1992; Hildebrandt *et al.*, 2003). Despite the fact that available pharmacokinetic evidence indicates that women should perhaps receive lower doses of antidepressants as compared to men, current guidelines do not suggest that men and women should be dosed in a sex-based manner (Kokras *et al.*, 2011).

The clinical finding of a sex-differentiated antidepressant response has also been validated in preclinical research (Dalla *et al.*, 2010; 2011). For instance, in a most recent study we reported that male rats may benefit to a greater extent when treated chronically with the TCA clomipramine (Pitychoutis *et al.* 2011). We further revealed that individual differences in response to novelty may predict differential responsiveness to clomipramine treatment and are associated with qualitative and quantitative sex-related behavioral and neurochemical alterations (Pitychoutis *et al.* 2011). Further, clomipramine treatment may induce sex-differentiated effects on cellular immunoreactivity in the chronic mild stress (CMS) model of depression, with female rats presenting a relatively immunosuppressed phenotype as compared to males (Pitychoutis *et al.*, 2009; Pitychoutis et al., 2010b). Moreover, 2 weeks of clomipramine treatment in the Flinders Sensitive Line (FSL) rats, a putative genetic model of depression, induced sex-related effects on behavioral despair, as assessed in the forced swim test (FST), that were accompanied by sexually dimorphic serotonergic alterations in several limbic brain regions (Kokras *et al.*, 2009).

4. Sex differences in the pharmacogenetics of antidepressants

Pharmacogenetics investigates how genes influence responsiveness to drugs, both in terms of efficacy and adverse effects. The ultimate goal of this scientific field is to provide "tailor-made" pharmacotherapies based on the genetic constitution of the individual. Importantly, genetic prediction of antidepressant response has the potential to facilitate an informed choice of agent and a patient-tailored dose in order for response rates to be significantly improved and adverse effects to be alleviated.

Recent pharmacogenetic research on the impact of sex on antidepressant treatment has focused mostly on SSRIs, because these drugs represent the first-choice of pharmacological intervention for the treatment of major depression worldwide. Given that not all patients respond sufficiently to the initial treatment with an SSRI, non-response has been associated with individual differences in pharmacodynamic processes and in this context has been partly attributed to the polymorphic nature of certain genes related to the metabolism of monoamines, to the serotonergic and other neurobiological systems (Steimer *et al.*, 2001). Multiple genes influencing central monoaminergic neurotransmission have served as targets of vast pharmacogenetic screening. Among these are the rate-limiting enzyme of 5-HT biosynthesis, tryptophan hydroxylase 1 & 2 (TPH1 & TPH2), inactivation enzymes monoamine oxidases A & B (MAO-A; MAO-B) and catechol-O-methyl-transferase (COMT), as well as 5-HT's protein-targets, such as the 5-HT$_{1A}$ receptor (Drago *et al.*, 2009). In humans, there are two distinct TPH genes located on chromosomes 11 and 12, coding for two different homologous enzymes, with TPH2 being the predominant isoform in the CNS (Walther & Bader, 2003).

Therefore, sedulous research on whether/which DNA polymorphisms are somehow involved in SSRI responsiveness and if these vary between the two sexes, is of great importance for improving the clinical care of depressed patients.

4.1 Genes related to the metabolism of monoamines

Three monoamine-related genes have been associated to date with a sex-dependent antidepressant response (Table 1). The MAO-A gene is located on the X chromosome in humans, is expressed on the outer mitochondrial membrane where it catabolizes the intraneuronal deamination of dopamine (DA), norepinephrine (NA), and 5-HT. A prominent variable number tandem repeat (VNTR) polymorphism consists of a 30 base pair repeated sequence present in 2, 3, 3.5, 4, or 5 repeats (R) at 1.2 kb upstream of the MAO-A gene and affects its enzymatic activity. Specifically, the 3.5R and 4R alleles transcribe 2–10 times more efficiently as compared to 2, 3, or 5R alleles (Muller *et al.*, 2002; Drago *et al.*, 2009). This polymorphism has been associated with the response rates of depressed women to the SSRI fluoxetine in a Chinese patient cohort. According to this study, women carriers of the shorter 3R-allele (low-transcribers of the MAO-A gene) responded better to 4-week fluoxetine treatment as compared to the longer 4R-allele carriers (high-transcribers of the MAO-A gene) (Yu *et al.*, 2005). Notably, no such association was observed among the male population included in this study. Similar findings were observed in a cohort of Caucasian depressed patients, who were treated with various antidepressant drugs (Domschke *et al.*, 2008b). Again, the longer MAO-A alleles were associated with a greater risk of slower and less efficient response in a sex-specific context (i.e. in female patients only). Noteworthy, other studies have failed to detect any effect of this variant on pharmacoresponse in major depression (Cusin *et al.*, 2002; Muller *et al.*, 2002; Peters *et al.*, 2004). A second MAO-A polymorphism (T941G) has been reported to affect treatment response to mirtazapine in a sex-specific manner. Mirtazapine-treated depressed women homozygous for the T-allele showed a faster and better response compared to patients carrying the TG or GG genotype, while in men no association was observed (Tadic *et al.*, 2007a). Another study provided evidence regarding the implication of the functional A644G SNP within intron 13 of the MAO-B gene, in the outcome of treatment with paroxetine only in women with major depression (Tadic *et al.*, 2007b). The aforementioned associations may not be unrelated to the fact that the genes encoding MAO-A and MAO-B are located on the short arm of the X chromosome (Yu *et al.*, 2005).

GENE	GENETIC VARIATION	DRUG	RESULT	REFERENCE
MAO-A	30 bp VNTR (promoter)	fluoxetine	Women with the "*shorter*" 3R/3R genotype responded better to fluoxetine treatment as compared to those with the "*longer*" 4R allele	Yu et al., 2005
MAO-A	30 bp VNTR (promoter)	mirtazapine, citalopram/ escitalopram, venlafaxine and combinations	In women, the "*longer*" alleles were associated with slower and less efficient response to antidepressant treatment	Domschke et al., 2008b
MAO-A	T941G (synonymous; Arg297)	mirtazapine or paroxetine	Women homozygous for the T-allele presented faster and better response to antidepressant treatment as compared to TG/GG-patients	Tadić et al., 2007a
MAO-B	A644G (intron 13)	mirtazapine or paroxetine	Women homozygous for the A-allele showed a clinically meaningful faster and more pronounced response to treatment with paroxetine	Tadić et al., 2007b
COMT	G472A (Val158Met)	fluoxetine	In men, the Val/Val genotype was associated with poorer response to antidepressant treatment	Tsai et al., 2009

Table 1. Sex differences in genetic variants implicated in the metabolism of monoamines.

Depressive symptomatology can be alleviated by SSRI treatment, partly due to the enhancement of the serotonergic tone that in turn enhances dopamine outflow in the reward system of the brain (Naranjo *et al.*, 2001). Given that the COMT enzyme degrades DA, it represents a promising candidate for pharmacogenetics screening. A functional SNP (G472A) that causes a substitution of Valine to Methionine in codon 158 (Val158Met) of the COMT gene results in a three- to four-fold decrement of the enzymatic activity of the membrane-bound isoform (Lachman *et al.*, 1996). Notably, a recent study by Tsai and colleagues (2009) conducted in Chinese depressed patients treated with fluoxetine revealed a sex-dependent association of the COMTVal/Val genotype with poorer antidepressant response, but only in male patients (Tsai *et al.*, 2009).

4.2 Genes specific to serotonergic neurotransmission

A battery of pharmacogenetic studies have focused on genetic variations of the 5-HT transporter (SLC6A4; 5-HTT) gene that is located on chromosome 17 in humans (Table 2; Drago *et al.*, 2009). Perhaps the most interesting is the functional polymorphism on the promoter of the 5-HTT gene, known as 5-HTT gene-linked polymorphic region (5-HTTLPR) that consists of 16 imperfect 22 base pair repeats. The polymorphic nature of this site regards the relative presence/absence of two of the repeats. Thus, their absence produces a shorter allele (S), whereas their presence produces a 44 base-pair longer allele (L). According to this "*bi-allelic scheme*", carriers of the L-allele are characterized by an enhanced expression rate of the 5-HTT, with the opposite holding true for the carriers of the S-allele. Most importantly, it has been hypothesized that L-allele carriers may benefit to a greater extent from antidepressant treatment. This notion has been attributed to a generalized responsiveness of the serotonergic system owing to the enhanced expression/activity of 5-HTT (Serretti *et al.*, 2007). Notably, the 5-HT$_{1A}$ receptor transcription rate is modulated by a variation (C1019G) in the upstream regulatory region of this gene. Indeed, the C-allele appears to be associated with the down-regulation of 5-HT$_{1A}$ receptor that may explain the better response rates to chronic antidepressant treatment (Parsey *et al.*, 2006; Drago *et al.*, 2009).

A recent study by Smits *et al.* (2008) screened the 5-HTTLPR polymorphism of the 5-HTT gene for associations with non-responsiveness to SSRI treatment (Smits *et al.*, 2008). According to these results, the response of male patients of a Caucasian cohort to SSRI treatment was independent of the studied polymorphisms in the 5-HTT locus, whereas in women the 5-HTLPR S-allele was associated with a less favorable response to treatment. These findings replicated in part an earlier study showing that paroxetine efficacy in patients with panic disorder was lower in women with the SS genotype compared to women carrying the L-allele (Perna *et al.*, 2005). Another study lent further support and extended the aforementioned associations; in depressed patients 4-week treatment with either SSRIs or non-SSRI drugs, the S-allele was associated with lower antidepressant efficacy in depressed women but not in men, with this result being significant for both types of medication (Gressier *et al.*, 2009). Importantly, in a follow-up study the same group reported that depressed women with the SS genotype responded poorly to antidepressant treatment as compared to women with LL/LS genotype, whereas no significant difference was detected in men (Gressier *et al.* 2011). Moreover, in the same study, the S-allele was associated with elevated concentrations of thyroid stimulating hormone (TSH) levels in depressed women, thus underlining the important interaction among sex, thyroid function and the serotonergic system (Gressier *et al.* 2011)

A study by Yu *et al.* (2006) further supported the impact of sex in the prediction of the effectiveness of SSRI treatment (Yu *et al.*, 2006). These authors reported that the C/C genotype of the C1019G polymorphism of the 5-HT$_{1A}$ receptor gene may be considered a sex-specific factor for the prediction of a beneficial outcome with fluoxetine treatment, only in female patients of a Chinese cohort.

GENE	GENETIC VARIATION	DRUG	RESULT	REFERENCE
5-HTT	5-HTTLPR (promoter)	SSRIs; paroxetine the most frequently prescribed	Women with the S-allele showed a less favourable response to SSRI treatment	Smits et al., 2008
5-HTT	5-HTTLPR (promoter)	SSRIs and non-SSRIs	The SS genotype was associated with lower antidepressant efficacy with both SSRI and non-SSRI drugs in depressed women but not in men	Gressier et al., 2009
5-HT1A	C1019G (promoter)	fluoxetine	Women with the C/C genotype showed a better response than G-allele carriers	Yu et al., 2006

Table 2. Sex differences in genetic variants that are specific to the serotonergic system.

4.3 Genes related to other neurobiological systems

Genetic variants associated with other neurobiological systems have also been implicated in patients' response to antidepressant agents (Table 3). For instance, the angiotensin I converting enzyme (ACE) gene is expressed in the brain where it degrades several neuropeptides, such as substance P (Skidgel & Erdos, 1987). The latter, has been strongly implicated in the neurobiology of major depression, while antagonists for this neuropeptide have been reported to significantly improve depressive symptoms (Kramer *et al.*, 1998; Nutt, 1998). Research on an insertion/deletion (I/D) polymorphism, represented by the presence/absence of a 287 base pair region within the ACE gene has indicated that the D-allele was associated with faster onset of antidepressant therapy (i.e. SSRIs, TCAs etc), but only in female depressed patients (Baghai *et al.*, 2004).

Preclinical research in animal models implicates the endocannabinoid system both in the pathogenesis of major depression and anxiety, as well as in the mediation of antidepressant response (Martin *et al.*, 2002). In a study conducted in a Caucasian cohort of depressed patients receiving various antidepressant medications, the G-allele of a synonymous polymorphism (G1359A) of the cannabinoid receptor CB1 (CNR1) gene was shown to confer a greater risk for resistance to antidepressant treatment, especially in depressed women with high comorbid anxiety (Domschke et al., 2008a).

Galanin (GAL) is a 30-aminoacid estrogen-inducible neuropeptide that derives from preprogalanin (PPGAL) (Evans & Shine, 1991). GAL is highly expressed in brain regions involved in the regulation of anxiety and depression (Kuteeva et al., 2008). In a recent study Unschuld et al. (2010) reported a female-specific association of symptom severity in premenopausal depressed women with the rare allele of the PPGAL SNP rs948854. In particular, premenopausal depressed women carriers of the G-allele of rs948854, presented more severe vegetative but not cognitive depressive symptomatology at discharge and worse response to antidepressant medication (Unschuld et al. 2010). According to the authors, these results may be related to the existence of several estrogen-response elements (ERE) in the promoter region of the PPGAL gene that have been held responsible for the estrogenic regulation of GAL expression (Unschuld et al. 2010; Kaplan et al., 1988; Howard et al., 1997).

GENE	GENETIC VARIATION	DRUG	RESULT	REFERENCE
CNR1	G1359A (synonymous; Thr453)	mirtazapine, citalopram/escitalopram, venlafaxine and combinations	In women the G-allele was associated with resistance to antidepressant treatment	Domschke et al., 2008a
ACE	287 bp Insertion/deletion (I/D) polymorphism (intron 16)	TCAs, or SSRIs or dual-acting antidepressants	In women the D-allele predicted faster onset of different antidepressant therapies	Baghai et al., 2004
PPGAL	rs948854 (promoter)	SSRIs, TCAs or mirtazapine	In women the G-allele was associated with worse response to antidepressant treatment	Unschuld et al., 2010

Table 3. Sex differences in genetic variants that are associated with other neurobiological systems.

4.4 Pharmacokinetics genes

Sex differences in antidepressant response have largely been attributed to sex-differentiated pharmacokinetic disposition of psychotropic agents. This notion is supported by the fact that hormonal fluctuations during the menstrual cycle may affect the pharmacokinetics of psychotropic medications (Hildebrandt et al., 2003). Importantly, cytochrome P450 (CYP)-

3A4, CYP2D6, CYP2C19 and CYP1A2 are important for the metabolism of antidepressant drugs (Staddon et al., 2002). Genetic polymorphisms in these CYP genes may account for inter-individual pharmacokinetic disposition of psychotropic medications. However, it is still not known whether these actually have the same effect in both sexes (Kokras *et al.*, 2011). Although sex differences in the pharmacokinetics of antidepressants have been shown to affect response, the clinical relevance of this sex-differentiated response remains to be elucidated (Meibohm *et al.*, 2002; Kokras *et al.*, 2011).

Notably, sex differences in human CYP-catalyzed drug metabolism are well-documented; for instance CYP3A4, the predominant CYP catalyst of oxidative metabolism in human liver, is expressed at a higher protein and mRNA levels in women *versus* men (Waxman & Holloway, 2009). Moreover, sex-differentiated genetic markers of CYP3A4 activity and expression have recently been reported in human liver microsomes (Schirmer et al., 2007). Of note, it is still not clear if sex influences CYP2C19 and CYP2D6 activity in a clinically meaningful way in humans (Scandlyn *et al.*, 2008; Borobia *et al.*, 2009). A recent study reported that both the CYP2D6 genotype and sex influenced the disposition of mirtazapine in a Spanish cohort of healthy volunteers; however, a sex x genotype interaction was not detected (Borobia et al., 2009). In support of the aforementioned findings, CYP2C19 and CYP2D6 polymorphisms were also shown to affect the disposition of citalopram similarly in men and women (Fudio *et al.* 2010).

5. Epimyth and future challenges

The studies reported herein tentatively indicate that variants in genes pertaining to a multitude of central processes may affect antidepressant response in a sex-dependent fashion. Among these are genes modulating the brain's monoaminergic systems (e.g. 5-HTT, 5-HT$_{1A}$ receptor and MAO-A) or even genes related to other fundamental neuromodulatory processes (e.g. ACE and GAL). These differences may stem from the complex crosstalk between sex hormones and genes modulating the monoaminergic systems by modifying gene expression or even epigenetic processes (Petronis, 2001; Damberg, 2005).

It is widely accepted that there is a substantial inter-individual variation in response to antidepressant drugs. Research on the pharmacogenetics of antidepressants aims to identify genetic variants implicated in antidepressant response, in order to both serve as predictor of the outcome and to decipher their complex mechanism of action. However, as noted in recent reviews on this subject-matter, despite the initial enthusiasm, the lack of consistent findings regarding genes regulating pharmacokinetic and pharmacodynamic processes has been frustrating (Keers & Aitchison, 2011). Notably, it is believed that the few phar-macogenetic associations that have been replicated explain only a small fraction of individual differences in response to antidepressant pharmacotherapies (Uher *et al.*, 2010). Still, when novel genetic targets were screened the results appeared to be modest and point to the notion that the genetic control of responsiveness to antidepressants is determined by multiple genetic loci (Keers & Aitchison, 2011).

To this direction, genome-wide association studies (GWAS) have revealed novel genetic variants and regulatory intergenic sequences that may be very important to the mechanism of action of antidepressant drugs. In the Genome-Based Therapeutic Drugs for Depression (GENDEP) project, previously unexpected genes related to neurogenetic and immune processes implicated in the pathophysiology of depression, appeared to serve as potent predictors of antidepressant response in patients treated for 12 weeks with escitalopram (SSRI; N=394) or nortriptyline (TCA; N=312) (Uher *et al.*, 2010). Pharmacogenomic analyses revealed a significant association between the uronyl 2-sulphotransferase (UST) gene and response to nortriptyline. On the other hand, response to escitalopram was predicted by a marker in the gene encoding interleukin-11 (IL-11), with this being further supported by a less robust association in the IL-6 gene (Uher *et al.*, 2010). In another GWAS study, Garriock *et al.* (2010) used the STAR*D sample in order to determine which DNA variations influenced response to citalopram treatment and also implicated novel genes in the mechanism of action of SSRIs (Garriock *et al.*, 2010). Despite the significance of these studies in the field, the role of sex was not determined.

Overall, despite the promising advances in this field, pharmacogenetics-driven, personalized antidepressant pharmacotherapies are still far from being introduced into the clinical practice (Drago *et al.*, 2009). Although it is still early for firm conclusions, the currently available evidence seems to suggest that an intriguing genetic x sex interplay may be associated with the differential responsiveness that the two sexes exhibit upon antidepressant treatment. Therefore, a profound analysis of the role of sex in the pharmacogenetics of depression is considered imperative in order for the clinical significance of this interaction to be determined.

6. Acknowledgment

This work was supported by the European Community's Seventh Framework Programme FP7/2007–2013 under grant agreement No. HEALTH-F2-2009-241526, EUTrigTreat.

7. References

Antonijevic, I.A. (2006). Depressive disorders - is it time to endorse different pathophysiologies? *Psychoneuroendocrinology*, Vol.31, No.1, pp. 1-15, ISSN 0306-4530

Baghai, T.C., Schule, C., Zill, P., Deiml, T., Eser, D., Zwanzger, P., Ella, R., Rupprecht, R. & Bondy, B. (2004). The angiotensin I converting enzyme insertion/deletion polymorphism influences therapeutic outcome in major depressed women, but not in men. *Neurosci Lett*, Vol.363, No.1, pp. 38-42, ISSN 0304-3940

Borobia, A.M., Novalbos, J., Guerra-Lopez, P., Lopez-Rodriguez, R., Tabares, B., Rodriguez, V., Abad-Santos, F. & Carcas, A.J. (2009). Influence of sex and CYP2D6 genotype on mirtazapine disposition, evaluated in Spanish healthy volunteers. *Pharmacol Res*, Vol.59, No.6, pp. 393-398, ISSN 1096-1186

Cusin, C., Serretti, A., Zanardi, R., Lattuada, E., Rossini, D., Lilli, R., Lorenzi, C. & Smeraldi, E. (2002). Influence of monoamine oxidase A and serotonin receptor 2A polymorphisms in SSRI antidepressant activity. *Int J Neuropsychopharmacol*, Vol.5, No.1, pp. 27-35, ISSN 1461-1457

Dalla, C., Pitychoutis, P.M., Kokras, N. & Papadopoulou-Daifoti, Z. (2010). Sex Differences in Animal Models of Depression and Antidepressant Response. *Basic & Clinical Pharmacology & Toxicology*, Vol.106, No.3, pp. 226-233, ISSN 1742-7835

Dalla, C., Pitychoutis, P.M., Kokras, N., Papadopoulou-Daifoti, Z., (2011) Sex differences in response to stress and expression of depressive-like behaviours in the rat. *Curr Top Behav Neurosci.* Vol.8 pp. 97-118, DOI: 10.1007/7854_2010_94

Damberg, M. (2005). Transcription factor AP-2 and monoaminergic functions in the central nervous system. *J Neural Transm*, Vol.112, No.10, pp. 1281-1296, ISSN 0300-9564

Domschke, K., Dannlowski, U., Ohrmann, P., Lawford, B., Bauer, J., Kugel, H., Heindel, W., Young, R., Morris, P., Arolt, V., Deckert, J., Suslow, T. & Baune, B.T. (2008a). Cannabinoid receptor 1 (CNR1) gene: impact on antidepressant treatment response and emotion processing in major depression. *Eur Neuropsychopharmacol*, Vol.18, No.10, pp. 751-759, ISSN 0924-977X

Domschke, K., Hohoff, C., Mortensen, L.S., Roehrs, T., Deckert, J., Arolt, V. & Baune, B.T. (2008b). Monoamine oxidase A variant influences antidepressant treatment response in female patients with Major Depression. *Prog Neuropsychopharmacol Biol Psychiatry*, Vol.32, No.1, pp. 224-228, ISSN 0278-5846

Drago, A., De Ronchi, D. & Serretti, A. (2009). Pharmacogenetics of antidepressant response: an update. *Hum Genomics*, Vol.3, No.3, pp. 257-274, ISSN 1479-7364

Evans, H.F. & Shine, J. (1991). Human galanin: molecular cloning reveals a unique structure. *Endocrinology*, Vol.129, No.3, pp. 1682-1684, ISSN 0013-7227

Fudio, S., Borobia, A.M., Pinana, E., Ramirez, E., Tabares, B., Guerra, P., Carcas, A. & Frias, J. (2010) Evaluation of the influence of sex and CYP2C19 and CYP2D6 polymorphisms in the disposition of citalopram. *Eur J Pharmacol*, Vol.626, No.2-3, pp. 200-204, ISSN 1879-0712

Garriock, H.A., Kraft, J.B., Shyn, S.I., Peters, E.J., Yokoyama, J.S., Jenkins, G.D., Reinalda, M.S., Slager, S.L., McGrath, P.J. & Hamilton, S.P. (2010). A Genomewide Association Study of Citalopram Response in Major Depressive Disorder. *Biological Psychiatry*, Vol.67, No.2, pp. 133-138, ISSN 0006-3223

Glassman, A.H., Perel, J.M., Shostak, M., Kantor, S.J. & Fleiss, J.L. (1977). Clinical implications of imipramine plasma levels for depressive illness. *Arch Gen Psychiatry*, Vol.34, No.2, pp. 197-204, ISSN 0003-990X

Gressier, F., Bouaziz, E., Verstuyft, C., Hardy, P., Becquemont, L. & Corruble, E. (2009). 5-HTTLPR modulates antidepressant efficacy in depressed women. *Psychiatr Genet*, Vol.19, No.4, pp. 195-200, ISSN 1473-5873

Gressier, F., Trabado, S., Verstuyft, C., Bouaziz, E., Hardy, P., Feve, B., Becquemont, L. & Corruble, E. Thyroid-stimulating hormone, 5-HTTLPR genotype, and antidepressant response in depressed women. *Psychiatr Genet*, Vol.21, No.5, pp. 253-256, ISSN 1473-5873

Grigoriadis, S. & Robinson, G.E. (2007). Gender issues in depression. *Ann Clin Psychiatry*, Vol.19, No.4, pp. 247-255, ISSN 1547-3325

Hasler, G., Drevets, W.C., Manji, H.K. & Charney, D.S. (2004). Discovering endophenotypes for major depression. *Neuropsychopharmacology*, Vol.29, No.10, pp. 1765-1781, ISSN 0893-133X

Hildebrandt, M.G., Steyerberg, E.W., Stage, K.B., Passchier, J. & Kragh-Soerensen, P. (2003). Are gender differences important for the clinical effects of antidepressants? *Am J Psychiatry*, Vol.160, No.9, pp. 1643-1650, ISSN 0002-953X

Howard, G., Peng, L. & Hyde, J.F. (1997). An estrogen receptor binding site within the human galanin gene. *Endocrinology*, Vol.138, No.11, pp. 4649-4656, ISSN 0013-7227

Kaplan, L.M., Gabriel, S.M., Koenig, J.I., Sunday, M.E., Spindel, E.R., Martin, J.B. & Chin, W.W. (1988). Galanin is an estrogen-inducible, secretory product of the rat anterior pituitary. *Proc Natl Acad Sci U S A*, Vol.85, No.19, pp. 7408-7412, ISSN 0027-8424

Keers, R. & Aitchison, K.J. (2011). Pharmacogenetics of antidepressant response. *Expert Review of Neurotherapeutics*, Vol.11, No.1, pp. 101-125, ISSN 1473-7175

Kessler, R.C., McGonagle, K.A., Zhao, S., Nelson, C.B., Hughes, M., Eshleman, S., Wittchen, H.U. & Kendler, K.S. (1994). Lifetime and 12-month prevalence of DSM-III-R psychiatric disorders in the United States. Results from the National Comorbidity Survey. *Arch Gen Psychiatry*, Vol.51, No.1, pp. 8-19, ISSN 0003-990X

Kokras, N., Antoniou, K., Dalla, C., Bekris, S., Xagoraris, M., Ovestreet, D.H. & Papadopoulou-Daifoti, Z. (2009). Sex-related differential response to clomipramine treatment in a rat model of depression. *J Psychopharmacol*, Vol.23, No.8, pp. 945-956, ISSN 1461-7285

Kokras, N., Dalla, C. & Papadopoulou-Daifoti, Z. (2011). Sex differences in pharmacokinetics of antidepressants. *Expert Opinion on Drug Metabolism & Toxicology*, Vol.7, No.2, pp. 213-226, ISSN 1742-5255

Kornstein, S.G., Schatzberg, A.F., Thase, M.E., Yonkers, K.A., McCullough, J.P., Keitner, G.I., Gelenberg, A.J., Davis, S.M., Harrison, W.M. & Keller, M.B. (2000a). Gender differences in treatment response to sertraline versus imipramine in chronic depression. *Am J Psychiatry*, Vol.157, No.9, pp. 1445-1452, ISSN 0002-953X

Kornstein, S.G., Schatzberg, A.F., Thase, M.E., Yonkers, K.A., McCullough, J.P., Keitner, G.I., Gelenberg, A.J., Ryan, C.E., Hess, A.L., Harrison, W., Davis, S.M. & Keller, M.B. (2000b). Gender differences in chronic major and double depression. *J Affect Disord*, Vol.60, No.1, pp. 1-11, ISSN 0165-0327

Kramer, M.S., Cutler, N., Feighner, J., Shrivastava, R., Carman, J., Sramek, J.J., Reines, S.A., Liu, G., Snavely, D., Wyatt-Knowles, E., Hale, J.J., Mills, S.G., MacCoss, M., Swain, C.J., Harrison, T., Hill, R.G., Hefti, F., Scolnick, E.M., Cascieri, M.A., Chicchi, G.G., Sadowski, S., Williams, A.R., Hewson, L., Smith, D., Carlson, E.J., Hargreaves, R.J. & Rupniak, N.M. (1998). Distinct mechanism for antidepressant activity by blockade of central substance P receptors. *Science*, Vol.281, No.5383, pp. 1640-1645, ISSN 0036-8075

Kuehner, C. (2003). Gender differences in unipolar depression: an update of epidemiological findings and possible explanations. *Acta Psychiatr Scand*, Vol.108, No.3, pp. 163-174, ISSN 0001-690X

Kuteeva, E., Hokfelt, T., Wardi, T. & Ogren, S.O. (2008). Galanin, galanin receptor subtypes and depression-like behaviour. *Cell Mol Life Sci*, Vol.65, No.12, pp. 1854-1863, ISSN 1420-682X

Lachman, H.M., Papolos, D.F., Saito, T., Yu, Y.M., Szumlanski, C.L. & Weinshilboum, R.M. (1996). Human catechol-O-methyltransferase pharmacogenetics: description of a functional polymorphism and its potential application to neuropsychiatric disorders. *Pharmacogenetics*, Vol.6, No.3, pp. 243-250, ISSN 0960-314X

Marcus, S.M., Young, E.A., Kerber, K.B., Kornstein, S., Farabaugh, A.H., Mitchell, J., Wisniewski, S.R., Balasubramani, G.K., Trivedi, M.H. & Rush, A.J. (2005). Gender differences in depression: findings from the STAR*D study. *J Affect Disord*, Vol.87, No.2-3, pp. 141-150, ISSN 0165-0327

Martin, M., Ledent, C., Parmentier, M., Maldonado, R. & Valverde, O. (2002). Involvement of CB1 cannabinoid receptors in emotional behaviour. *Psychopharmacology (Berl)*, Vol.159, No.4, pp. 379-387, ISSN 0033-3158

Meibohm, B., Beierle, I. & Derendorf, H. (2002). How important are gender differences in pharmacokinetics? *Clin Pharmacokinet*, Vol.41, No.5, pp. 329-342, ISSN 0312-5963

Muller, D.J., Schulze, T.G., Macciardi, F., Ohlraun, S., Gross, M.M., Scherk, H., Neidt, H., Syagailo, Y.V., Grassle, M., Nothen, M.M., Maier, W., Lesch, K.P. & Rietschel, M. (2002). Moclobemide response in depressed patients: association study with a functional polymorphism in the monoamine oxidase A promoter. *Pharmacopsychiatry*, Vol.35, No.4, pp. 157-158, ISSN 0176-3679

Naranjo, C.A., Tremblay, L.K. & Busto, U.E. (2001). The role of the brain reward system in depression. *Prog Neuropsychopharmacol Biol Psychiatry*, Vol.25, No.4, pp. 781-823, ISSN 0278-5846

Nutt, D. (1998). Substance-P antagonists: a new treatment for depression? *Lancet*, Vol.352, No.9141, pp. 1644-1646, ISSN 0140-6736

Oldehinkel, A.J. & Bouma, E.M. (2011). Sensitivity to the depressogenic effect of stress and HPA-axis reactivity in adolescence: A review of gender differences. *Neurosci Biobehav Rev*, Vol.35, No.8, pp. 1757-1770, ISSN 1873-7528

Paine, M.F., Ludington, S.S., Chen, M.L., Stewart, P.W., Huang, S.M. & Watkins, P.B. (2005). Do men and women differ in proximal small intestinal CYP3A or P-glycoprotein expression? *Drug Metab Dispos*, Vol.33, No.3, pp. 426-433, ISSN 0090-9556

Parsey, R.V., Olvet, D.M., Oquendo, M.A., Huang, Y.Y., Ogden, R.T. & Mann, J.J. (2006). Higher 5-HT1A receptor binding potential during a major depressive episode predicts poor treatment response: preliminary data from a naturalistic study. *Neuropsychopharmacology*, Vol.31, No.8, pp. 1745-1749, ISSN 0893-133X

Perna, G., Favaron, E., Di Bella, D., Bussi, R. & Bellodi, L. (2005). Antipanic efficacy of paroxetine and polymorphism within the promoter of the serotonin transporter gene. *Neuropsychopharmacology*, Vol.30, No.12, pp. 2230-2235, ISSN 0893-133X

Peters, E.J., Slager, S.L., McGrath, P.J., Knowles, J.A. & Hamilton, S.P. (2004). Investigation of serotonin-related genes in antidepressant response. *Mol Psychiatry*, Vol.9, No.9, pp. 879-889, ISSN 1359-4184

Petronis, A. (2001). Human morbid genetics revisited: relevance of epigenetics. *Trends Genet*, Vol.17, No.3, pp. 142-146, ISSN 0168-9525

Pitychoutis, P.M., Griva, E., Ioannou, K., Tsitsilonis, O.E. & Papadopoulou-Daifoti, Z. (2009). Chronic antidepressant treatment exerts sexually dimorphic immunomodulatory effects in an experimental model of major depression: do females lack an advantage? *International Journal of Neuropsychopharmacology*, Vol.12, No.9, pp. 1157-1163, ISSN 1461-1457

Pitychoutis, P.M., Pallis, E.G., Mikail, H.G. & Papadopoulou-Daifoti, Z. (2011) Individual differences in novelty-seeking predict differential responses to chronic antidepressant treatment through sex- and phenotype-dependent neurochemical signatures. *Behav Brain Res*, , Vol.223, pp. 154-168 ISSN 1872-7549

Pitychoutis, P.M. & Papadopoulou-Daifoti, Z. (2010). Of depression and immunity: does sex matter? *International Journal of Neuropsychopharmacology*, Vol.13, No.5, pp. 675-689, ISSN 1461-1457

Pitychoutis, P.M., Zisaki, A., Dalla, C. & Papadopoulou-Daifoti, Z. (2010a). Pharmacogenetic Insights into Depression and Antidepressant Response: Does Sex Matter? *Current Pharmaceutical Design*, Vol.16, No.20, pp. 2214-2223, ISSN 1381-6128

Pitychoutis, P.M., Tsitsilonis, O.E. & Papadopoulou-Daifoti, Z. (2010b). Antidepressant pharmacotherapy: focus on sex differences in neuroimmunopharmacological crossroads. *Future Neurology*, Vol.5, No.4, pp. 581-596, ISSN

Prange, A.J., Jr., Wilson, I.C., Rabon, A.M. & Lipton, M.A. (1969). Enhancement of imipramine antidepressant activity by thyroid hormone. *Am J Psychiatry*, Vol.126, No.4, pp. 457-469, ISSN 0002-953X

Quitkin, F.M., Stewart, J.W., McGrath, P.J., Taylor, B.P., Tisminetzky, M.S., Petkova, E., Chen, Y., Ma, G. & Klein, D.F. (2002). Are there differences between women's and men's antidepressant responses? *The American journal of psychiatry*, Vol.159, No.11, pp. 1848-1854, ISSN 0002-953X

Rosenzweig-Lipson, S., Beyer, C.E., Hughes, Z.A., Khawaja, X., Rajarao, S.J., Malberg, J.E., Rahman, Z., Ring, R.H. & Schechter, L.E. (2007). Differentiating antidepressants of the future: efficacy and safety. *Pharmacol Ther*, Vol.113, No.1, pp. 134-153, ISSN 0163-7258

Rubinow, D.R., Schmidt, P.J. & Roca, C.A. (1998). Estrogen-serotonin interactions: implications for affective regulation. *Biol Psychiatry*, Vol.44, No.9, pp. 839-850, ISSN 0006-3223

Rush, A.J. (2007). STAR*D: what have we learned? *Am J Psychiatry*, Vol.164, No.2, pp. 201-204, ISSN 0002-953X

Rush, A.J., Fava, M., Wisniewski, S.R., Lavori, P.W., Trivedi, M.H., Sackeim, H.A., Thase, M.E., Nierenberg, A.A., Quitkin, F.M., Kashner, T.M., Kupfer, D.J., Rosenbaum, J.F., Alpert, J., Stewart, J.W., McGrath, P.J., Biggs, M.M., Shores-Wilson, K., Lebowitz, B.D., Ritz, L. & Niederehe, G. (2004). Sequenced treatment alternatives to relieve depression (STAR*D): rationale and design. *Control Clin Trials*, Vol.25, No.1, pp. 119-142, ISSN 0197-2456

Scandlyn, M.J., Stuart, E.C. & Rosengren, R.J. (2008). Sex-specific differences in CYP450 isoforms in humans. *Expert Opin Drug Metab Toxicol*, Vol.4, No.4, pp. 413-424, ISSN 1742-5255

Schirmer, M., Rosenberger, A., Klein, K., Kulle, B., Toliat, M.R., Nurnberg, P., Zanger, U.M. & Wojnowski, L. (2007). Sex-dependent genetic markers of CYP3A4 expression and activity in human liver microsomes. *Pharmacogenomics*, Vol.8, No.5, pp. 443-453, ISSN 1744-8042

Serretti, A., Kato, M., De Ronchi, D. & Kinoshita, T. (2007). Meta-analysis of serotonin transporter gene promoter polymorphism (5-HTTLPR) association with selective serotonin reuptake inhibitor efficacy in depressed patients. *Mol Psychiatry*, Vol.12, No.3, pp. 247-257, ISSN 1359-4184

Skidgel, R.A. & Erdos, E.G. (1987). The broad substrate specificity of human angiotensin I converting enzyme. *Clin Exp Hypertens A*, Vol.9, No.2-3, pp. 243-259, ISSN 0730-0077

Sloan, D.M. & Kornstein, S.G. (2003). Gender differences in depression and response to antidepressant treatment. *Psychiatr Clin North Am*, Vol.26, No.3, pp. 581-594, ISSN 0193-953X

Smits, K.M., Smits, L.J., Peeters, F.P., Schouten, J.S., Janssen, R.G., Smeets, H.J., van Os, J. & Prins, M.H. (2008). The influence of 5-HTTLPR and STin2 polymorphisms in the serotonin transporter gene on treatment effect of selective serotonin reuptake inhibitors in depressive patients. *Psychiatr Genet*, Vol.18, No.4, pp. 184-190, ISSN 1473-5873

Sobocki, P., Jonsson, B., Angst, J. & Rehnberg, C. (2006). Cost of depression in Europe. *Journal of Mental Health Policy and Economics*, Vol.9, No.2, pp. 87-98, ISSN 1091-4358

Staddon, S., Arranz, M.J., Mancama, D., Mata, I. & Kerwin, R.W. (2002). Clinical applications of pharmacogenetics in psychiatry. *Psychopharmacology (Berl)*, Vol.162, No.1, pp. 18-23, ISSN 0033-3158

Steimer, W., Muller, B., Leucht, S. & Kissling, W. (2001). Pharmacogenetics: a new diagnostic tool in the management of antidepressive drug therapy. *Clin Chim Acta*, Vol.308, No.1-2, pp. 33-41, ISSN 0009-8981

Tadic, A., Muller, M.J., Rujescu, D., Kohnen, R., Stassen, H.H., Dahmen, N. & Szegedi, A. (2007a). The MAOA T941G polymorphism and short-term treatment response to mirtazapine and paroxetine in major depression. *Am J Med Genet B Neuropsychiatr Genet*, Vol.144B, No.3, pp. 325-331, ISSN 1552-4841

Tadic, A., Rujescu, D., Muller, M.J., Kohnen, R., Stassen, H.H., Dahmen, N. & Szegedi, A. (2007b). A monoamine oxidase B gene variant and short-term antidepressant treatment response. *Prog Neuropsychopharmacol Biol Psychiatry*, Vol.31, No.7, pp. 1370-1377, ISSN 0278-5846

Thiels, C., Linden, M., Grieger, F. & Leonard, J. (2005). Gender differences in routine treatment of depressed outpatients with the selective serotonin reuptake inhibitor sertraline. *Int Clin Psychopharmacol*, Vol.20, No.1, pp. 1-7, ISSN 0268-1315

Tsai, S.J., Gau, Y.T., Hong, C.J., Liou, Y.J., Yu, Y.W. & Chen, T.J. (2009). Sexually dimorphic effect of catechol-O-methyltransferase val158met polymorphism on clinical response to fluoxetine in major depressive patients. *J Affect Disord*, Vol.113, No.1-2, pp. 183-187, ISSN 0165-0327

Uher, R., Perroud, N., Ng, M.Y.M., Hauser, J., Henigsberg, N., Maier, W., Mors, O., Placentino, A., Rietschel, M., Souery, D., Zagar, T., Czerski, P.M., Jerman, B., Larsen, E.R., Schulze, T.G., Zobel, A., Cohen-Woods, S., Pirlo, K., Butler, A.W., Muglia, P., Barnes, M.R., Lathrop, M., Farmer, A., Breen, G., Aitchison, K.J., Craig, I., Lewis, C.M. & McGuffin, P. (2010). Genome-Wide Pharmacogenetics of Antidepressant Response in the GENDEP Project. *American Journal of Psychiatry*, Vol.167, No.5, pp. 555-564, ISSN 0002-953X

Unschuld, P.G., Ising, M., Roeske, D., Erhardt, A., Specht, M., Kloiber, S., Uhr, M., Muller-Myhsok, B., Holsboer, F. & Binder, E.B. Gender-specific association of galanin polymorphisms with HPA-axis dysregulation, symptom severity, and antidepressant treatment response. *Neuropsychopharmacology*, Vol.35, No.7, pp. 1583-1592, ISSN 1740-634X

Walther, D.J. & Bader, M. (2003). A unique central tryptophan hydroxylase isoform. *Biochem Pharmacol*, Vol.66, No.9, pp. 1673-1680, ISSN 0006-2952

Waxman, D.J. & Holloway, M.G. (2009). Sex differences in the expression of hepatic drug metabolizing enzymes. *Mol Pharmacol*, Vol.76, No.2, pp. 215-228, ISSN 1521-0111

WHO (2005). Gender and women's mental health (http://www.who.int/mental_health/prevention/genderwomen/en/)

Yonkers, K.A., Kando, J.C., Cole, J.O. & Blumenthal, S. (1992). Gender differences in pharmacokinetics and pharmacodynamics of psychotropic medication. *Am J Psychiatry*, Vol.149, No.5, pp. 587-595, ISSN 0002-953X

Young, M.A., Scheftner, W.A., Fawcett, J. & Klerman, G.L. (1990). Gender differences in the clinical features of unipolar major depressive disorder. *J Nerv Ment Dis*, Vol.178, No.3, pp. 200-203, ISSN 0022-3018

Young, E.A., Kornstein, S.G., Marcus, S.M., Harvey, A.T., Warden, D., Wisniewski, S.R., Balasubramani, G.K., Fava, M., Trivedi, M.H. & John Rush, A. (2009). Sex differences in response to citalopram: a STAR*D report. *J Psychiatr Res*, Vol.43, No.5, pp. 503-511, ISSN 0022-3956

Yu, Y.W., Tsai, S.J., Hong, C.J., Chen, T.J., Chen, M.C. & Yang, C.W. (2005). Association study of a monoamine oxidase a gene promoter polymorphism with major depressive disorder and antidepressant response. *Neuropsychopharmacology*, Vol.30, No.9, pp. 1719-1723, ISSN 0893-133X

Yu, Y.W., Tsai, S.J., Liou, Y.J., Hong, C.J. & Chen, T.J. (2006). Association study of two serotonin 1A receptor gene polymorphisms and fluoxetine treatment response in Chinese major depressive disorders. *Eur Neuropsychopharmacol*, Vol.16, No.7, pp. 498-503, ISSN 0924-977X

9

Pharmacogenomics in Gastroenterology

Maria Ana Redal[1], Waldo Horacio Belloso[2],
Paula Scibona[2], Leonardo Garfi[2] and Santiago Isolabella[2,3]
[1]*Molecular Medicine and Genomics Unit, Institute for Basic Sciences and Experimental Medicine, and Department of Cellular and Molecular Biology, Hospital Italiano de Buenos Aires School of Medicine, Buenos Aires, [2]Clinical Pharmacology Section, Internal Medicine Service, and Department of Pharmacology and Toxicology, Hospital Italiano de Buenos Aires School of Medicine [3]Central Pharmacy Service, Hospital Italiano de Buenos Aires Argentina*

1. Introduction

The prescription of drugs is an instrumental practice of modern therapeutics. According to the definition of the World Health Organization, the adequate prescription involves the selection of the correct drug, dose and duration of administration. In this sense, it is known that drugs that are prescribed for certain indications cannot produce the desired therapeutic effect in approximately 30 to 60% of the cases (Wang et al., 2011).

The pharmacological effects of most drugs depend on the result of a series of pharmacokinetic processes, which determine the amount of drug that reaches the biophase (target tissues), as well as on pharmacodynamics, involving the interaction between the drug and its site of action. These processes occur at variable levels in different individuals, and one of the major determinants of this variability is genetics. The structure, function and expression of most enzymes involved in drug transport and metabolism as well as the specific drug receptors may be affected by the presence of genetic variants, which may in turn modify the intended therapeutic effect or the appearance of adverse effects. In cases in which polymorphisms or mutations affect the structure or expression of these proteins, with corresponding implications in their function, genomic analyses can be applied to predict the patient's response prior to treatment. This concept represents the central aim of pharmacogenomics (Weinshilboum & Wang, 2006).

Importantly, pharmacogenomic analyses do not explain all of the variability in drug responses. The new paradigm of individualized therapy must combine genetic information and non-genetic factors, such as sex, age, diet, environmental factors, drug interactions, demographics and clinical observations to determine the best treatment for a patient, both in the selection of drugs and in the dosage; the aim is to optimize the patient's therapeutic experience (Belloso & Redal, 2010). As with other areas of modern therapeutics, pharmacogenomics is gaining a place in the treatment of gastroenterological diseases.

Some gastroenterological diseases, such as gastroesophageal reflux and peptic ulcer disease, are among the most frequent and relevant pathologies in adult patients. In addition, inflammatory bowel disease, hepatitis C and postoperative or cancer-associated nausea and vomiting are conditions in which pharmacological therapy does not show a universal response. Interestingly, genetic factors may partially explain this variability of therapeutic efficacy for most drugs that are used in the treatment of these important gastroenterologic disorders.

In this chapter, we evaluate the major polymorphisms that are associated with the effectiveness or toxicity of drugs that are commonly used in gastroenterology.

2. Genes and polymorphisms

The magnitude of the expression of transporters, metabolizing enzymes and receptors depend primarily on genetic factors. Among these factors, different types of inherited genetic variants may be found, such as deletions, insertions and the multiplication or repetition of sequences, which may involve large portions of DNA. However, the most frequent variants and the most common targets of pharmacogenetic tests are the single nucleotide polymorphisms (SNPs). SNPs are modifications of a single base in the nucleotide sequence.

Studies of the human genome sequence have established that there are more than 15 million SNPs, of which only a small minority appear to have any impact on the kinetics or dynamics of drugs. Different approaches of pharmacogenomic study can range from purely genetic to the identification of those SNPs that confer clinical impacts; conversely, they can include the identification of specific sequences of nucleotides to recognize individuals with particular behaviors in relation to metabolism or drug responses (*The International HapMap Consortium: A haplotype map of the human genome*, 2005; Redon et al., 2006).

The genes that encode metabolic proteins, transporters or receptors may have different polymorphisms, and some of these polymorphisms will confer a particular impact on the magnitude of the expression of the gene products (Leucuta & Viase, 2006).

A polymorphism is considered when an allelic variant appears in more than 1% of the general population. These variants may be associated with a deficient expression or, in a minority of the cases, the overexpression of the enzyme, transporter or receptor.

For most drugs, the genotypic study of its metabolizing enzymes does not exhaust the potential sources of genetic variability. By accounting for the overall potential polymorphisms of transporters and receptors that are involved in the pharmacology of drugs, it may be possible to characterize multiple SNPs from multiple genes, which would refine our understanding of the impact of pharmacogenomics in the selection of therapeutic agents.

3. Peptic ulcer disease by Helicobacter pylori infection and gastro esophageal reflux disease

3.1 Clinical characteristics

Helicobacter pylori (HP) infection is associated with chronic gastritis, peptic ulcer disease, gastric mucosal associated lymphoid tissue (MALT) lymphoma and gastric cancer. The eradication of bacterial infection provides an effective means of curing or preventing these HP-associated diseases.

Gastroesophageal reflux disease (GERD) is noted by its prevalence, variety of clinical presentations and under-recognized morbidity. In general, GERD is considered for patients who demonstrate symptoms that are suggestive of reflux or complications thereof and with or without esophageal inflammation.

The most common symptoms of GERD are heartburn (or pyrosis), regurgitation and dysphagia. In addition, a variety of extraesophageal manifestations have been described including bronchospasm, laryngitis, and chronic cough.

A possible role for HP in the pathogenesis of GERD has also been suggested. However, the link between GERD and HP is complex and remains poorly defined.

3.2 Pharmacological treatment

The current treatment strategies for the cure of HP infection are based on a triple therapy that includes a proton pump inhibitor (PPI) and two antibiotics, which are usually amoxicillin and/or clarithromycin or metronidazole. These regimens are effective in 70-90% of patients. Treatment failures have been attributed to bacterial resistance to the antibiotics.

PPIs also constitute the standard treatment for GERD; in fact, the introduction of PPIs for the management of acid-peptic disorders constitutes one of the great success stories in gastroenterology because of their efficacy and safety. Nevertheless, the treatment response is not uniform, and in fact, the average response to treatment may actually hamper the identification of two different populations of patients, which include those who respond almost completely and those who have a consistently suboptimal response.

3.3 Pharmacogenomic considerations

Among the mechanisms of drug metabolism in the body, the most important is cytochrome P450. The complex enzymes that are involved in the metabolism of drugs include CYP2C19, CYP2D6, CYP2C9 and CYP3A4/5/7.

The CYP2C19 isoenzyme metabolizes all of the PPIs that are currently available, some antidepressant drugs, the antifungal voriconazole, thalidomide and the antiplatelet clopidogrel.

The gene that encodes CYP2C19 has been mapped to chromosome 10 (10q24.1-q24.3). At least 21 variants of CYP2C19, from *1 to *20, have been identified. CYP2C19*1 is the wild-type allele. The variant allele CYP2C19*2, which contains 681G>A on exon 5 that causes a splicing defect, which is the major genetic defect that is responsible for the polymorphism of S-mephenytoin metabolism in humans. *CYP2C19*3 carries the 636G>A SNP, which results in a premature stop codon in exon 4. Both *CYP2C19*2* and **3* are null alleles, which result in the absence of enzymatic activity (de Morais et al., 1994). The majority of the PMs of CYP2C19 are due to these two variant alleles (Desta et al., 2002).

It has been described that approximately 3-5% of the Caucasian population has a total absence of enzymatic activity that is primarily associated with the gene variant CYP2C19*2, and it is associated to a lesser extent with CYP2C19*3. The frequency of these polymorphisms is highly variable among different populations (Goldstein et al., 1997). Likewise, the CYP2C19 * 17 variant (I331V) was identified more recently, and it is found in ultra-rapid metabolizers (UMs) (Sim, 2006). The alleles *2 and *3, which are associated with poor metabolizers (PMs), have been found in approximately 85% of the Caucasian population and nearly 100% of the Asian population. If the alleles *4 and *6 are included, the prevalence of the PM phenotype in Caucasians is 92%.

The biotransformation of PPI occurs primarily through CYP2C19, and the study of polymorphisms for these drugs has a specific application. CYP2C19 is responsible for the initial hydroxylation of omeprazole and lanzoprazole and, to a lesser extent, the demethylation of pantoprazole and rabeprazole, which are the steps that produce metabolites without antacid activity (figure 1). The ability of these drugs to reduce gastric acidity depends largely on the concentration that is reached in the plasma after absorption. Therefore, those who rapidly metabolize the drugs ,rapid metabolizers (RMs) have significantly lower gastric pH values than those who are "extensive metabolizers", "intermediate metabolizers" (IMs) or PMs. The PMs have inherited variations in both of the alleles and therefore cannot express the functional enzyme. The differences in the area under the curve (AUC), which is a variable that quantifies the exposure of the subject to the current drug, can be up to 13-fold higher for the PM in the case of omeprazole.

In addition, it has been observed that these pharmacokinetic and pharmacodynamic differences result in diverse clinical outcomes by using proton- pump inhibitor therapies, which are primarily used in the treatment of gastroesophagic reflux disease (GERD) and the eradication of HP (Furuta, 2005).

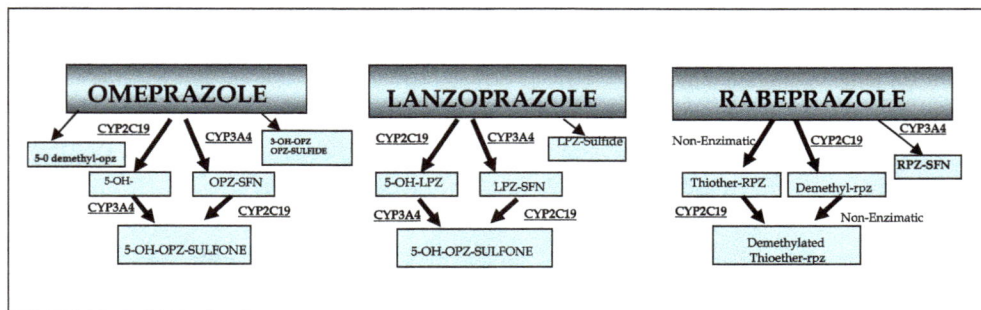

Fig. 1. Metabolism of omeprazole, lanzoprazole and rabeprazole

3.4 Pharmacogenomic influences in the treatment of GERD with PPIs

In recent years, it has been established that one of the causes of GERD that is refractory to PPI therapy, which occurs in approximately 10% of patients, is related to differences in the efficiency of the metabolism of the drug. Endoscopic cure rates are much lower in RMs than in IMs, and higher cure rates are observed in the PMs, which display a poorer outcome in relation to the severity of the injury (less than 17% for RM C or D lesions, Los Angeles classification). It was established that the genotype is also crucial for the nocturnal acid bouts, which are episodes in which the pH falls below 4 for more than an hour and are considered to be an influential factor in the treatment outcome. These intrusions are much more frequent in RMs than in the other two types of metabolizing patterns. This result suggests that patients who are refractory to standard doses of PPI should be offered an increased dose or frequency on the premise that they are RMs (Kawamura et al., 2007; Egan et al., 2003).

The safety profile of PPIs also seems to be influenced by pharmacogenetics, which is illustrated in the case of GERD treatments that require long treatment periods. There is some evidence that IMs and, to a larger extent, PMs, have a higher risk of hyperplasia of enterochromaffin-like cells, which is related to the development of carcinoid tumors, than their RM counterparts (Rosemary & Adithan, 2007). Likewise, the first two groups have higher rates of megaloblastic anemia by vitamin B12 deficiency, which arises from the neutralization of the gastric pH for extended periods; these groups also suffer from atrophic gastritis, which is especially likely if it coexists with HP infection (Kang, 2008).

3.5 Pharmacogenomic influences on the eradication of Helicobacter pylori

To eradicate and as a part of the therapeutic strategy for managing patients with various conditions, such as peptic ulcer disease or MALT, PPIs are a central part of the scheme that also require the addition of antibiotics. The suppression of gastric acidity is also crucial for the bioavailability and stabilization of the plasma concentration of antibiotics, which can force HP to its growth phase, which is where it is most responsive to treatment, increase the intragastric concentrations of antibiotics and provide some intrinsic actions against HP.

Response rates in the eradication of HP are also influenced by the genotype of the patient (figure 2), such that the PMs are able to achieve 100% eradication with the standard dose of PPIs and with the addition of 500 mg of amoxicillin and omeprazole four times a day for two weeks. In this scheme, the eradication rate for IMs is 60%, and that for RMs is only 30% (Kang, 2008). In addition, adequate results have been reported with dual schemes that utilize 10 mg of rabeprazole twice per day, which has a greater ability to suppress gastric acidity than omeprazole that is combined with amoxicillin, and has reached 90% eradication in both PMs and IMs (Furuta, 2005). Therefore, in a large number of cases, the use of a second antibiotic may be avoided. Moreover, in the cases of eradication failure, an attempt can be made by doubling the dose of rabeprazole with amoxicillin before a third antibiotic is added; the intention of this treatment is to achieve effectiveness in the case of RMs. This differential approach that permits the individualization of PPI treatment according to the CYP2C19 genotype constitutes a real breakthrough, and it facilitates the avoidance of the addition of clarithromycin or metronidazole, which are not exempt from adherence problems, cost, resistance and adverse effects.

The addition of clarithromycin to the regimen of PPIs and amoxicillin has a pharmacokinetic basis: clarithromycin inhibits another cytochrome, CYP3A4, which is an alternative pathway for the metabolism of PPIs. Therefore, PPI concentrations are extremely high when PMs are exposed concomitantly to these drugs and clarithromycin, although the rise of the plasma concentration has been observed with all of the genotypes (Furuta, 1999).

This technique may represent one mechanism to increase the effectiveness of the triple scheme regardless of the CYP2C19 genotype. Nevertheless, the RMs cure rates are lower than the IMs and PMs cure rates, which is probably because the RMs receive insufficient doses of PPIs in accordance with the enzyme expression. It is believed that in the case of the triple scheme, prior knowledge of CYP2C19 genotype may help to optimize the dose of PPI to minimize the possibility of therapeutic failures. It is recommended that the dose and the dosing interval, up to four times daily, should be increased to ensure a gastric pH that is close to 7 for the majority of the day (Chaudhry & Kochhar, 2008).

Finally, in patients for whom therapy has been individualized but fails to eradicate the disease, a consideration should be made regarding the possibility of an infection by a HP strain that is resistant to clarithromycin (Furuta & Graham, 2006).

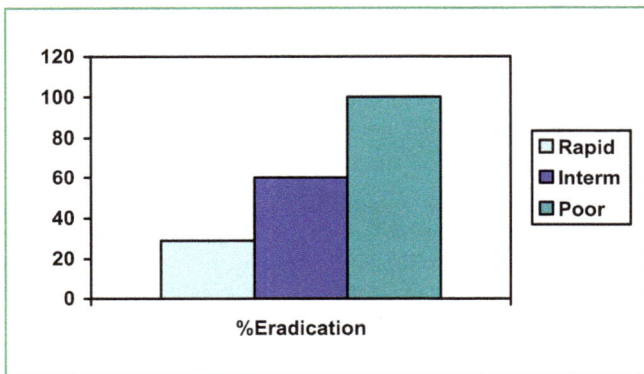

Fig. 2. Omeprazole metabolism by CYP2C19. (Furuta et al, 1998)
The percent of HP eradication is dependent upon the metabolizer phenotype.

4. Inflammatory Bowel Disease

4.1 Clinical characteristics

Inflammatory bowel disease (IBD) is a chronic, disabling disease that generally presents with flares and remissions. Ulcerative colitis (UC) and Crohn's disease constitute the most frequent forms of presentation.There are remarkable differences between both conditions regarding the clinical presentation, extension and extra-intestinal manifestations of the disease. The precise etiology of IBD is unknown, but both ambient and genetic factors may play a significant role.

4.2 Pharmacological treatment

The clinical course of this condition has changed substantially since immune modulator therapies and monoclonal antibodies were introduced to the therapeutic armamentarium; as a result, the extent of the remission periods has increased. However, a curative pharmacological approach is not yet available.

In addition, considerable variability exists regarding the efficacy and toxicity of the treatment. Multiple factors may influence the response to treatment, which include disease severity and complications; environmental factors, such as smoking; and genetic factors. It is estimated that between 20% and 95% of the variability in the toxicity and the treatment response may be explained by polymorphisms. The overall response rate to the treatment is more difficult to estimate than toxicity because there are multiple confounding factors, such as the concomitant use of other drugs, which may influence outcomes. The polymorphism of the enzyme thiopurine methyl transferase (TPMT) (figure 3) and its influence on treatment with Azathioprine (AZA) and 6-mercaptopurine (6-MP) is the best example of how genotyping can help to optimize therapy in inflammatory bowel disease (Hindorf et al., 2002), (table 1).

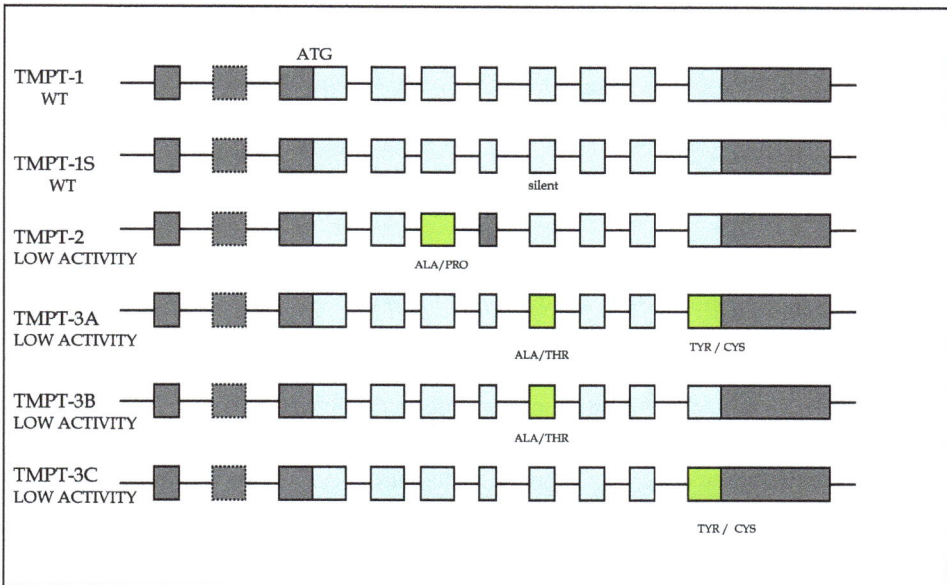

Fig. 3. Allelic variant of the TMPT locus. The boxes depict exons in the TMPT gene. The grey boxes are the untranslated region and blue boxes represent exons in the open reading frame. The green boxes are exons that contain mutations resulting in amino acid changes.

Genotype	Phenotype / Activity	AZA dose
TMPT*1/*1	High	Standard doses
TMPT*1/*2 TMPT*1/*3 (A,B or C)	Intermediate	Half dose
TMPT*2/*3 (A,B or C) TMPT*3/*3 (A,B or C)	Deficient/ Null	Avoid AZA. Alternative treatment recommended.

Table 1. Relationship between genotype and phenotype in TPMT and doses of AZA in patients with IBD

AZA is a thiopurine derivative with immunosuppressive properties that has been available on the market for almost 40 years. It is widely used in the treatment of rheumatic diseases of children and adults, transplantation and inflammatory bowel disease, and it is used in different treatment combinations. However, approximately 40% of IBD patients do not respond to AZA treatment, and 10-25% must discontinue treatment because of adverse reactions, being either major (leukopenia, pancreatitis and hepatitis) or minor (rash, nausea, flu-like syndrome and diarrhea) Adverse reactions, which include liver, gastrointestinal and bone marrow toxicity are present in approximately 15-28% of patients.

Hematologic toxicity occurs in approximately 2-9% of patients, and it can, in extreme cases, lead to death (Pierik et al., 2006).

AZA is a pro-drug that is administered orally in doses of approximately 2.5 mg/kg per day. Fifteen to sixty percent of the drug is absorbed in the intestine, and after it enters the body, it is converted to 6-MP by a non-enzymatic reaction. 6-MP is also a pro-drug that undergoes a series of enzymatic reactions to form thioguanide nucleotides (6-TGNs), which are active metabolites that antagonize the metabolism of purines; inhibit the synthesis of DNA, RNA and proteins; and may also interfere with cellular metabolism and prevent mitosis. 6-TGNs are responsible for the immunosuppressive activity and the myelosuppressive action of AZA.

The inactivation of AZA and 6-MP depend primarily on two metabolic pathways; one pathway utilizes xanthine oxidase, producing 6-thiouric acid, and the other utilizes TPMT, which converts the original drug to 6-methylmercaptopurine. Both of the metabolites are inactive.

In myelopoietic precursors, no xanthine oxidase activity is observed; therefore, TPMT expression and function are vital for the inactivation of thiopuric derivatives.

However, the accumulation of active metabolites also depends on the activity of these enzymes. In this regard, the toxicity of both AZA and 6-MP are strongly related to the TMPT activity. The decreased activity or deficiency of TMPT causes 6-MP to be preferentially metabolized to 6-TGNs, which are responsible for much of the toxicity of 6-MP.

Following the introduction of the pharmacogenetic test for TPMT, there have been major changes in the prescription patterns of AZA in the last decade. The choice to use or not use AZA in accordance with the TPMT genotype offers the possibility of a safer and more effective treatment.

Several studies have shown that 80-90% of patients who have at least one of the aforementioned variants will have to discontinue AZA treatment due to adverse effects, which primarily include neutropenia (Evans & McLeod, 2003).

4.3 Pharmagenomic considerations

Supporting evidence currently exists for the pre-treatment genetic testing of TPMT in the reduction of neutropenic episodes in patients receiving azathioprine, although the evidence regarding its contribution in increasing drug efficacy is not as strong (Lakatos, 2010). A recent survey in the UK showed that 67% of gastroenterologists used TPMT testing before prescribing AZA (Payne et al., 2007). In 2004, the US Food and Drug Administration (FDA) approved TPMT testing in the US and made the recommendation to include this information in the drug prescription brochure; however, no formal recommendation was made for mandatory testing.

A socio-economic study of IBD has demonstrated that TPMT genotyping is a cost-effective method that can identify patients with active low/absent enzyme to avoid treatment with AZA and its subsequent severe hematologic complications (van den Akker, 2006)

It is now recommended that patients with IBD who have low or intermediate enzyme activity should receive a starting dose of 50% of the usually prescribed does, and treatment with AZA should be avoided in patients with null enzymatic activity to prevent toxicity (Pierik et al., 2006; Lakatos, 2010)

5. Gilbert Meulengracht syndrome and irinotecan

5.1 Clinical characteristics

Gilbert syndrome is characterized by the presence of unconjugated hyperbilirubinemia, which is usually moderate, transient or intermittent; has a non-obstructive origin without liver inflammation or fibrosis; and is not associated with changes in histology.

The occurrence of this syndrome is primarily related to the genetic variability in a family of enzymes (UDP-glucuronyltranferase (UGTs)) that are part of a detoxification system against endogenous toxins and xenobiotic chemicals. These membrane enzymes catalyze the glucuronidation of different substances by making them more polar to facilitate their excretion through bile or urine.

This is a route of detoxification that is used for substances that are taken with meals, tobacco smoke, or drugs; however, this route is primarily involved in the maintenance of the homeostasis of endogenous substances, such as bilirubin, steroids, thyroid hormones and bile acids (Strassbourg, 2008).

5.2 Pharmacogenomic considerations

Different polymorphisms are associated with the variable activity of these enzymes, which affects their ability to detoxify substances. Subsequently, the glucuronidated products are recognized by transport systems for organic anions, and they are secreted in urine or bile.

From a pharmacogenetic standpoint, the primary current use of the identification of alleles of UGT1A1 is focused on the ability to adequately predict the occurrence of severe hematologic toxicity (grade 3 or 4) in cytostatic treatment combinations, which include high doses of irinotecan.

The UGT1A1 enzyme is the only enzyme that is relevant in the metabolism of bilirubin. At least 113 variants have been identified, but very few are common in the general population. One hundred ninety-five SNPs have been identified in the UGT1A1 gene. Among these, there are 11 SNPs in exons 1-5. The UGT1A1*6 (211 G>A) in exon 1 is the most common SNPs that is found in the East Asian population (15.7%), but it is not common in the Caucasian population (0.7%) (Bernabeu et al., 2010). It has been suggested that the allele *6 contributes to the high incidence of neonatal hyperbilirubinemia in Asian children (Akaba et al., 1999). Exon 1 is unique for each member of the UGT1A1 subfamily, whereas exons 2 to 5 are common to all of the members of the subfamily. The variants in the 3´UTR of UGT1A1 in exon 5, therefore, may have distinct effects on all of the members of the UGT1A1 subfamily.

Polymorphism in the promoter region of the UGT1A1 gene is caused by variability in the number of TA repeats in the TATA-box that is located upstream of UGT1A1. The presence of seven TA repeats (UGT1A1*28) is associated with reduced UGT1A1 expression compared to the wild type allele (UGT1A1*1), which contains six TA repeats. Homozygous individuals who carry the A $(TA)_7$ TAA allele show significantly higher plasma levels of unconjugated bilirubin caused by a 30% reduction in the transcription of UGT1A1 (Lyer et al., 2002). There are interethnic differences in the frequency of the UGT1A1*28 allele, which has an approximate incidence of 6-12% in the Caucasian population, 0-3% in the Asian population and 16-19% in the African population (Shu-Feng Zhou et al., 2008).

However, there are other polymorphisms, such as UGT1A1*36, which contains 5 TA; UGT1A1*37, which contains 8 TA; and other polymorphisms that are not linked to the TATA-box region, such as the variant UGT1A1*7 (1456T>G, mutation in exon 1); UGT1A1*27 (686C>A), which is very rare in all of the ethnic groups that were examined; and the variant UGT1A1*62, which is found exclusively in Asians and is not present in either Caucasians or Africans.

Because haplotypes with UGT1A1 variants may coexist in the same person, the scenario is actually more complex. This may help to explain why there is hyperbilirubinemia in 5-9% of Caucasians, while 10-16% are homozygous for the UGT1A1*28 variant (Strassburg, 2010).

Irinotecan is a derivative of camptothecin. Camptothecins interact specifically with the enzyme topoisomerase I, which relieves DNA torsional strain by inducing reversible single-strand breaks. Irinotecan and its active metabolite SN-38 bind to the topoisomerase I-DNA complex and prevent the relegation of these single-strand breaks. Current research suggests that the cytotoxicity of irinotecan is related to double-strand DNA damage that is produced during DNA synthesis, when replication enzymes interact with the ternary complex that is formed by topoisomerase I, DNA, and either irinotecan or SN-38. Mammalian cells cannot efficiently repair these double-strand breaks. The irinotecan metabolite SN-38 is conjugated by UGT1A1. The presence of seven TA repeats, rather than the wild type number of six, in the UGT1A1 promoter reduces enzyme expression and consequently the expression of SN-38; this also confers a higher chance of developing diarrhea and/or leukopenia during irinotecan therapy when compared to patients with a wild type genotype. Gilbert´s syndrome is also associated with the TA_7/TA_7 genotype, and these patients may have an increased risk of irinotecan-induced toxicity (Côté et al., 2007).

In the same way, the recognition of patients with UGT1A1 deficiency may contribute to the prediction of the development of severe hyperbilirubinemia in patients with HIV infection who are treated with atazanavir, which is an enzyme blocker, and increased plasma concentrations of the integrase inhibitor raltegravir.

Irinotecam is primarily converted to its active metabolite SN-38 by liver carboxylesterases. UGT 1A1 inactivates SN-38 into the more polar SN-38 glucuronide, which is further eliminated in bile and urine (figure 4).

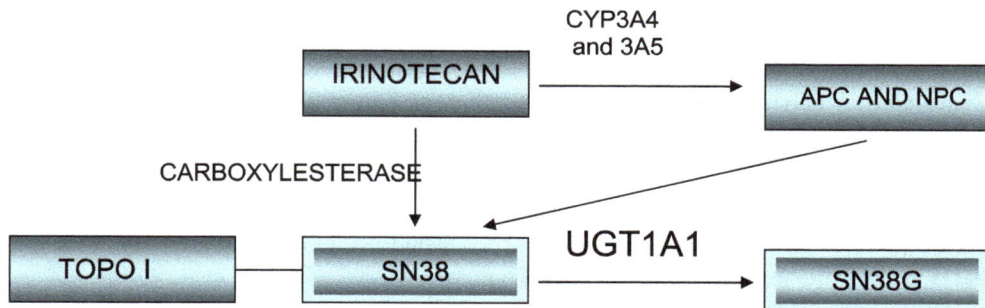

Fig. 4. Metabolic pathway of irinotecan

6. Hepatitis C infection

6.1 Clinical characteristics

The hepatitis C virus (HCV) infection affects over 170 million people worldwide; it causes chronic hepatitis, which may, in turn, lead to cirrhosis and hepatocellular carcinoma (HCC). There are six different genotypes whose prevalence varies geographically. Genotype I is responsible for most of the infections in North America, South America and Europe. Direct contact with blood (as in uncontrolled transfusions) or the use of parenteral drugs constitute the most common method of transmission, while unprotected sex is a secondary risk factor.

A patient's immune response will determine whether HCV is eventually eliminated or remains, which can produce a persistent infection; this latter outcome occurs in the majority of cases. The course of HCV infection is variable, although in most patients, it will progress toward cirrhosis.

The hepatitis C virus is a flavivirus. The HCV genome is a positive-sense RNA molecule of approximately 9500 nucleotides and encodes a polyprotein precursor of approximately 3000 amino acids.

The observation of nucleotide and amino acid mutations that are specifically segregated in groups or subgroups in almost all of the regions of the HCV genome has permitted the classification of HCV genotypes and subtypes whose sequences differ from each other by 30% and 20%, respectively. Currently, we accept the existence of at least 6 genotypes that are divided, in turn, into more than 84 subtypes. These genotypes were identified by a number (1 through 6), and the subtypes were identified by a lowercase letter in the order of their discovery (e.g., 1a, 1b, 2a, 3a, etc.).

After they bind to the cell surface, HCV particles enter the cell by receptor-mediated endocytosis. The cytosolic recognition of specific motifs in viral products induces the production of interferons and proinflammatory cytokines, which leads to the recruitment of a signaling complex that activates transcription factors. The subsequent expression of interferon alpha regulatory factor 3 (IRF-3) target genes, and likely lambda (type III) interferons induces innate immune programs and drives the maturation of adaptive immunity for infection control. The coordinated activities of CD4+ T cells and cytotoxic CD8+ T cells, which are primed in the context of HLA class II and I alleles, respectively, on antigen presenting cells, are critically important for the control of acute HCV infection. Mutations in viral epitopes that are targeted by cytotoxic CD8+ T cells can permit the virus to escape immunomediated clearance. The up-regulation of inhibitory receptors on exhausted (functionally impaired) T cells is another mechanism of T-cell dysfunction during chronic infection.

The host immune response determines whether the HCV persists or is eradicated spontaneously.

One of the most influential factors appears to be related to certain polymorphisms of a site that is in close proximity to the IL28B gene (Thomas et al., 2009; Grebely et al., 2010).

The risk of chronic infection that follows an acute episode of hepatitis C is high. In most studies, 80% to hundred percent of patients remain HCV RNA-positive, and 60 to 80 percent have persistently elevated liver enzymes (Chu et al., 1999; Farci et al., 1991). The mechanism that is responsible for the high prevalence of chronic infection is unclear. This mechanism may be related to the genetic diversity of the virus and its tendency toward rapid mutation, which allows HCV to constantly escape immune recognition. Most patients with chronic infection are asymptomatic or have only mild, nonspecific symptoms. The most frequent complaint is fatigue; other less common manifestations include nausea, anorexia, myalgia, arthralgia, weakness, and weight loss.

Cirrhosis occurs in up to 50 percent of chronically infected patients (Tong et al., 1995; Takahashi et al., 1993; Yano et al., 1996). Complications of hepatitis C are mostly confined to patients who have developed cirrhosis. The development of cirrhosis is silent in the majority of patients in whom it occurs. The progression to fibrosis and later to cirrhosis depends on many factors, such as the duration of infection, advanced age, male sex, co-infection with other viruses (HIV or HBV), or alcohol intake. HCC in patients with hepatitis C occurs almost exclusively in those with cirrhosis, which suggests that this is the major risk factor. The deaths that are associated with chronic hepatitis C are more likely to be related to end-stage liver disease rather than hepatocellular carcinoma (HCC). However, HCV accounts for approximately one-third of HCC cases in the United States. Estimations of the risk of developing HCC after the development of cirrhosis have varied from 0 to 3 percent per year in various reports. The risk appears to be greater with genotype 1b when compared with genotype 2a/c (Fattovich et al., 1997; Hu & Tong , 1999; Planas et al., 2004; Bruno et al., 2007).

Once the complications of cirrhosis have occurred, liver transplantation is the only effective therapy. Recurrent HCV infection of the graft occurs in almost all patients, although the long-term survival following transplantation for HCV is similar to the survival that is related to other causes of hepatic failure (60 to 80 percent). Several factors may be important determinants of disease progression in individual patients; these factors include age, ethnic background, gender, HCV-specific cellular immune response, viral diversity, alcohol use, daily use of marijuana, viral coinfection, environmental factors and geography.

6.2 Pharmacological treatment

The decision to treat a patient with chronic HCV infection is based upon several factors, which include the natural history of the disease, the stage of fibrosis, and the efficacy and adverse effects that are related to the therapy. For patients with clinically significant hepatic fibrosis, there is widespread agreement that antiviral therapy is indicated because of the high risk of cirrhosis.

Currently, the standard treatment for HCV infection is ribavirin in combination with peg-interferon (INF), but unfortunately, approximately 50% of patients with genotype I do not respond to the treatment (Liapiakis & Jacobson , 2010). In contrast, 70-80% of patients with genotypes II or III have sustained virological response (SVR) that is defined as undetectable HCV RNA 6 months after the treatment. Although the treatment response rate depends on several factors, such as patient age, sex, viral genotype, viral load at the start of treatment and the liver fibrosis rate, genetic factors that may be related with the rate of response to treatment and disease progression have been recently identified (table 2).

Ribavirin is a nucleoside analogue. The mechanism by which ribavirin contributes to its clinical antiviral efficacy is not fully understood. Ribavirin has direct antiviral activity in tissue culture against many RNA viruses. Ribavirin increases the mutational frequency in the genomes of several RNA viruses, and ribavirin triphosphate inhibits HCV polymerase in a biochemical reaction. Ribavirin is generally well tolerated. The major adverse effects include hemolysis, nonspecific fatigue, depression, insomnia, vertigo, anorexia, nausea, nasal congestion, and pruritus. As a result of hemolysis, ribavirin treatment may be associated with a mild reversible increase in serum bilirubin and uric acid.

Peg-INF is derived from the recombinant human interferon Alpha2a. Alpha interferons possess potent antiviral activity.

General characteristics	• Non I HCV Genotype • Low viral load • Caucasian descent • IL28B Genotype • Absence of fibrosis • Weight < 85kg • Age< 40 years • Female gender
Before treatment initiation	• Absence of insulin resistance • Absence of liver steatosis • Use of statins
During treatment	• Rapid virological response (at week 4 of treatment) • Adherence to treatment • Standard dose of ribavirin.

Table 2. Predictors of adequate responses to treatment with ribavirin and INF in HCV

They induce interferon-stimulated genes (ISGs) that help to establish an antiviral status milieu within cells, although the response is not virus-specific. Alpha interferons act by binding to cell surface receptors, which activates a response cascade that culminates in the expression of multiple ISGs, some of which block viral protein synthesis. Peg-INF binds the human type I INF receptor, which leads to receptor dimerization. Receptor dimerization activates multiple intracellular signal transduction pathways that are initially mediated by the JAK/STAT signal cascade. A combination therapy with ribavirin and interferon may be associated with an increased risk of side effects (such as nausea, rash, and dyspnea) when compared to the treatment with interferon alone (table 2). However, a meta-analysis and the large studies that were discussed above have suggested that the incidence of serious side effects of these treatments are not significantly different (Schalm et al., 1997; Mc Hutchison et al., 1998).

6.3 Pharmacogenomic considerations

As aforementioned, the efficacy of INF treatment is determined by a number of factors. Among these factors, genetic variance has been established as an important predictor of treatment response and viral clearance.

Four independent genetic studies (Genome Wide Association Study (GWAS)) have identified a polymorphism in the IL28B gene on chromosome 19 that encodes IFN-λ that has a strong association with the response rate to combination therapy with peg-INF and ribavirin (Ge et al., 2009; Suppiah et al., 2009; Tanakah et al., 2009; Rauch et al., 2010).

Using a GWAS, several investigators from the US and the UK identified a SNP on chromosome 19, rs12979860. The rs12979860 SNP is 3 kb upstream of the aforementioned IL-28B gene (Brian, 2011). Ge et al. identified rs1297960 as the variant that is most strongly associated with SVR in European–American, African-American and Hispanic populations.

Their study showed an association of the CC genotype with a greater rate of SVR than the TT genotype. The frequency of the CC genotype was 39%, 16% and 35% in European-American, African- American and Hispanic populations, respectively.

Suppah et al. and Rauch et al. -in a European cohort- and Tanaka et al. -in Japanese patients- found the strongest association with rs8099917 (located 8 kb upstream of IL28B), which is in linkage disequilibrium with rs12979860. The TT genotype of rs8099917 was significantly associated with the presence of a sustained virological response (SVR) following treatment with peg-IFN and ribavirin in patients who were chronically infected with genotype 1, while the minor allele G is associated with the absence of the response and the increased risk of progression to chronic states.

A higher prevalence of the T allele in the HIV-negative control population was also found, which suggests that this allele may be associated with the possibility of the clearance of the hepatitis C virus (Thomas et al., 2009; Aparicio et al., 2010).

These findings may impact the prognosis and treatment of HCV infection. Furthermore, the ability to identify patients with a risk allele, particularly in homozygosity, in which the response to treatment would be very poor, would make them candidates for alternative therapies.

7. Postoperative and cancer-associated nausea and vomiting

7.1 Clinical characteristics

Postoperative nausea and vomiting is a frequent experience for patients who are subjected to surgery with general anesthesia. Twenty to forty percent of surgical patients may display this disorder, and in certain high-risk groups, the incidence is even higher (Candiotti et al., 2005). In addition, nausea and vomiting is one of the most distressful side effects of cytotoxic drugs that are administered to patients with oncologic conditions. There are multiple factors related to the individual risk of developing nausea and vomiting, such as female sex, young age, alcohol consumption, preexisting nausea, and the emetogenic potential of the chemotherapeutic agents that are used (Perwitasari et al., 2011).

7.2 Pharmacological treatment

Among the most commonly used drugs, the receptor antagonists of serotonin type 3 (5HT3), such as ondansetron, granisetron and tropisentron, are widely used as antiemetics to primarily prevent nausea and vomiting that are associated with chemotherapy and postoperative conditions. These drugs provide a substantial contribution toward the prevention and the treatment of nausea and vomiting in these scenarios. However, 20-30% of patients do not respond to treatment with 5HT3 antagonists.

7.3 Pharmacogenomic considerations

One reason that may explain these interindividual differences in the response to treatment is the variation in the hepatic biotransformation of the drug, which, in turn, could be genetically determined by polymorphic variants of the gene that encodes CYP2D6. All of the 5HT3 antagonists are metabolized by the CYP450 complex, and they are primarily metabolized by the CYP2D6 isoenzyme.

The CYP2D6 gene is mapped to chromosome 22q13.1 and encompasses nine exons with an open reading frame of 1383 base pairs that encode 461 amino acids (Eichelbaum et al., 1987). More than 63 different CYP2D6 variants have been identified by the human cytochrome P450 allele nomenclature. Relative to the wild type CYP2D6 allele, different variants of the CYP2D6 gene may result in the complete absence of enzyme activity, reduced activity, normal activity or even increased activity. Null alleles of CYP2D6 do not encode a functional protein, and there is no detectable residual enzymatic activity. These null alleles are responsible for the PM phenotype when they are present in homozygosity or compound heterozygosity. The mechanisms by which there variants are leading to a total loss of function include the following: a) single-base changes or small insertions/deletions that interrupt the reading frame or interfere with the correct splicing, which leads to a prematurely terminated protein or stop codon (e.g., CYP2D6*3, *4, *6, *8, *11, *15, *19, *20, *38, *40, *42, and *44) (Kagimoto et al., 1990); b) nonfunctional full-length coded alleles (e.g., CYP2D6*5, *12, *14 and *18) (Evert. et al., 1997); and c) the deletion of the entire CYP2D6 gene as a result of large sequence deletions (e.g., CYP2D6*5, *13, and *16) (Gaedigk et al., 1991). However, extremely high CYP2D6 activity results from the gene duplication of functional alleles *1 and *2 that are fused in a head-to-tail orientation as a result of unequal crossover events and other mechanisms. This was noted by a molecular characterization of the CYP2D6 locus in patients with extremely rapid metabolism (Bertilsson et al., 1993). Approximately 5-10% of the Caucasian population has no activity of the enzyme (PMs) and approximately 2% are UMs. These patients have two active gene copies resulting in the production of enzymes with increased activity which will rapidly decrease the plasma concentration of the substrate drug with subsequent treatment failure (Lewis et al., 2010; Ho et al., 2006; Vermiere et al., 2010).

Therefore, antiemetic treatment may be optimized through CYP2D6 genotyping prior to chemotherapy or surgical treatment by identifying the patients that will behave as PMs or UMs for these drugs; this analysis can specifically identify which patients would require a dose adjustment (Perwitasari et al., 2011).

Because the CYP2D6 polymorphism explains only a proportion of the therapeutic failures in these patients, it has been postulated that changes in both the dopamine receptor and serotonin receptor may also be related to the antiemetic treatment response (Perwitasari, 2011). Interestingly, it has also been postulated that CYP2D6 polymorphisms may be related to the predisposition to the development of dyskinesias with the use of metoclopramide, but the confirmation of these findings has not yet been provided (van der Padt et al., 2006). In summary, genetic variants may help in the individualization of drug dosing and the prediction of treatment outcome with the use of 5HT3 antagonists, although its routine use in therapeutics will require further confirmation by larger studies.

8. Resume

In table 3 major gastroenterological diseases are described as well as the drugs available for pharmacological treatment and the enzymes involved in their metabolism.

DISEASE	ENZYME	DRUGS
Peptic Ulcer	CYP2C19	Proton Pump Inhibitors
Inflammatory Bowel Disease	TMPT	Azathioprine 6-Mercaptopurine
Gilbert Meulengracht syndrome	UGT1A1	Irinotecan
Hepatitis C	IL28B	Peg-IFN
Nausea and vomiting associated with chemotherapy and postoperative states.	CYP2D6	Type 3 serotonin receptor (5HT3) antagonists

Table 3. Gastroenterological diseases, drug and associated metabolic enzyme

In table 4, the genes involved in the pharmacogenomic studies for gastroenterological diseases are summarized, as well as their effects in the enzymatic activities and phenotypic consequences.

GENE	POLIMORPHISM	EFFECT	CONSEQUENCES
CYP2C19	SNPs-Alleles: *2, *3, *4, *6	Decrease activity	Poor metabolizers
	SNPs-Allele: *17	Increase activity	Ultrarapid Metabolizers
TMPT	SNPs-Alleles: *2, *3ª, *3B, *3C	Decrease activity	Toxicity
UGT1A1	STRs -Short Tandem Repeats-:113 Alleles	Different activity levels	Predict the occurrence of severe hematologic toxicity with irinotecan
IL28B	SNPs: TT variant	Associated with the sustained virological response (SVR)	Impact on the prognosis and treatment of Hepatitis C with interferon
CYP2D6	SNPs: more than 50 alleles	Different activity levels	Poor to Ultrarapid Metabolizers

Table 4. The most important genes, variants and their effects on the enzymatic activities involved in pharmacological treatment of gastroenterological diseases.

9. Conclusions

In some of the most important areas of gastroenterological therapy, the relevance of pharmacogenomic analysis has been already demonstrated or is in the process of confirmation for both the identification of the proper dosage for a particular patient and the prevention of significant toxicity.

The major polymorphisms (*2 and *3) of CYP2C19 associated with the phenotype of poor metabolizers in certain drugs, can identify patients who will achieve higher plasma concentrations of the main proton-pump inhibitors with the use of standard doses. Because this particular therapeutic group has a wide therapeutic range, the presence of higher concentrations is associated with higher treatment success rates for the treatment of Helicobacter pylori in either peptic ulcer disease or gastroesophagic reflux disease. The knowledge of these associations is particularly useful in populations with a higher prevalence of these polymorphisms. The analysis of variants in the promoter region of the UGT1A1 enzyme coding gene facilitates the identification of patients with Gilbert Meulengracht syndrome, although its pharmacogenetic relevance is currently limited to the cytostatic irinotecan. The experience that has been gained with the use of pharmacogenomic studies in the context of inflammatory bowel disease is currently limited to the analysis of variants of the TMPT coding gene. These variants are associated with the risk of the hematologic adverse effects of azathioprine, and its analysis has resulted in favourable pharmacoeconomic evaluations.

Other polymorphisms, such as the ones in the intracellular glucocorticoid receptor, the MDR1 gene that encodes P-glycoprotein and the TNF receptor, warrant further evaluation. However, to date there is no incontrovertible evidence regarding their clinical usefulness. The identification of polymorphisms in IL28 likely represents a potential new paradigm in the treatment of Hepatitis C infection. Genetic testing for antiemetic drugs will likely show great potential are expected to be developed in the near future, although their final usefulness will only be established after the acquisition of more clinical data.

Currently, pharmacogenomics only constitutes a tool that can be utilized for personalized medicine, and it provides a concrete potential to predict therapeutic responses beyond the population level. Because it has been recently developed, it also benefits from the interest that is generated by its novelty. In the next few years, it will become more clear which aspects of this method can offer specific advantages regarding the efficacy and safety of the patients when compared to the aspects that are only of an academic interest.

However, given the fact that the therapeutic experience with the use of drugs in gastroenterology is far from satisfactory, any firm step in the direction of individualizing drug treatment will facilitate better patient care.

10. References

Akaba, K.; Kimura, T.; Sasaki, A.; Tanabe, S.; Wakabayashi, T.; Hiroi, M.; Yasumura, S.; Maki, K.; Aikawa, S.; Hayasaka,K. (1999) Neonatal hyperbilirubinemia and a common mutation of the bilirubin uridine diphosphate-glucuronosyltransferase gene in Japanese. *J. Hum. Genet.*, 44(1), 22-25.

Aparicio E, Parera M, Franco S, y col. IL28 SNP rs8099917 is strongly associated with Pegylated Interferon-alpha and ribavirin therapy treatment failure in HCV/HIV-1 coinfected patients. *PloS One* 2010; 5(10):e13771

Belloso WH, Redal MA. La farmacogenómica y el camino hacia la medicina personalizada. *Medicina* (Bs As) 2010; 70: 265-74.

Bernabeu I, Marazuela M, Lucas T, Loidi L, Alvarez-Escolá C, Luque-Ramírez M, Fernandez-Rodriguez E, Paniagua AE, Quinteiro C, Casanueva FF.Pegvisomant-induced liver injury is related to the UGT1A1*28 polymorphism of Gilbert`s Syndrome. *J clin endocrinol metab.* 2010, 95 (5): 2147:2154.

Bertilsson, L.; Dahl, M. L.; Sjoqvist, F.; Aberg-Wistedt, A.; Humble, M.; Johansson, I.; Lundqvist, E.; Ingelman-Sundberg,M. (1993) Molecular basis for rational megaprescribing in ultrarapid hydroxylators of debrisoquine. *Lancet*, 341(8836), 63.

Brian L. Pearlman (2011). The IL-28 Genotype: How It Will Affect the Care of Patients with Hepatitis C Virus Infection *Curr Gastroenterol Rep* 13:78–86

Bruno S, Crosignani A, Maisonneuve P, et al. Hepatitis C virus genotype 1b as a major risk factor associated with hepatocellular carcinoma in patients with cirrhosis: a seventeen-year prospective cohort study. *Hepatology* 2007; 46:1350.

Candiotti KA, Birnbach DJ, Lubarsky DA, Nhuch F, Kamat A, Koch WH, Nikoloff M, Wu L, Andrews D. The impact of pharmacogenomics on postoperative nausea and vomiting. *Anesthesiology* 2005; 102(3):543-9

Chaudhry A.S, Kochhar R. Indian Genetic polymorphism of CYP2C219 and therapeutic response to proton pump inhibitors. *J med Res* 127, june 2008 p521-530

Chu CM, Yeh CT, Liaw YF. Fulminant hepatic failure in acute hepatitis C: increased risk in chronic carriers of hepatitis B virus. *Gut* 1999; 45:613./

Côté Jean-François, Sylvain Kirzin, Andrew Kramar, et al. *UGT1A1* Polymorphism Can Predict Hematologic Toxicity in Patients Treated with Irinotecan *Clin Cancer Res* 2007;13:3269-3275.

De Morais, S. M.; Wilkinson, G. R.; Blaisdell, J.; Meyer, U. A.;Nakamura, K.; Goldstein, J. A. (1994) Identification of a new genetic defect responsible for the polymorphism of (S)-mephenytoin metabolism in Japanese. *Mol. Pharmacol.*, 46(4), 594-598.].

De Morais, S. M.; Wilkinson, G. R.; Blaisdell, J.; Nakamura, K.;Meyer, U. A.; Goldstein, J. A. (1994) The major genetic defect responsible for the polymorphism of S-mephenytoin metabolism in humans. *J. Biol. Chem.*, 269(22), 15419-15422.].

Desta, Z.; Zhao, X.; Shin, J. G.; Flockhart, D. A. (2002) Clinical significance of the cytochrome P450 2C19 genetic polymorphism. *Clin. Pharmacokinet.*, 41(12), 913-958.].

Egan LJ, Myhre GM, Mays DC, y col. CYP2C19 pharmacogenetics in the clinical use of proton-pump inhibitors for gastroesophageal reflux disease: varian alleles predict gastric acid suppression but not oesophageal acid exposure or reflux symptoms. *Aliment Pharmacol Ther* 2003; 17:1521-8.

Eichelbaum, M.; Baur, M. P.; Dengler, H. J.; Osikowska-Evers, B. O.; Tieves, G.; Zekorn, C.; Rittner, C. (1987) Chromosomal assignment of human cytochrome P-450 (debrisoquine/sparteine type) to chromosome 22. *Br. J. Clin. Pharmacol.*, 23(4), 455-458.

Evans WE, McLeod HL. Pharmacogenomics-drugs disposition, drug targets, and side effects. *N Engl j Med* 2003; 348: 538-549

Evert, B.; Eichelbaum, M.; Haubruck, H.; Zanger, U. M. (1997) Functional properties of CYP2D6 1 (wild-type) and CYP2D6 7 (His324Pro) expressed by recombinant baculovirus in insect cells. *Naunyn. Schmiedebergs. Arch. Pharmacol.*, 355(3), 309-318.

Farci P, Alter HJ, Wong D, et al. A long-term study of hepatitis C virus replication in non-A, non-B hepatitis. *N Engl J Med* 1991; 325:98.)

Fattovich G, Giustina G, Degos F, et al. Morbidity and mortality in compensated cirrhosis type C: a retrospective follow-up study of 384 patients. *Gastroenterology* 1997; 112:463.

Furuta T, Ohashi K, Kamata T, Takashima M, Kosuge K, Kawasaki T, Hanai H, Kubota T, Ishizaki T, Kaneko E. Effect of genetic differences in omeprazole metabolism on cure rates for Helicobacter pylori infection and peptic ulcer. *Ann Intern Med.* 1998 Dec 15; 129(12):1027-30.

Furuta T, Ohashi K, Kobayashi K, Iida I, Yoshida H, Shirai N, Takashima M, Kosuge K, Hanai H, Chiba K, Ishizaki T, Kaneko E. Effects of clarithromycin on the metabolism of omeprazole in relation to CYP2C19 genotype status in humans. *Clinical pharmacology and therapeutics* 1999; Sep;66(3):265-74.

Furuta T, Shirai N, Ohashi K, Ishizaki T. Therapeutic impact of CYP2C19 pharmacogenetics o proton-pump inhibitor-based eradication therapy for Helicobacter pylori. *Methods Find Exp Clin Pharmacol* 2003; 25(2):131-43.

Furuta T, Graham DY. Pharmacologic aspect of eradication therapy for Helicobacter pylori infection. *Gastroenterol Clin North Am* 2010; 39(3):465-80.

Gaedigk, A.; Blum, M.; Gaedigk, R.; Eichelbaum, M.; Meyer, U. A. (1991) Deletion of the entire cytochrome P450 CYP2D6 gene as a cause of impaired drug metabolism in poor metabolizers of the debrisoquine/sparteine polymorphism. *Am. J. Hum. Genet.*, 48(5), 943-950.

Ge D, Fellay J, Thompson AJ, y col. Genetic variation in interleukin 28B predicts hepatitis C treatment-induced viral celarance. *Nature* 2009; 461:399-401

Goldstein JA, Ishikazi T, Chiba K, y col. Frequencies of the defective CYP2C19 alleles responsibles for the mephenytoin poor metabolizer phenotype in various Oriental, Caucasian, Saudi arabian and American Black populations. *Pharmacogenetics* 1997; 7:59-64.

Grebely J, Petoumenos K, Hellard M, et al. Potential role for interleukin-28B genotype in treatment decision-making in recent hepatitis C virus infection. *Hepatology* 2010; 52:1216.

Hindorf U, Lindqvist M, Peterson C, et al.. Pharmacogenetics Turing standardised initiation of thiopurine treatment in inflammatory bowel disease. *Gut* 2006; 55:1423-31.

Ho KY, Gan TJ. Pharmacology, pharmacogenetics and clinical efficacy of 5-hydroxytryptamine type 3 receptorantagonists for postoperative nausea and vomiting. *Curr Opin Anesthesiol* 2006; 19(6):606-11.

Hu KQ, Tong MJ. The long-term outcomes of patients with compensated hepatitis C virus-related cirrhosis and history of parenteral exposure in the United States. *Hepatology* 1999; 29:1311.

Jung Mook Kang. Effect of the CYP2C19 polymorphism on the erradication rate of helicobacter pylori infection by 7 day triple therapy eith regular proton pump inhibitor dosage. *Journal of Gastroenterology and Hepatology* 2008; 23: 1287-1291)

Kagimoto, M.; Heim, M.; Kagimoto, K.; Zeugin, T.; Meyer, U. A. (1990) Multiple mutations of the human cytochrome P450IID6 gene (CYP2D6) in poor metabolizers of debrisoquine. Study of the functional significance of individual mutations by expression of chimeric genes. *J. Biol. Chem.*, 265(28), 17209-17214.

Kang JM, Kim N, Lee DH y col. Effect of the CYP2C19 polymorphism on the eradication rate of Helicobacter pylori infection by 7-day triple therapy with regular proton-pump inhibitor dosage. *J Gastroenterol Hepatol* 2008; 23:1287-91.

Kawamura M, Ohara S, Koike T, y col. Cytochrome P450 2C19 polymorphism influences the rpeventive effect of lanzoprazole on the recurrence of the erosive reflux esophagitis. *J Gastroenterol Hepatol* 2007; 22:222-6.

Lakatos P. Role of genetics in prediction of disease course and response to therapy. *World J gastroenterol* 2010. 16(21): 2609-2615

Lakatos Peter L. Role of genetics in prediction of disease course and response to therapy. *World Journal of Gastroenterology.* 2010 June 7: 16 (21): 2609-2615

Leucuta SE, Viase L. Pharmacokinetics and metabolic drug interactions. *Curr Clin Pharmacol* 2006; 1:5-20.

Lewis DF, Ito Y, Eddershaw PJ, y col. An evaluation of ondansetron binding interactions with human cytochrome P450 enzymes CYP3A4 and CYP2D6. *Drug Metab Lett* 2010; 4(1):25-30.

Liapiakis AM, Jacobson I. Pharmacogenetics of Hepatitis C therapy. *Pharmacogenomics* 2010; 11(2):135-9.

Lyer L, Das S, Janisch L, Wen M, Ramírez J, Karrison T, Fleming GF, Vokes EE, Schilsky RL, Ratain MJ. UGT1A1*28 polymorphism as a determinant of irinotecan disposition and toxicity. *The Pharmacogenomics Journal* 2002; 2, 43–47.

McHutchison JG, Gordon SC, Schiff ER, et al. Interferon alfa-2b alone or in combination with ribavirin as initial treatment for chronic hepatitis C. Hepatitis Interventional Therapy Group. *N Engl J Med* 1998; 339:1485.)

Payne K, Newman W, Fargher E, Tricker K, Bruce IN, Ollier WE. TPMT testing in rheumatology: any better than routine monitoring? *Rheumatology (Oxford)*. May 2007;46(5):727-729.

Perwitasari DA, Gelderblom H, Attohari J, Mustofa M, Dwiprahasto I, Nortier JWR, Guchelaar H-J. Anti-emetic drugs in oncology: pharmacology and individualization by pharmacogenetics. *Int J Clin Pharm* 2011; 33:33-43.

Pierik M, Rutgeerst P, Vlietinck R, Vermeire, S. Pharmacogenomics in inflammatory bowel disease. *World Gastroenterol* 2006. 12(23); 3657-3667

Pierik M., Rutgeerts P.,Vlientinck R., Vermeire S. Pharmocogenetics in inflamatory bowel disease.*World J Gastroenterol*. 2006; June21;12 (23) 3657-3667

Planas R, Ballesté B, Alvarez MA, et al. Natural history of decompensated hepatitis C virus-related cirrhosis. A study of 200 patients. *J Hepatol* 2004; 40:823.

Rauch A, Kutalik Z, Descombes P, y col. Genetic variation in interleukin 28B is associated with chronic hepatitis C and treatment failure: gemome-wide association study. *Gastroenterology* 2010; 138:1338-45.

Redon R, Ishikawa S, Fitch KR y col. Global variation in copy number in the human genome. *Nature* 2006; 80:444-54.

Rosemary J. and Adithan C. The Pharmacogenetics of CYP2C9 and CYP2C19: Ethnic variation and clinical significance.. *Current Clinical Pharmacology* 2007; 2, 93_109.

Schalm SW, Hansen BE, Chemello L, et al. Ribavirin enhances the efficacy but not the adverse effects of interferon in chronic hepatitis C. Meta-analysis of individual patient data from European centers. *J Hepatol* 1997; 26:961.

Shu-Feng Zhou, Yuan Ming Di1, Eli Chan, Yao-Min Du, Vivian Deh-Wei Chow, Charlie Changli Xue, Xinsheng Lai, Jian-Cheng Wang, Chun Guang Li1, Min Tian and Wei Duan (2008) Clinical Pharmacogenetics and Potential Application in Personalized Medicine *Current Drug Metabolism, 9*, 738-784.

Sim SC, Risinger C, Dahl ML, Aklillu E, y col. A common novel CYP2C19 gene variant causes ultrarapid drug metabolism relevant for the drug response to the proton-pump inhibitors and antidepressants. *Clin Pharmacol Ther* 2006; 79: 103-13.

Strassburg CP. Gilbert-Meulengracht's syndrome and pharmacogenetics: is jaundice just the tip of the iceberg? *Drug Metab Rev.* 2010;42(1):162-75.

Strassburg CP. Pharmacogenetics of Gilbert's syndrome. *Pharmacogenomics* 2008; 9(6):703-15.

Suppiah V, Moldovan M, Ahlenstiel G, y col. Interleukin 28B is associated with response to Hepatitis C interferon-alpha and ribavirin therapy. *Nat Genet* 2009; 41:1100-4

Takahashi M, Yamada G, Miyamoto R, et al. Natural course of chronic hepatitis C. *Am J Gastroenterol* 1993; 88:240

Tanaka Y, Nishida N, Sugiyama M, y col. Genome-wide association of Interleukin 28B with response to interferon alpha and ribavirin therapy for chronic hepatitis C. *Nat Genetic* 2009; 41:1105-9.

Tashica Furuta. Influence of CYP2C19 polymorphism on proton pump inhibitor based therapies. *Drug Metab.* 2005; 20(3) 153-167

The International HapMap Consortium: A haplotype map of the human genome. *Nature* 2005; 437:1299-320.

Thomas DL, Thio CL, Martin MP, et al. Genetic variation in IL28B and spontaneous clearance of hepatitis C virus. *Nature* 2009; 461:798.

Thomas DL, Thio CL, Martin MP, y col. Genetic variation of IL28B and spontaneous clearance of hepatitis C virus. *Nature* 461; 2009: 198-802

Tong MJ, el-Farra NS, Reikes AR, Co RL. Clinical outcomes after transfusion-associated hepatitis C. *N Engl J Med* 1995; 332:1463.

van den Akker Elske -van Marle, David Gurwitz Symone B Detmar, Christine M Enzing, Michael M Hopkins, Emma Gutierrez de Mesa & Dolores Ibarreta. Cost-effectiveness of pharmacogenomics in clinical practice: a case study of thiopurine methyltransferase genotyping in acute lymphoblastic leukemia in Europe. *Pharmacogenomics* 2006; July, Vol. 7, No. 5, Pages 783-792.

Van der Padt A, van Schaik RHN, Sonneveld P. Acute dystonic reaction to metoclopramide in patients carrying homozygous cytochrome P450 2D6 genetic polymorphisms. *The Netherlands J Med* 2006; 64(5):160-2

Vermeire S, Van Assche G, Rutgeerts P. Role of genetics in prediction of disease course and response to therapy. *World J Gastroenterol* 2010, June 7; 16(21):2609-15.

Wang L, McLeod HL, Weinshilboum RL. Genomics and drug response. *N Engl J Med* 2011; 364:1144-53.

Weinshilboum RM, Wang L. Pharmacogenetics and pharmacogenomics: development, science and translation. *Annu Rev Genomics Hum Genet* 2006;7:223-45.

Winter J, Walker A, Shapiro D, y col. Cost-efectiveness of thiopurine-methyltransferase genotype screening in patients about to commence azathioprine therapy for treatment of inflammatory bowel disease. *Aliment Pharmacol Ther* 2004; 20:904-15.

Yano M, Kumada H, Kage M, et al. The long-term pathological evolution of chronic hepatitis C. *Hepatology* 1996; 23:1334.)

10

The Pharmacogenetics
of the Antimalarial Amodiaquine

José Pedro Gil[1,2,3]
1Department of Physiology and Pharmacology, Drug Resistance Unit,
Division of Pharmacogenetics, Karolinska Institutet, Stockholm,
2Department of Biomedical Sciences, University of Algarve
IBB-Institute for Biotechnology and Bioengineering,
The Centre for Molecular and Structural Biomedicine, Gambelas,
3Department of Biological Sciences, The Harpur College of Arts and Sciences,
Binghamton University, Binghamton, the New York State University, NY,
1Sweden
2Portugal
3USA

1. Introduction

Malaria is globally the most lethal parasitic disease. With an annual number of new cases reaching hundreds of millions and a mortality of *circa* 800.000 (WHO, 2010), this disease represents a worldwide major public health concern.

Malaria generally occurs in tropical and subtropical areas, with most of the lethality focused in the African continent, particularly among children under five. The disease further commands a major economic impact in the Developing World estimated as a Gross Internal Product reduction of more than US$ 6 billion for the year 2010 alone (Sachs and Malaney, 2002)(WHO, 2010). Such burden has significantly slowed down the social development of these regions in the last decades.

Malaria is caused by an intracellular Protozoan belonging to the *genus Plasmodium*. *P. falciparum*, *P. vivax*, *P. ovale*, *P. malariae* and *P. knowlesi* are the five different species able to infect humans (Levine, 1988)(Cox-Singh *et al.*, 2008). *P. falciparum* is responsible for the most severe forms of the disease, and hence the near totality of the mortality.

The parasites are transmitted through an arthropod vector, the dynamics of the disease being the result of a complex interplay between the human host, the parasite and its mosquito vector.

2. *Plasmodium falciparum* – A brief reference to its life-cycle

As a referential example, the 48-hour life cycle of *P. falciparum*, the major malaria pathogen – and the principal target of complex chemotherapeutic measures – is herein presented.

We assume as an arbitrary starting point the moment when a female *Anopheles* mosquito infected with *P.falciparum* penetrates the human skin to obtain a blood meal. If the mosquito saliva is infected with parasite sporozoites, these will be injected into the bloodstream of the host. These forms travel in the bloodstream to the liver where they invade hepatocytes. In this intracellular environment it rapidly divides asexually, generating the next life cycle stage form, the merozoites. These, following the rupture of the hepatocyte, are released in the bloodstream. Here, they invade erythrocytes. Once inside the erythrocyte, the merozoite develops towards the mature trophozoite stage. After these, the parasite undergoes a series of asexual divisions to produce a large segmented schizont filled with mono-nucleated merozoites. The erythrocyte then ruptures releasing the merozoites, a clinically important event associated to the characteristic malaria peaks of fever and chills. These merozoites swiftly reinvade new red blood cells, reinitiating the intra-eryrthocytic cycle. In parallel, a small proportion of merozoites take a new development route towards becoming sexual forms: the male and female gametocytes. These can reinvade the mosquito vector during its blood meal. Inside the mosquito, zygotes will form after meiotic events. Further development will lead to the formation of oocysts. These, after repeated mitotic divisions, produce a large number of sporozoites, which actively migrate to the salivary glands of the mosquito, ready to be injected into the bloodstream of a human. The cycle is hence restarted.

3. Malaria chemotherapy

Chemotherapy has been the mainstay for the clinical control of malaria for hundreds of years. Starting with the introduction of artemisinin rich teas in China 1500 years ago (Hsu, 2009) and the use of barks containing quinine in South America in the XVII Century (Peters, 1970), the XX Century saw the development of several synthetic and semi-synthetic compounds. Quinine prevailed as the major antimalarial drug used worldwide for near 300 years, until the advent of the Second World War. The extension of this conflict drove the search for alternative synthetic variants. Derived from these efforts, chloroquine (CQ), a highly effective 4-aminoquinoline, emerged in the immediate post-War as the global mainstay for the treatment and control of malaria (Coatney *et al.*, 1963). By the end of the 1950s the next major malaria challenge emerged: *P. falciparum* have been able to develop resistance to this drug (Young and Moore, 1961). From two main *foci* in South East Asia and South America, resistance parasites invaded most of the other malaria-affected regions. In the late 1970s reached Africa. By the end of the Century the burden of malaria topped in a calculated multi-million death toll and an uncontrolled situation in large regions, particularly in the African Continent (Marsh, 1998).

The severity of the situation demanded a change in concept. This came from South East Asia. In the late 1980s, Thailand - a region known to be a major cradle for the development of drug resistance - was fighting with a steep decrease of efficacy of their main national control programme drug, mefloquine (Nosten *et al.*, 1991). A strategy of combining this long half-life drug with the fast acting/short half-life antimalarials of the artemisinin class (re-discovered in China during the 1970s) saved the former during the next decade (Nosten *et al.*, 2000).

The success of artemisinin combination therapy (ACT) in the Thai national malaria programme drove the rapid adoption, and progressive worldwide implementation of this strategy for the treatment of uncomplicated malaria.

This relatively new antimalaria strategy is based on the powerful pharmacodynamic action of the artemisinin derivatives (ARTs). These, typically artesunate or artemether, are known to have a Parasite Reduction Ratio of 1:10.000 (i.e., a reduction towards 0.01% of the initial parasitaemia in 48 hours of treatment), orders of magnitude above the typically found with long lasting quinoline drugs (White, 1997). This effect is short-lived, due to the characteristic very short half live of the ARTs, typically 20 minutes to 2-3 hours (Gautam *et al.*, 2009). Upon this first impact, the long-standing partner is expected to handle more efficiently the remaining parasite population. The association of drugs with different expected mechanisms of action and associated modes of parasite resistance has been deemed as a strong deterrent for the development of the latter (Eastman and Fido, 2009).

The two global main ACTs in use are artemether-lumefantrine and artesunate-amodiaquine. (WHO, 2010). The latter represents the main drive for this review.

4. Amodiaquine

Amodiaquine (AQ) emerged in the shadow of CQ success, in the late 1940s (Burckhalter *et al.*, 1948). Similar to CQ, AQ has a core 4-aminoquinoline structure. Contrarily to CQ it also represents a Mannich base.

AQ was never used to the same extent as CQ due to the large prevalence of the latter in the global malaria control programmes until the end of the XX Century. Also, its use was severely curtailed in the beginning of the 1990s, upon its removal from the WHO list of recommended antimalarials for the treatment of uncomplicated malaria (WHO, 1990). This decision followed the emergence of a number of clinical reports on rare (*ca.* 1:2000) but life-threatening secondary events associated to its use in prophylaxis regimens among Caucasian travellers (Larrey *et al.*, 1986)(Rouveix *et al.*, 1989)(Neftel *et al.*, 1986)(Hatton *et al.*, 1986). These included in most cases acute agranulocytosis, but also severe liver damage. During the 1990s, research - mainly based on *in vitro* approaches and the use of animal models - have pointed for the causing agent to be a toxic short lived quinone-imine (QI) metabolite of AQ (Jewell *et al.*, 1995)(Tingle *et al.*, 1995)(Naisbitt *et al.*, 1997). The mode of action of this putative metabolite is still under discussion, but it is generally accepted that it operates by binding covalently to cell structures or/and as an hapten associated to a specific anti-AQ IgG antibody driven immunological response (Clarke *et al.*, 1990).

The described prophylaxis effects were never formally confirmed in circumstances of the regular treatment of uncomplicated malaria. This lack of confirmatory data has raised some criticisms concerning a possible over-cautious decision at WHO (Olliaro *et al.*, 1996). In fact, the actual usefulness of this decision in a time when the efficacy of CQ was collapsing worldwide is still open to discussion. Nevertheless, AQ as a monotherapy kept being used in many African and South American regions for decades, both in the public and in the private sector.

Interestingly, the fact that AQ has not been as intensively used as CQ possibly slowed down the development of parasite resistance against this drug. AQ was recovered for global use in the XXI Century as combination therapy partner, due its low price and capacity to handle CQ resistance parasites. Two combinations are available, artesunate-AQ (an ACT), and AQ-sulfadoxine-pyrimethamine, although the latter has been recently considered to be withdrawn from the WHO list of recommended drugs for the treatment of uncomplicated malaria (WHO,

2010). Artesunate-AQ (AS-AQ) is particularly prevalent in the African continent, the epicentre of malaria mortality and morbidity. The combination represents the first or second line antimalarial treatment for uncomplicated malaria in more then twenty sub-Saharan countries (www.who.int/entity/malaria/am_drug_policies_by_region_afro/en/).

AS-AQ is administrated orally in one daily dose, for three days. The present guideline is: 4mg/Kg/day artesunate + 10mg/Kg/day AQ (WHO, 2010). Contrarily to other antimalarials (e.g. lumefantrine, CQ, piperaquine), the age of the patient does not seem to affect the plasma concentrations of AQ. The present dosing has shown to be effective in areas where resistance to AQ monotherapy was not widespread (<20% of the infections). In the event of rising resistance, changes in the formulation might be necessary, namely increasing the dosing in AQ. Such changes in the dosing have been applied in the past, e.g. with CQ (Peters, 1970) and mefloquine (Carrara et al., 2009).

Presently, AS-AQ is available as a fixed formulation in three tablet options: 25 mg AS/67.5 mg AQ, 50 mg AS/135 mg AQ or 100 mg AS/270 mg AQ (Coarsucam®/Winthrop®,Sanofi-Aventis, Paris; DNDi, Geneva).

Both AQ and desethylamodiaquine (DEAQ, AQ main active metabolite) show significant inter-individual variation on their pharmacokinetic parameters. AQ has a relatively short half-life of 4-12 hours (Giao and de Vries., 2000), being readily biotransformed in the liver towards DEAQ. DEAQ is a fully active antimalarial that, albeit less potent then AQ (Gerstner et al., 2003)(Echeverry et al., 2007) is the main responsible for the long pharmacodynamic effect of AQ therapy (Winstanley et al., 1990). DEAQ has a longer half-life of 3-20 days (Hombhanje et al., 2005)(Hietala et al., 2007). Although AQ has been even considered as a pro-drug due to its short half-life, circumstances of extreme AQ exposure have been documented where this drug was detected in the urine of patients, months after its administration (Winstanley et al., 1987).

AQ has been associated with both mild and severe adverse events. Mild events include mainly gastro-intestinal effects, particularly vomiting (Brasseur et al., 1999)(Adjuik et al., 2002)(Cairns et al., 2010)(Nankabirwa et al., 2010) and self-reported abdominal pain (Parikh et al., 2007)(Bojang et al., 2010), both frequently observed in amodiaquine efficacy clinical trials. Most importantly, several studies have noted situations of (clinically asymptomatic) neutropenia upon AQ therapies in subsets of the treated population (Staedke et al., 2001)(Adjuik et al., 2002). Although this relatively common drop in neutrophil count is not an exclusive effect of this drug (Nankabirwa et al., 2010), it is possibly linked with the rare severe adverse events observed in AQ prophylaxis. Accordingly, in this (now abandoned) higher dose regimens of typically 400 mg/week, the most documented serious adverse event was agranulocytosis (~1:2000 prevalence), followed by hepatic toxicity (~1:16000)(Phillips-Howard and West, 1990)(Hatton et al., 1986).

The few data available suggest that the AQ adverse events are drug dose dependent (Hatton et al., 1986)(Cairns et a., 2010). Although drug associated severe and lethal reactions have not been generally observed in AQ regimens for the treatment of uncomplicated malaria (Olliaro et al., 1996)(Olliaro and Mussano, 2003), mild events are relatively frequent, being a threat for full regimen compliance (e.g. Gerstl et al., 2010), leading to incomplete cure and potential selection of resistant parasites. This effect can be decreased through genetic evidence-based adjustment of the dose, at a personalized level.

In addition, the knowledge of the frequencies of rare genetic variants associated with documented AQ-driven adverse events in certain ethnic groups and regions under AQ exposure can be useful as a pharmacovigilance tool. As an example, and taking in account the surpassing of a specific (evidence-based) threshold of allele frequency, the use of alternative first line ACTs (e.g aminoalcohol quinoline based, as artemether-lumefantrine) for those regions could be decided. Such type of measures - although not totally preventing - have the potential of decreasing the occurrence of serious events.

It should be noted that such a population pharmacogenetics approach can be of great importance: the effect of fatal adverse events in the public opinion can be very significant, especially after the 1990s temporary withdrawal of AQ from the WHO list of recommended antimalarials. Such dramatic events - in particular involving the typical children under five - could lead to a further mistrust of the public about a drug that is pivotal in a large number of national malaria control programmes.

5. The main players of AQ disposition

As previously mentioned, upon oral absorption AQ is readily metabolized towards the pharmacologically active DEAQ. This biotransformation occurs mostly in the liver and is almost exclusively performed by the cytochrome P450 (CYP) 2C8 (Li et al., 2002). The high specificity of CYP2C8 for this reaction has even led to the proposal of AQ as a specific probe drug for this P450 isoform (Walsky et al., 2004). Besides this main step, other putative AQ metabolites have been proposed and at least partially confirmed (figure 1). These include 2-hydroxy-DEAQ (Churchill et al., 1985), N-Bis-DEAQ (Mount et al., 1986) and M2, the latter initially detected in the microsome-based seminal studies of Li et al (2002), and recently confirmed through in vitro electrochemical approaches (Johansson et al., 2009). A fraction of DEAQ itself is believed to also be transformed in 2-hydroxy-DEAQ through P450 action. Several of these post-CYP2C8 action steps are catalyzed by members of the CYP1 sub-family (Li et al., 2002)(Gil and Gil-Berglund, 2007)(Johansson et al., 2009).

Most importantly, both AQ and DEAQ are able to generate the highly reactive quinone-imine (QI) metabolite responsible for the described serious side affects of AQ therapies. DEAQ is considered less prone to create QIs (Tingle et al., 1995), reinforcing the action of CYP2C8 over AQ as a protective event. The generation of these compounds has been previously proposed to occur spontaneously, but recent investigations have pointed to a fundamental role of CYP1A1 and CYP1B1 as well as the family of myeloperoxidases in the process. In this processes, the M2 metabolite initially identified by Li et al. has been proposed to be a central player in the generation of the toxic QIs (Johansson et al., 2009).

Taking in account the fact that these species are most likely short-lived, it is expected that the enzymes involved in its generation will be present in the location of its toxic action. Suggestively, CYP1A1 and CYP1B1 are essentially extra-hepatic P450 isoforms, with confirmed expression in several blood cell types (e.g. leukocyes)(Furukawa et al., 2004), the most frequent location for these fatal toxicities (neutropenia).

Scarce information is available concerning other ADME phases in AQ metabolism. The analysis of QI adducts in animal models have pointed for the presence of glutathione conjugates, although no specific isoform has ever been determined (Masubuchi et al., 2007). The potential production of phase II metabolites further points to the likely involvement of phase III (transport) systems. The most common phase III glutathione conjugate transporters are the members of the ATP binding cassette (ABC) superfamily of proteins, and more specifically of the ABCC (also referred as MRP) type of transporters.

A summarized proposal of the complex metabolism of AQ is presented in figure 1.

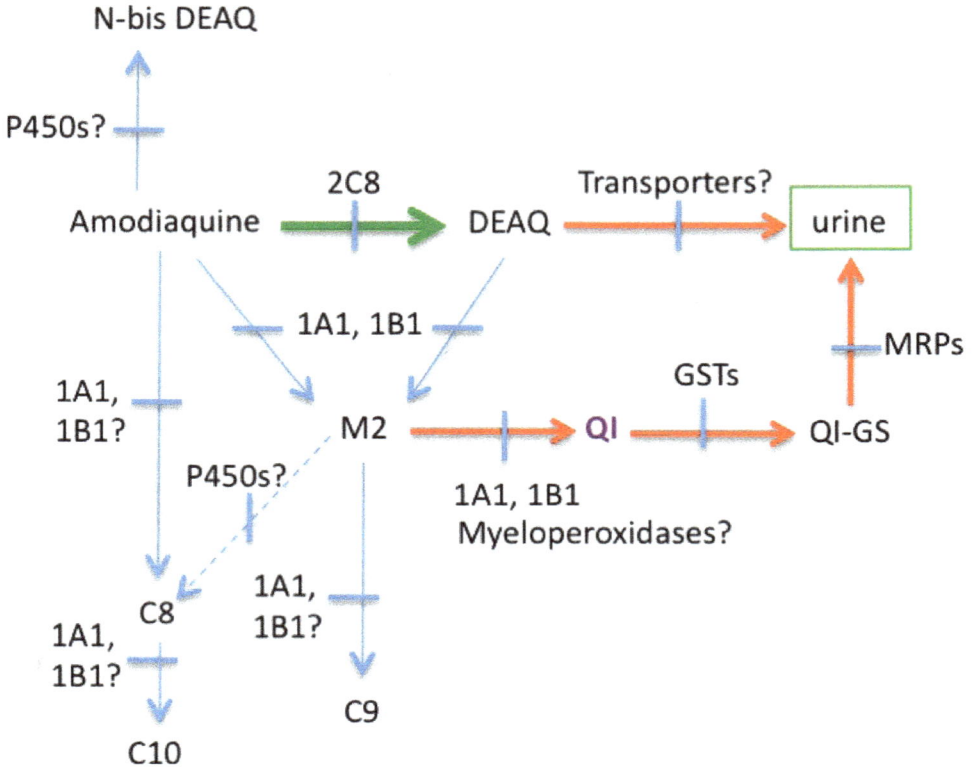

Abbreviations - 1A1: CYP1A1; 1B1: CYP1B1; DEAQ:desethylAQ; QI: quinoneimine; N-bis DEAQ: bis-desethylAQ; C8: compound 8; C9: compound 9; C10: compound 10; QI-GS: quinoneimine-glutathione conjugates; GST: glutathione S-transferase; MRPs: multidrug resistance proteins.

Fig. 1. The metabolism of AQ. Although the main biotransformation in this process is the synthesis of DEAQ, a constellation of minor – but most likely non-negligible – metabolites have been proposed to result in parallel (Churchill *et al.*, 1985)(Mount *et al.*, 1986)(Li *et al.*, 2002). Most importantly, events leading to the formation of the toxic QIs, involving both AQ and DEAQ are included among them. The presented scheme represents a summary of the available data from *in vitro* studies with microsomes, animal models, the few available human *in vivo* data, as well as the most recent information utilizing electrochemical approaches to simulate drug oxidation *in vitro* (Harrison *et al.*, 1992)(Jewell *et al.*, 1995)(Tingle *et al.*, 1995)(Naisbitt *et al.*, 1997)(Li *et al.*, 2002)(Johansson *et al.*, 2009).

The previously identified M2 metabolite (Li *et al.*, 2002) seems to be a central component in the generation of the QIs from both AQ and DEAQ, with CYP1A1 and CYP1B1 being the main enzymes involved in the process (Johansson *et al.*, 2009). The QIs have been proposed to result from the action of myeloperoxidases, an event that is herein tentatively proposed to involve the M2 metabolite, although a direct action of these enzymes in both AQ and DEAQ cannot be disregarded.

In vitro electrochemical approaches have generated a number of putative compounds, the most relevant being indicated here (C8, C9 and C10). This complex of compounds, due to its expected hydroxylated structures has been proposed to most likely represent the previously reported 2-hydroxy-DEAQ (Churchill *et al.*, 1985).

6. The pharmacogenetics of AQ metabolism

As described, based on current knowledge, three main drug metabolizing enzymes are involved in the biotransformation of AQ: CYP2C8 (the main one), CYP1A1 and CYP1B1. All of them harbour significant genetic polymorphisms, some with marked effects in the catalytic activities of the respectively coded proteins.

6.1 CYP2C8

The *CYP2C8* comprises nine exons. 14 alleles have been annotated in the gene coding for this 490 amino acid enzyme (http://www.cypalleles.ki.se/cyp2c8.htm), most of them rare. Apart from the most prevalent alleles, 2C8*1 (wild type), 2C8*2, 2C8*3, and 2C8*4, the majority of the remaining ones (2C8*5 - 2C8*12, see figure 2) have been identified only in the Japanese population (Soyama *et al.*, 2001)(Nakajima *et al.*, 2003). Few works have evaluated the presence of these minor alleles in other regions (Cavaco *et al.*, 2006)(Suarez-Kurtz *et al.*, 2010), although the output of large consortium projects (e.g. HapMap, www.sanger.ac.uk/resources/downloads/human/hapmap3.html) supports the view of these alleles being specific among the Japanese. On the other hand, 2C8*2, 2C8*3 and 2C8*4 are rare in this population. (Nakajima *et al.*, 2003)(table 1).

African settings represent the major context where AQ therapy is practiced, both in combination with artesunate or sulfadoxine-pyrimethamine. The first CYP2C8 pharmacogenetic study in endemic African populations was performed in East African populations, in the islands of Zanzibar (Cavaco *et al.*, 2005)(table 1). In this population all the most studied mutant alleles, namely 2C8*2, 2C8*3 and 2C8*4, were detected. Further studies in other regions of the continent have confirmed 2C8*2 as the main allele among the native populations (see table 1). Interestingly, outside Zanzibar, 2C8*3 (when found) has been documented at lower frequencies, while 2C8*4 has not been detected at all. These results point to the populations of Zanzibar as somewhat particular, perhaps due to the historical/migration influences from the Arabian Peninsula (Low and Smith, 1976).

The data from native African populations was consistent with previous reports in African-American, where the 2C8*2 allele represents the main mutant allele in Black populations (table 1), with the non-active 2C8*3 mostly present among Caucasians (Cavaco *et al.*, 2006).

A number of *in vitro* studies have been performed to characterize the phenotypic effect of the CYP2C8 polymorphisms.

Region (n*)	2C8*2	2C8*3	2C8*4	Reference
Zanzibar (Unguja and Pemba)(n= 165)	13.9%	2.1%	0.6%	Cavaco et al., 2005
Ghana (Accra)(n= 204)	17.9%	0%	0%	Kudzi et al., 2009
Ghana (n= 92)	17.9%	n/t[a]	n/t[a]	Adjei et al., 2008
Ghana (Tamale) (n= 200)	16.8%	0.0%	0.0%	Rower et al., 2005
Burkina Faso (Bobo-Dioulasso) (n=275)	11.5%	0.4%	n/t	Parikh et al., 2007
Southern India (n=245)	0.8%	2.9%	n/t	Arun Kumar et al., 2011
Malaysia[b] (n= 57)	0.8%	1.2%	0%	Muthiah et al., 2005
South East Asia (n= 20) [c]	0.0%	5.0%	0%	Solus et al, 2004
Papua-New Guinea (Madang) (n = 305)	0%	0%	0%	Hombhanje et al., 2005
Brazil (scattered regions)(n= 1034)[d]	6.4%	8.6%	3.4%	Suarez-Kurtz et al., 2010

*number of subjects analysed; n/t (non tested)
[a] Any 2C8*3 or 2C8*4 alleles present confounded in the 2C8*1 group.
[b] Indian ethnic group
[c] Derived from a commercial repository – no specific origin disclosed.
[d] Ethnically mixed populations, originated from several scattered regions of the country. The sample is claimed by the authors to be representative of the present day Brazilian population; when considering self-reporting ethnic origin, the 2C8*3 frequency increased among "White" subjects, while the *2 among "Black" individuals.
(note: this compilation is intended to be a representative sample of the published information and not an exhaustive collection of the available data)
Abbreviation – CYP2C8: 2C8

Table 1. CYP2C8 main allele frequencies in populations from malaria endemic regions (Africa, Asia, Oceania and South America).

The CYP2C8*2 allele is characterized by the presence of an I269F SNP. Quantitative HPLC/UV analysis of the DEAQ resulting from in vitro incubations of recombinant CYP2C8*2 enzyme with AQ pointed to a significant decrease of approximately 30% in the V_{max}, (maximum substrate transformation rate) as compared with the wild-type (2C8*1) reference (0.16 ± 0.06 μmol/min/μmol P450 vs 0.23 ± 0.09 μmol/min/μmol P450). In parallel, the mutant allele was associated with a three-fold increase in its Km (substrate concentration at which the reaction reaches half of the V_{max} value) (2.55 ± 1.06 μM vs 0.81 ± 0.23 μM) (Parikh et al., 2007). This decreased performance was reflected in a significantly lower intrinsic clearance (V_{max}/K_m) of AQ (2C8*2: 0.05 l/min/μmol P450 vs 2C8*1: 0.30 l/min/μmol P450). As for the CYP2C8*3, the presence of the two linked mutations characterizing this protein (R139K and R399K) had a marked effect on its catalytic capacities, with no AQ metabolism detected at any of the tested substrate concentrations (Parikh et al., 2007). It was concluded that the 2C8*3 protein has very low AQ metabolism activity. These results obtained with AQ are supported by data from previous studies using the CYP2C8 probe drug paclitaxel (Dai et al., 2001).

As for 2C8*4, *in vitro* experiments by Singh *et al.* have reported this protein as having a 10 fold decrease in paclitaxel 6-alpha hydroxylase activity. The associated SNP (I264M, see figure 2) was proposed to affect heme insertion and the correct folding of the protein (Singh *et al.*, 2008). It is expectable that this also represents a low activity allele as for the biotransformation of amodiaquine.

More recently, Gao and collaborators performed tests based on the heterologous expression of *2C8*2*, *2C8*3* and *2C8*4* in *Saccharomyces cerevisae*. Microsomes prepared from the transfected yeast cells were incubated with different concentrations of AQ. The experiments showed a decrease in the overall activity of the mutant alleles towards ~ 45-75% of the wild type values (Gao *et al.*, 2010). The reasons behind the observed large differences in the capacities of these alleles between the microsome based systems and the *in vitro* based ones (i.e. reconstituted protein) are not fully clear.

Some of the remaining minor alleles have been studied in some detail in Japan. The *2C8*5* allele carries a 475delA mutation causing a frameshift effect leading to a premature translation termination at residue 177, and hence no functional protein (Soyama *et al.*, 2002). Using microsomes obtained from *CYP2C8* transfected COS-1 cells, the 2C8*6, 2C8*9 and 2C8*10 proteins were shown not to significantly differ from the wild type (2C8*1) on paclitaxel 6-alpha hydroxylase activity. As for 2C8*8, this allele showed more than ten fold decrease in catalytic activity, associated with a less stable protein. As expected, 2C8*7 – involving the introduction of a translational stop codon - had no detectable enzyme activity (Hichiya *et al.*, 2005). Finally, Hanioka and collaborators have recently used the same yeast system for testing the *2C8*13* and *2C8*14* alleles. While 2C8*13 did not show significant differences in V_{max} and K_m for paclitaxel 6-alpha hydroxylation as compared with 2C8*1, 2C8*14 showed a 3 fold higher K_m, albeit with no changes in the V_{max}.

A summary of relevant *CYP2C8* SNPs and the associated phenotype characteristics is presented in figure 2.

In vivo, there is limited information on the impact of *CYP2C8* polymorphisms in AQ therapy, both in terms of efficacy and risk of adverse events.

Parikh and collaborators have performed a retrospective analysis of an AQ monotherapy efficacy trial searching for *in vivo* phenotype/2C8 genotype associations (Parikh *et al.*, 2007). The study involved 275 uncomplicated malaria patients from the region of Bobo-Dioulasso, southwest Burkina Faso. No associations were found between the clinical success of AQ therapy and the presence of minor *CYP2C8* alleles (*2C8*2* and *2C8*3*). This is probably due to the fact that DEAQ, the main AQ metabolite, also represents a fully active antimalarial entity, i.e. enhanced AQ metabolism does not lead to an inactive metabolite that would decrease the clinical (pharmacodynamic) success of the therapy. More importantly, Parikh *et al* found a positive correlation between harbouring a *2C8*2* allele and events of mild side effects, mainly abdominal pain (self reported): 52% of occurrences among the *2C8*2* carriers *versus* 30% for the *2C8*1/*1* subjects. This is until now the only reported association between the patient *CYP2C8* status and effects of AQ therapy. Another trial, performed in Ghana did not report such an association (Adjei *et al.*, 2008). It also did not find clear associations between the pharmacokinetic parameters of AQ and the presence of less active alleles, although a trend for decreased DEAQ plasma concentrations among the *2C8*2* carriers was noted. It must be noted however, that the smaller size of this study (n=92) might have prevented the detection of such associations.

These are the only two published studies exploring the impact of the *CYP2C8* polymorphism in AQ based therapies, while near 100 million treatments performed in the last five years (WHO, 2010). It is evident that there is an urgent need of further research in this area, in order to guarantee the longest "useful life" for this drug, presently a cornerstone in the global control of malaria.

6.2 CYP1A1

CYP1A1 represents a 512 amino acid cytochrome P450 enzyme mainly expressed in extra-hepatic tissues, including the lungs (Willey *et al.*, 1997), intestine (Paine *et al.*, 1999)(Paine *et al.*, 2006), placenta (Hakkola *et al.*, 1996) and, importantly, lymphocytes (Dey *et al.*, 2001, van Duursen *et al.*, 2005). It is usually present at low constitutive baseline levels. The gene is readily inducible through the AHR (Aryl Hidrocarbon Receptor) regulatory pathway, typically by exposure to PAHs (polycyclic aromatic hydrocarbons, e.g. components of tobacco smoke). Upon induction, CYP1A1 can also be found in the liver, where it usually is at very low (pre-induction) baseline levels. CYP1A1 is able to metabolize a number of clinically relevant drugs, including the calcium blocker flunarizine, the anticancer drug toremifene and the cardiovascular disease drug fluvastatin. Significant inter-individual variability in the elimination of these drugs has been described. This variability is probably of minor clinical concern, due to the non-hepatic patterns of expression of the gene. In the context of this review, the importance of CYP1A1 is mainly focused in its probable involvement in the generation of short lived but toxic AQ metabolites (Johansson *et al.*, 2009).

The *CYP1A1* gene (15q24.1) is organized in 7 exons. It harbours significant polymorphisms, comprising eleven established alleles (figure 2), as well as a number of SNPs with haplotype associations still to be assigned (http://www.cypalleles.ki.se/cyp1a1.htm). A significant portion of the non-synonymous polymorphisms is concentrated at exon 7 (figure 2)(table 2).

The *CYP1A1*2* allele has been documented *in vitro* to represent a more drug responsive gene upon exposure to the prototype inducer 2,3,7,8-tetrachlorodibenzo-para-dioxin (TCDD)(studies with the *1A1*2A* and *1A1*2B* haplotypes)(Spurr *et al.*, 1987)(Landi *et al.*, 1994). Also, at least in the case of *1A1*2B* and *1A1*2C*, this allele was shown to code for more active enzymes (Cosma *et al.*, 1993). The increased transcriptional response is related to the presence of a T3801C transition in the gene's 3' UTR, while the referred enhanced enzymatic activity (reflected specifically in an increased V_{max}) is linked with a non-synonymous I462V SNP at exon 7 (Cosma *et al.*, 1993). This enhanced activity of the proteins harbouring 462V (1A1*2B and 1A1*2C) was also confirmed in terms of estrone and 17 ß-estradiol 2-hydroxylation, as a 5-10 fold increase in comparison to the wild type (Kisselev *et al.*, 2005).

The T461N SNP (defining *1A1*4*) was shown not to alter significantly the behaviour of its coded enzyme (Kisselev *et al.*, 2005). As for the 3' UTR T3204C transition defining the *1A1*3* allele (proposed to be specific of African populations) it does not seem to influence the levels of *CYP1A1* expression (Smart and Daly, 2000). *1A1*7* represents a frameshift mutation leading to the generation of a stop codon and hence precluding the production of an active enzyme. Finally, alleles *1A1*8* (T448N), *1A1*9* (R464C) and *1A1*10* (R477W) carry non-synonymous SNPs located close to the protein heme binding protein, and are hence expected to affect the activity of the enzyme (Saito *et al.*, 2003).

Region (n*)	1A1*2	1A1*7	1A1*3	1A1*4	Reference
Namibia[a] (n= 134)	14.9%[b]	n/t	n/t	n/t	Fujihara *et al.*, 2009
Southwest Libya (El Awaynat and Tahala)[c] (n=129)	6.5%[d]	n/t	0%	18.1%	Martinez-Labarga *et al.*, 2007
Midwest and Southeast Nigeria (n= 250)	24.2%[e]	n/t	13%	0%	Okobia *et al.*, 2005
South Africa[f] (n= 96)	0%[g]	n/t	n/t	n/t	Dandara *et al.*, 2002
Zimbabwe (n= 148)	0%[g]	n/t	n/t	n/t	Dandara *et al.*, 2002
Tanzania (n= 114)	1.3%[g]	n/t	n/t	n/t	Dandara *et al.*, 2002
Mali (n=116)	24.0%[g]	n/t	n/t	n/t	Garte *et al.*, 1998
East India (Chennai) (n=150)	33%[g]	n/t	n/t	n/t	Suneetha *et al.*, 2011
Southwest India (Kerala) (n = 146)	20.9%	n/t	n/t	n/t	Sreeja *et al.*, 2005
Northern India (Delhi) (n= 309)	71.4%[h]	n/t	n/t	0%	Kumar *et al.*, 2010
Northern Thailand (Lampang)(n= 287)	84.9%[h,i]	n/t	n/t	n/t	Pisani *et al.*, 2006
China (Peking)(n= 284)[j]	28.2%[h]	n/t	n/t	0%	Zhang *et al.*, 2010

* number of subjects analyzed; n/t: not tested
[a] Bantu (Ocambo) ethnicity
[b] T3798C tested, defining the presence of *1A1*2A* or *1A1*2B*. As the I462V was not determined (*1A1*2C* contribution not included) it is not possible to distinguish between these two forms.
[c] Although these are regions not directly affected by malaria, the nomadic characteristics of the Tuareg populations under study puts them in risk when travelling to sub-Saharan areas (e.g. Northern Mali, Mauritania)
[d] *1A1*2A*= 4.5%, *1A1*2B*= 0.2%, *1A1*2C*=1.8%
[e] *1A1*2A*= 24%, *1A1*2C*= 0.2%. Data on *1A1*2B* not available.
[f] Venda ethnicity
[g] Only T3798C tested, so the data should be considered as the result of the *1A1*2A* + *1A1*2B* composite.
[h] T3798C and I462V tested but no information on the composite of the two giving rise to *2B*
[i] 286 subjects analysed for *1A1*2A*
[j] Only the I462V analysed so *1A1*2A* not included and *1A1*2B* contribution not available
(*note*: this compilation is intended to be a representative sample of the published information and not an exhaustive collection of the available data).
Abbreviation - *CYP1A1: 1A1*

Table 2. *CYP1A1* allele frequencies of population from malaria affected regions of Africa and Asia.

6.3 CYP1B1

Similarly to CYP1A1, the expression of the CYP1B1 isoform is also predominantly extra-hepatic, including peripheral blood cells (Hanaoka *et al.*, 2002)(Furukawa *et al.*, 2004), and it is inducible by exposure to several xenobiotics, namely PAHs (Nebert *et al.*, 2004).

Null alleles are rare in the general population. Most were identified among patients with glaucoma, for which these alleles are an established risk factor (Stoilov et al., 1998), and are not a major concern in the context of this review. The main polymorphic positions in this gene are summarized in figure 2.

The functional consequence of the major CYP1B1 alleles has been studied in vitro upon heterologous expression in E. coli and the quantification of the enzyme's capacity of catalyzing the 4- and 2- hydroxylation of estradiol. The introduction of the R48G, A119S and N453S SNPs did not significantly change the V_{max} and K_m of the resulting proteins, as compared with the wild type (1B1*1) (Li et al., 2000). The L432V SNP was on the other hand associated increased of circa 3 fold in the K_m. Later works using Saccaromyces cervisae heterologous expression systems supported the view of L432V carrier proteins as less active (>K_m values <V_{max} values). Interestingly, in these works this effect was only observed in the context of a SNP haplotype including other polymorphic positions (R48G + A119S + L432V)(Aklillu et al., 2002). Finally, several minor allele of this SNP (present in the 1B1*3, 1B1*5, 1B1*6 and 1B1*7 alleles) have been proposed as associated with a transcriptionaly less active gene (Helmig et al., 2009, 2010).

Presently there is still scarce information available concerning the CYP1B1 allele frequencies in populations living in malaria regions (table 3).

Region (n*)	1B1*2	1B1*3	1B1*4	1B1*5	1B1*6	1B1*7	Reference
Ethiopia (Adis Ababa) (n=150)	36.7%	39.0%	2.0%	0.7%	6.3%	7.0%	Aklillu et al., 2002
North India (Lucknow) (n=200)	33.0%	21.3%	18.3%	n/t	n/t	n/t	Shah et al., 2008
South Central Chin (Chengdu) (N= 400[a])	n/t	57.5%[b]	n/t	n/t	n/t	n/t	Wang et al., 2011
Northeast China (Nanjing) (N= 227)	n/t	15.1%[c]	n/t	n/t	n/t	n/t	Liang et al., 2005

* number of subjects analyzed; n/t: not tested.
[a] Only women were included in the study.
[b] Only the L432V SNP was analysed, meaning that the declared frequency for 1B1*3, also is likely to include also the 1B1*5, 1B1*6 and 1B1*7 alleles.
[c] Only women included in the study. The sole analysis of the A119S does not distinguish between the 1B1*2, 1B1*6 and 1B1*7.
(note: this compilation is intended to be a representative sample of the published information and not an exhaustive collection of the available data).
Abbreviation – CYP1B1: 1B1

Table 3. CYP1B1 allele frequencies of population from malaria affected regions in Africa and Asia.

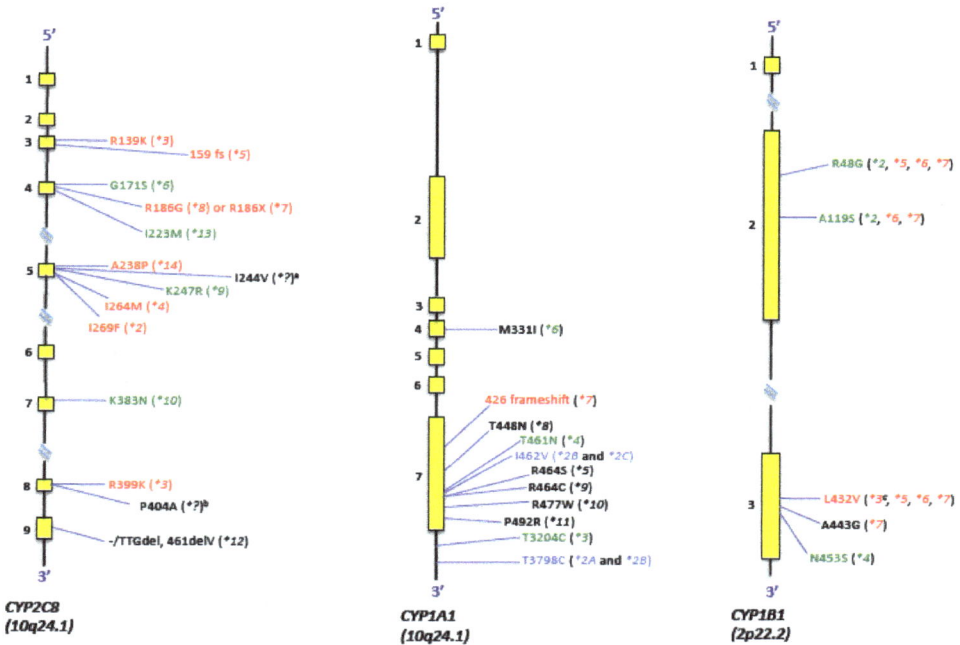

CYP2C8
(10q24.1)

CYP1A1
(10q24.1)

CYP1B1
(2p22.2)

[a] Haplotype not determined yet (reference SNP: rs11572102, NCBI
(http://www.ncbi.nlm.nih.gov/SNP/snp_ref.cgi?rs=11572102);
[b] Discovered by Soyama et al., 2001 and phenotypically characterized by reduced catalytic activity
(Soyama et al., 2002)(Jiang et al., 2011).
[c] The colour code was herein applied according to the data of Aklillu et al. (2002). It is to note that initial
studies by Li et al (2000) noticed a significant decrease in the activity of the protein.

Fig. 2. Genetic diversity of *CYP2C8*, *CYP1A1* and *CYP1B1*, the main polymorphic genes
involved in AQ phase I metabolism. Although the gene structures are represented, the
locations of established polymorphisms are presented using the amino acid nomenclature as
this is more relevant for the present review. For the sake of clarity, only the most studied
alleles, with established haplotype structures are presented. Alleles shown in red color
indicate protein products reported to be less active than the reference wild type (*1). Alleles
in green do not have a significant differences as compared with *1, whereas alleles flagged
in blue have higher activity than the wild type. For alleles in black there is currently no
experimental information available. In the case of the *CYP1B1* the use of the colors is restricted
to alleles (and not SNPs) due to the availability of haplotype data (Akillilu et al., 2002).

7. The CYP2C8, CYP1A1, CYP1B1 trio - Potential implications

In terms of therapeutic efficacy, since DEAQ is a powerful and clinically valuable
antimalarial, variations in the CYP2C8 enzymatic capacity are not expected to have
significant pharmacodynamic consequences. As mentioned, this expectation is in line with
observations by Parikh et al in Burkina-Faso, where the presence of *CYP2C8*2* did not
influence the treatment outcome of AQ monotherapy. On the other hand, pharmacogenetics
might be of particular importance in the identification of individuals in higher risk of

developing AQ-related adverse events. This is supported by the observation in the same study that the presence of *CYP2C8*2* (still an allele associated with significant catalytic capacity, as compared with the much less functional 2C8*3 and 2C8*4) can influence the individual risk for mild adverse events, *even* in heterozygous form could.

Recently *in vitro* evidence was published supporting the involvement of CYP1A1 and CYP1B1 in the generation of toxic QIs from AQ (and DEAQ) (Johansson *et al.*, 2009). This confirmation of preliminarily reports (Li *et al.*, 2002, I. Cavaco, Universidade do Algarve, unpublished) has opened a new perspective towards individualization of AQ therapy to minimize adverse events. In fact, contrarily to the previous view of a spontaneous formation of QIs (Tingle *et al.*, 1995), the involvement of these polymorphic P450s reinforces a broader genetic basis for the phenomenon, which was until now almost exclusively focused on *CYP2C8 (Cavaco et al.*, 2005*)*. The now recognized more extensive genetic background of AQ adverse drug events underlines the importance of individualized medicine and the possibility to identify appropriate molecular markers for predicting response to treatment/risk of adverse reactions.

With this new data, the hypothetical characterization of the sub-group of subjects in higher risk is starting to emerge. The first assumption is that such individuals carry a deficient *CYP2C8* gene (*2C8*2*, ideally the very low active *2C8*3* or *2C8*4*), allowing an extended half-life for AQ (Parikh *et al.*, 2007). This will probably represent the group with $T_{1/2}$ values >12 hours (Giao and de Vries, 2001), as well as the observed outliers showing very long exposure to the drug (Winstanley *et al.*, 1987). With this increased pool of circulating AQ (as previously referred, a compound more prone than DEAQ for the formation of the QI reactive species (Tingle *et al.*, 1995)), the drug will have higher chances to be extra-hepatically catalysed by CYP1A1 and CYP1B1 - both present in leucocytes, where AQ tends to accumulate (Naisbitt *et al.*, 1997). The rate of QI formation is expected to be further enhanced if particularly efficient versions of CYP1A1 and CYP1B1 are present, namely the CYP1A1*2, and CYP1B1*1 (wild type) enzymes. The resulting enhanced generation of QIs in the blood, coupled with the referred low CYP2C8 activity could be the basis of the previously documented AQ induced severe agranulocytosis.

Interestingly, the involvement of CYP1A1 and CYP1B1 has another implication: In adult patients whom are smokers, both genes are likely to be induced by the polycyclic aromatic hydrocarbons (PAHs), which is present in tobacco smoke, through the activation of the aryl hydrocarbon receptor (AhR) based pathway (Nebert *et al.*, 2004). This will also lead to the expression of these genes in the liver, another location for fatal AQ induced toxicity. Adult patients are characteristic of areas of low transmission, where the low exposure during the earlier periods of life does not allow the development of natural immunity to the diseases as an adult (premunition, frequent in the African continent (Struik and Riley, 2004)). Such malaria settings are the norm in South America regions, where populations carry a significant Caucasian genetic background and hence, an expected high frequency of the *CYP2C8*3* allele. This has been confirmed in a pilot screening study conducted in populations of Northern Colombia where the frequency of this allele was *ca.* 7% (I. Cavaco, Universidade do Algarve, unpublished). In such areas it would be worthwhile to conduct trials in order to understand the influence that tobacco habits might have in the incidence of mild and serious adverse events associated to AQ treatments. Its connection with the *CYP2C8/CYP1A1/CYP1B1* polymorphic set would be of interest, e.g. identifying patients that should be advised to decrease their smoking rate in time periods relevant for treatment.

Currently the epicentre of AQ use is in the Africa where the *2C8*3* and *2C8*4* alleles seem to be rare in the native populations. However, this observation is based on a very limited number of small studies, surely not representative of the overall population of the continent, the genetically most diverse on the planet (Lambert and Tishkoff, 2009). In addition, even though these alleles are considered "rare", one has to take into account the dimensions of the malaria control challenge. A frequency of 1% for the *2C8*3* allele in a universe of at least 20 million AS-AQ treatments performed per year (WHO, 2010 - just the public sector, and not counting with the SP-AQ combination), would translate to ~2,000 homozygotes for *2C8*3* patients per year. Secondly, AQ resistance, although still not globally prevalent, is slowly increasing (Holmgren *et al.*, 2006). Its potential expansion might lead to the need for increased drug dosage, as previously decided in the cases of CQ (Peters, 1970)(Ursing *et al.*, 2009, 2011) and mefloquine (Carrara *et al.*, 2009). By approaching the top of the AQ therapeutic window, the risks of toxicity will increase to a point when serious side effects might be "under the reach" of the less compromised *2C8*2* allele.

8. The *CYP2C8, CYP1A1, CYP1B1* trio - Potential applications

Pharmacogenetic markers in AQ therapies are expected to serve mostly as surveillance tools of adverse events of the drug. The identification of individuals with a genetic predisposition to AQ side effects (e.g. a *2C8*2/*2* carrier) would prompt the direct diversion of this patient towards different doses or the available second line treatment (e.g. artemether-lumefantrine or artesunate-mefloquine).

An alternative therapeutic strategy could be the use of a more personalized (i.e. more optimized) AQ dosing, with values below the conventional 10 mg/Kg, or through a different regimen schedule. As the incidence of side effects is dose dependent (Cairns *et al.*, 2010), individualized treatment would be expected to reduce those events. The success of such strategies could boost the patient's (and specially their guardians) trust on the treatment, leading to increased compliance to the full dosing regimen. This effect has been witnessed with the anti-HIV drug abacavir, where the application of pharmacogenetic testing has increased the use of this drug (Ingelman-Sundberg, 2008)(Chaponda and Pirmohamed, 2011). Unfortunately, clinical studies to support future guidelines concerning the ideal dose for certain pharmacogenetic configurations are clearly missing. Initiatives to address this issue, such as the WANECAM Consortium in East Africa, are presently under way (see: www.edctp.org/annualreport2010/EDCTP_Annual_Report_2010_English.pdf).

The application of pharmacogenetics can contribute to an extended useful life of AQ, through its better use. Chemotherapy represents a central strategy for the long desired global elimination of the disease (malERA Consultative Group on Drugs, 2011), an event fundamental for the social-economical development of the Developing World. AQ is one of its central tools in these efforts (Bhattarai *et al.*, 2007) – its safer and consequently longer use can be pivotal in this process.

But, although promising, are these pharmacogenetic applications possible in the present context of the Developing World health systems? In short, no. The prices of pharmacogenetic testing are still very high, totally eclipsing the costs of the therapy itself. A complete AS-AQ treatment in Africa will cost below US$5, already taking in consideration a price of US$ 0.5-1 for the Coarsucam®/Winthorp® fixed combination supplied by Sanofi-Aventis (Shillcutt *et al.*, 2008). As previously calculated (Ferreira *et al.*, 2008), the analysis of the *CYP2C8*3* allele alone will demand a minimum of US$50, taking in account the local costs of human resources and reagents. An upgrade towards the determination of the *CYP2C8*2* allele, plus *CYP1B1*2* and *CYP1A1*2*, would increase the financial burden per patients to values well above US$ 100 per patient, the equivalent of more than one hundred treatments. Besides, the maintenance of a system with the required quality standards for molecular diagnostic analysis would be in the order of many tens of thousands of US$/year. All this has to be put further in the context of populations with an available national health expenditure of less then US$25/year/citizen. The pharmacogenetic testing for AQ therapy alone would consume the funds of four years of health care.

So, what is the translational value of pharmacogenetics in such scenario? In fact there are at least two venues of development.

The first is what will be called here as "population pharmacogenetics". As explained, the application of individual dose adjusted AQ therapies based on pharmacogenetics is essentially not viable. Alternatively, the study of the allele frequencies of pivotal markers in representative samples of specific populations/regions can be of considerable interest for national and regional health programmes, particularly in countries with a rich ethnic diversity, as it is frequent in the African continent. This would define the populations where therapeutics based in AQ would be safe, and the ones where an alternative antimalarial (like artemether-lumefantrine) would be the better choice. In a way, it would be the equivalent of rationally deciding not to introduce AQ in Europe, due to the high prevalence of the *CYP2C8*3* allele (Cavaco *et al.*, 2006). Several malaria endemic countries have more than one first line recommended treatment (e.g. Burkina Faso, Mali, Colombia, Peru (http://www.who.int/malaria/publications/treatment-policies/en/index.html), having as such a start up capacity for implementing region-specific policies. Such a programme could be centralized taking advantage of pre-existing molecular technology facilities used e.g. for molecular parasitology. In this context it is worth mentioning that new techniques are surfacing for the extraction of DNA from Rapid Diagnostic Tests (P. Ferreira, Karolinska Institutet, pers. commun)(Alam *et al.*, 2011). These can be further coupled with novel inexpensive amplification-free genotyping approaches (Aw *et al.*, 2011), allowing the ready molecular characterization of the patient in field settings.

Such an application of pharmacogenetics would aid evidence-based decisions for optimized antimalarial use, at a population level. This would allow the use of safer ACT alternatives for the benefit of specific populations.

The second venue has to do with the target country. Malaria is a significant public health concern in three of the "BRIC" emerging economies: Brazil, India and China. These large countries are rapidly developing economic capacity compatible with a first large scale application of personalised anti-infection therapies. In this context, it should be noted that the populations of Brazil and India (incidentally, the ones with larger malaria burden) have been shown to harbour non-negligible *CYP2C8*3* frequencies (Arun Kumar *et al.*, 2011)(Suarez-Kurtz *et al.*, 2010)(table 1). In these countries the resources for personalized medicine as previously described are potentially available.

9. Conclusions

Although tens of millions of AQ doses are prescribed per year, the knowledge of the pharmacogenetics of this drug is still limited. In particular, stronger *in vivo* phenotype/genotype associations are needed for the definition of genetic markers of AQ overexposure risk.

This must be obtained through several venues. A basic need is the performance of clinical trials designed for the detection of adverse events, mild or eventually serious. These are needed to be relatively large (>500 subjects), due to the non-precise nature of the former (e.g. self reported abdominal pain in children under five), and the rarity of the latter. Such studies must include a long follow up for the detection of possible late onset events, as well as the reaction of the subject upon repetitive treatments. Also, the inclusion of full sequencing approaches in such reference studies would be fundamental, especially in cases of particularly relevant phenotypes. As previously mentioned, studies of this type are presently undergoing. Such trials will allow the establishment of better phenotype/genotype associations that can be further explored in the context of health structures integrated in national malaria programmes. In this second step, technologies like the DNA extraction from Rapid Diagnostic Test devices, coupled with novel simple genotyping methods with applications in the field can be used in order to further establish polymorphisms in CYP2C8, CYP1A1, CYP1B1 or other relevant genes (e.g. myeloperoxidases) as risk markers of AQ over-exposure.

With true personalized medicine being presently out of reach in most malaria affected countries, population pharmacogenetics of such markers will supply information for the use of the best available chemotherapy option, at a public health level. An example of such application would be the use of an alternative second line treatment (e.g. artemether-lumefantrine) as first liner for certain regions and/or populations of a country. Such a strategy would optimize the use of the available antimalarial arsenal in the national control programmes. A more personalized analysis could be potentially applied in the much less frequent (< 10%) situations of AS-AQ use as second liner.

A population-based approach, as described, can offer true benefits for the optimization of national malaria treatment, in particular when integrated in malaria elimination efforts, where the maintenance of the useful life of well established and effective therapies is key. Once the incidence of malaria decreases, as for example witnessed in the Zanzibari islands (Bhattarai *et al.*, 2007), countries will be able to start supporting more personalized application of pharmacogenetics. In conclusion, upon the solid establishment of pharmacogenetics markers, the success of their application at a population level can lay the basis for a future more personalized pharmacogenetics, once the countries would be able to finance it. By the same token, the Developing World would not be left behind in this area of translational medicine.

10. Acknowledgments

This work was partially supported by The Karolinska Institutet Fond.

11. References

Adjei GO; Kristensen K; Goka BQ; Hoegberg LC; Alifrangis M; Rodrigues OP & Kurtzhals
    JA (2008). Effect of concomitant artesunate administration and cytochrome

P4502C8 polymorphisms on the pharmacokinetics of amodiaquine in Ghanaian children with uncomplicated malaria. *Antimicrob Agents Chemother.*, 52(12):4400-4406.

Adjuik M, Agnamey P, Babiker A, Borrmann S, Brasseur P, Cisse M, Cobelens F, Diallo S, Faucher JF, Garner P, Gikunda S, Kremsner PG, Krishna S, Lell B, Loolpapit M, Matsiegui PB, Missinou MA, Mwanza J, Ntoumi F, Olliaro P, Osimbo P, Rezbach P, Some E, Taylor WR (2002). Amodiaquine-artesunate versus amodiaquine for uncomplicated Plasmodium falciparum malaria in African children: a randomised, multicentre trial. *Lancet.*, 359(9315):1365-1372.

Aklillu E; Oscarson M; Hidestrand M; Leidvik B; Otter C; & Ingelman-Sundberg M. Functional analysis of six different polymorphic CYP1B1 enzyme variants found in an Ethiopian population (2002). *Mol Pharmacol.*, 61(3):586-594.

Alam MS; Mohon AN; Mustafa S; Khan WA; Islam N; Karim MJ; Khanum H; Sullivan DJ Jr & Haque R. (2011). Real-time PCR assay and rapid diagnostic tests for the diagnosis of clinically suspected malaria patients in Bangladesh. *Malar J.*, 10:175.

Arun Kumar AS; Chakradhara Rao US; Umamaheswaran G; Ramu P; Kesavan R; Shewade DG; Balachandar J & Adithan C (2011). Haplotype structures of common variants of CYP2C8; CYP2C9; and ADRB1 genes in a South Indian population. *Genet Test Mol Biomarkers.*, 15(6):407-413.

Aw W; Lezhava A; Hayashizaki Y & Ishikawa T (2011). A new trend in personalized medicine: rapid detection of SNPs in drug transporter genes by the SmartAmp method. *Clin Pharmacol Ther.*, 89(4):617-620.

Bhattarai A, Ali AS, Kachur SP, Mårtensson A, Abbas AK, Khatib R, Al-Mafazy AW, Ramsan M, Rotllant G, Gerstenmaier JF, Molteni F, Abdulla S, Montgomery SM, Kaneko A, Björkman A. Impact of artemisinin-based combination therapy and insecticide-treated nets on malaria burden in Zanzibar (2007). *PLoS Med.*, 4(11):e309.

Bojang K, Akor F, Bittaye O, Conway D, Bottomley C, Milligan P, Greenwood B (2010). A randomised trial to compare the safety, tolerability and efficacy of three drug combinations for intermittent preventive treatment in children. *PLoS One.*, 5(6):e11225.

Brasseur P, Guiguemde R, Diallo S, Guiyedi V, Kombila M, Ringwald P, Olliaro P (1999). Amodiaquine remains effective for treating uncomplicated malaria in west and central Africa. *Trans R Soc Trop Med Hyg.*, 93(6):645-650.

Cairns M, Cisse B, Sokhna C, Cames C, Simondon K, Ba EH, Trape JF, Gaye O, Greenwood BM, Milligan PJ (2010). Amodiaquine dosage and tolerability for intermittent preventive treatment to prevent malaria in children. Antimicrob Agents Chemother., 54(3):1265-1274.

Carrara VI; Zwang J; Ashley EA; Price RN; Stepniewska K; Barends M; Brockman A; Anderson T; McGready R; Phaiphun L; Proux S; van Vugt M; Hutagalung R; Lwin KM; Phyo AP; Preechapornkul P; Imwong M; Pukrittayakamee S; Singhasivanon P; White NJ & Nosten F (2009). Changes in the treatment responses to artesunate-mefloquine on the northwestern border of Thailand during 13 years of continuous deployment. *PLoS One.*, 4(2):e4551.

Cavaco I; Strömberg-Nörklit J; Kaneko A; Msellem MI; Dahoma M; Ribeiro VL; Bjorkman A & Gil JP (2005). CYP2C8 polymorphism frequencies among malaria patients in Zanzibar. *Eur J Clin Pharmacol.*, 61(1):15-18.

Cavaco I; Piedade R; Gil JP & Ribeiro V (2006). CYP2C8 polymorphism among the Portuguese. *Clin Chem Lab Med.*, 44(2):168-170.

Chaponda M & Pirmohamed M (2011). Hypersensitivity reactions to HIV therapy. *Br J Clin Pharmacol.*, 71(5):659-671.

Churchill FC; Patchen LC; Campbell CC; Schwartz IK; Nguyen-Dinh P & Dickinson CM (1985). Amodiaquine as a prodrug: importance of metabolite(s) in the antimalarial effect of amodiaquine in humans. *Life Sci.*, 36(1):53-62.

Clarke JB; Maggs JL; Kitteringham NR & Park BK (1990). Immunogenicity of amodiaquine in the rat. *Int Arch Allergy Appl Immunol.*, 91(4):335-342.

Coatney GR (1963). Pitfalls in a discovery: the chronicle of chloroquine. *Am J Trop Med Hyg.*, 12:121-128.

Cosma G; Crofts F; Taioli E; Toniolo P & Garte S (1993). Relationship between genotype and function of the human CYP1A1 gene. *J Toxicol Environ Health.*, 40(2-3):309-316.

Cox-Singh J; Davis TM; Lee KS; Shamsul SS; Matusop A; Ratnam S; Rahman HA; Conway DJ & Singh B (2008). Plasmodium knowlesi malaria in humans is widely distributed and potentially life threatening. *Clin Infect Dis.*, 46(2):165-171.

Dai D; Zeldin DC; Blaisdell JA; Chanas B; Coulter SJ; Ghanayem BI & Goldstein JA (2001). Polymorphisms in human CYP2C8 decrease metabolism of the anticancer drug paclitaxel and arachidonic acid. *Pharmacogenetics.*, 11(7):597-607.

Dandara C; Sayi J; Masimirembwa CM; Magimba A; Kaaya S; De Sommers K; Snyman JR & Hasler JA (2002). Genetic polymorphism of cytochrome P450 1A1 (Cyp1A1) and glutathione transferases (M1; T1 and P1) among Africans. *Clin Chem Lab Med.*, 40(9):952-957.

Dey A; Parmar D; Dayal M; Dhawan A; & Seth PK (2001). Cytochrome P450 1A1 (CYP1A1) in blood lymphocytes evidence for catalytic activity and mRNA expression. *Life Sci.*, 69(4):383 393.

Eastman RT & Fidock DA (2009). Artemisinin-based combination therapies: a vital tool in efforts to eliminate malaria. *Nat Rev Microbiol.*, 7(12):864-874.

Echeverry DF; Holmgren G; Murillo C; Higuita JC; Björkman A; Gil JP & Osorio L (2007). Short report: polymorphisms in the pfcrt and pfmdr1 genes of Plasmodium falciparum and *in vitro* susceptibility to amodiaquine and desethylamodiaquine. *Am J Trop Med Hyg.* ,77(6):1034-1038.

Ferreira PE; Cavaco I & Gil JP (2008). Pharmacogentic tools for malaria and TB in the Developing World. *Personalized Med.*, 5(6): 627-639.

Fujihara J; Yasuda T; Iida R; Takatsuka H; Fujii Y & Takeshita H (2009). Cytochrome P450 1A1; glutathione S-transferases M1 and T1 polymorphisms in Ovambos and Mongolians. Leg Med (Tokyo)., Suppl 1:S408-410.

Furukawa M; Nishimura M; Ogino D; Chiba R; Ikai I; Ueda N; Naito S; Kuribayashi S; Moustafa MA; Uchida T; Sawada H; Kamataki T; Funae Y & Fukumoto M. (2004) Cytochrome p450 gene expression levels in peripheral blood mononuclear cells in comparison with the liver. *Cancer Sci.*, 95(6): 520-529.

Gao Y; Liu D; Wang H; Zhu J & Chen C (2010). Functional characterization of five CYP2C8 variants and prediction of CYP2C8 genotype-dependent effects on *in vitro* and *in vivo* drug-drug interactions. *Xenobiotica.*, 40(7):467-475.

Garte S (1998). The role of ethnicity in cancer susceptibility gene polymorphisms: the example of CYP1A1. *Carcinogenesis.*, 19(8):1329-1332.

Gautam A; Ahmed T; Batra V & Paliwal J (2009). Pharmacokinetics and pharmacodynamics of endoperoxide antimalarials. *Curr Drug Metab.*, 10(3):289-306.

Gerstl S, Dunkley S, Mukhtar A, Baker S, Maikere J (2010). Successful introduction of artesunate combination therapy is not enough to fight malaria: results from an adherence study in Sierra Leone. *Trans R Soc Trop Med Hyg.*, 104(5):328-35.

Gerstner U; Prajakwong S; Wiedermann G; Sirichaisinthop J; Wernsdorfer G & Wernsdorfer WH (2003). Comparison of the in-vitro activity of amodiaquine and its main metabolite; monodesethyl-amodiaquine; in Plasmodium falciparum. *Wien Klin Wochenschr.*, 115 (Suppl) 3:33-38.

Giao PT & de Vries PJ (2001). Pharmacokinetic interactions of antimalarial agents. *Clin Pharmacokinet.*, 40(5):343-373.

Gil JP; & Gil Berglund E (2007). CYP2C8 and antimalaria drug efficacy. *Pharmacogenomics,* 8(2):187-198.

Hakkola J; Pasanen M; Hukkanen J; Pelkonen O; Mäenpää J; Edwards RJ; Boobis AR & Raunio H. Expression of xenobiotic-metabolizing cytochrome P450 forms in human full-term placenta. *Biochem Pharmacol.*, 51(4):403-411.

Hanaoka T; Yamano Y; Pan G; Hara K; Ichiba M; Zhang J; Zhang S; Liu T; Li L; Takahashi K; Kagawa J; & Tsugane S (2002). Cytochrome P450 1B1 mRNA levels in peripheral blood cells and exposure to polycyclic aromatic hydrocarbons in Chinese coke oven workers. *Sci Total Environ.*, 296(1-3):27-33.

Harrison AC, Kitteringham NR, Clarke JB, Park BK (1992). The mechanism of bioactivation and antigen formation of amodiaquine in the rat. *Biochem Pharmacol.*, 43(7):1421-1430.

Hatton CS; Peto TE; Bunch C; Pasvol G; Russell SJ; Singer CR; Edwards G & Winstanley P (1986). Frequency of severe neutropenia associated with amodiaquine prophylaxis against malaria. *Lancet,* 1(8478):411-414.

Helmig S; Hadzaad B; Döhrel J & Schneider J (2009). Influence of the Cyp1B1 L432V gene polymorphism and exposure to tobacco smoke on Cyp1B1 mRNA expression in human leukocytes. *Drug Metab Dispos;* 37(7):1490-1495.

Helmig S; Seelinger JU; Philipp-Gehlhaar M; Döhrel J & Schneider J (2010). Cyp1B1 mRNA expression in correlation to cotinine levels with respect to the Cyp1B1 L432V gene polymorphism. *Eur J Epidemiol.;* 25(12):867-873.

Hichiya H; Tanaka-Kagawa T; Soyama A; Jinno H; Koyano S; Katori N; Matsushima E; Uchiyama S; Tokunaga H; Kimura H; Minami N; Katoh M; Sugai K; Goto Y; Tamura T; Yamamoto N; Ohe Y; Kunitoh H; Nokihara H; Yoshida T; Minami H; Saijo N; Ando M; Ozawa S; Saito Y & Sawada J (2005). Functional characterization of five novel CYP2C8 variants; G171S; R186X; R186G; K247R; and K383N; found in a Japanese population. *Drug Metab Dispos.*, 33(5):630-636.

Hietala SF; Bhattarai A; Msellem M; Röshammar D; Ali AS; Strömberg J; Hombhanje FW; Kaneko A; Björkman A & Ashton M (2007). Population pharmacokinetics of amodiaquine and desethylamodiaquine in pediatric patients with uncomplicated falciparum malaria. *J Pharmacokinet Pharmacodyn.*, 34(5):669-686.

Holmgren G; Gil JP; Ferreira PM; Veiga MI; Obonyo CO & Björkman A (2006). Amodiaquine resistant Plasmodium falciparum malaria *in vivo* is associated with selection of pfcrt 76T and pfmdr1 86Y. *Infect Genet Evol.*, 6(4):309-314.

Hombhanje FW; Hwaihwanje I; Tsukahara T; Saruwatari J; Nakagawa M; Osawa H; Paniu MM; Takahashi N; Lum JK; Aumora B; Masta A; Sapuri M; Kobayakawa T; Kaneko A & Ishizaki T (2005). The disposition of oral amodiaquine in Papua New Guinean children with falciparum malaria. *Br J Clin Pharmacol.*, 59(3):298-301 (2005).

Hsu E (2009). Diverse biologies and experiential continuities: did the ancient Chinese know that qinghao had anti-malarial properties? *Can Bull Med Hist.*, 26(1):203-213.

Ingelman-Sundberg M (2008). Pharmacogenomic biomarkers for prediction of severe adverse drug reactions. *N Engl J Med.*, 358(6):637-639.

Jewell H; Maggs JL; Harrison AC; O'Neill PM; Ruscoe JE & Park BK (1995). Role of hepatic metabolism in the bioactivation and detoxication of amodiaquine. *Xenobiotica.*, 25(2):199-217.

Jiang H; Zhong F; Sun L; Feng W; Huang ZX & Tan X (2011). Structural and functional insights into polymorphic enzymes of cytochrome P450 2C8. *Amino Acids.*, 40(4):1195-1204.

Johansson T; Jurva U; Grönberg G; Weidolf L & Masimirembwa C (2009). Novel metabolites of amodiaquine formed by CYP1A1 and CYP1B1: structure elucidation using electrochemistry; mass spectrometry; and NMR. *Drug Metab Dispos.*, 37(3):571-579.

Kisselev P; Schunck WH; Roots & Schwarz D (2005). Association of CYP1A1 polymorphisms with differential metabolic activation of 17beta-estradiol and estrone. *Cancer Res.*, 65(7):2972-2978.

Kudzi W; Dodoo AN; Mills JJ (2009). Characterisation of CYP2C8; CYP2C9 and CYP2C19 polymorphisms in a Ghanaian population. *BMC Med Genet.*; 10:124.

Kumar V; Singh S; Yadav CS; Ahmed RS; Gupta S; Pasha ST; Tripathi AK & Banerjee BD (2010). CYP1A1 and CYP3A4 polymorphic variations in Delhi population of Northern India. *Environ Toxicol Pharmacol.*, 29(2):126-130.

Lambert CA, Tishkoff SA (2009). Genetic structure in African populations: implications for human demographic history. *Cold Spring Harb Symp Quant Biol.* 274:395-402.

Landi MT; Bertazzi PA; Shields PG; Clark G; Lucier GW; Garte SJ; Cosma G & Caporaso NE (1994). Association between CYP1A1 genotype; mRNA expression and enzymatic activity in humans. *Pharmacogenetics.*, 4(5):242-246.

Larrey D; Castot A; Pёssayre D; Merigot P; Machayekhy JP; Feldmann G; Lenoir A; Rueff B & Benhamou JP (1986). Amodiaquine-induced hepatitis. A report of seven cases. *Ann Intern Med.*, 104(6):801-803.

Levine ND (1988). Progress in taxonomy of the Apicomplexan protozoa. *J Protozool.*, (4):518 520.

Li DN; Seidel A; Pritchard MP; Wolf CR & Friedberg T (2000). Polymorphisms in P450 CYP1B1 affect the conversion of estradiol to the potentially carcinogenic metabolite 4-hydroxyestradiol. *Pharmacogenetics.*, 10(4):343-353.

Li XQ; Bjorkman A; Andersson TB; Ridderstrom & Masimirembwa CM (2002). Amodiaquine clearance and its metabolism to N-desethylamodiaquine is mediated by CYP2C8: a new high affinity and turnover enzyme-specific probe substrate. *J Pharmacol Exp Ther.*, 300(2):399-407.

Liang G; Pu Y & Yin L (2005). Rapid detection of single nucleotide polymorphisms related with lung cancer susceptibility of Chinese population. *Cancer Lett.*, 223(2):265-274.

Low DA & Smith A (1976). *History of East Africa.* Oxford University Press; Oxford, UK.

malERA Consultative Group on Drugs (2011). A research agenda for malaria eradication: drugs. *PLoS Med.*, 8(1):e1000402.

Martinez-Labarga C; Lelli R; Tarsi T; Babalini C; De Angelis F; Ottoni C; Giambra V; Pepe G; Azebi E; Frezza D; Biondi G; & Rickards O (2007). Polymorphisms of the COL1A2; CYP1A1 and HS1;2 Ig enhancer genes in the Tuaregs from Libya. *Ann Hum Biol.*, 34(4):425-436.

Masubuchi N; Makino C; Murayama N (2007). Prediction of *in vivo* potential for metabolic activation of drugs into chemically reactive intermediate: correlation of *in vitro* and *in vivo* generation of reactive intermediates and *in vitro* glutathione conjugate formation in rats and humans. *Chem Res Toxicol.*, 20(3):455-464.

Marsh K (1998). Malaria disaster in Africa. *Lancet.*, 352(9132):924.

Mount DL; Patchen LC; Nguyen-Dinh P; Barber AM; Schwartz IK & Churchill FC (1986). Sensitive analysis of blood for amodiaquine and three metabolites by high-performance liquid chromatography with electrochemical detection. *J Chromatogr.*, 383(2):375-386.

Muthiah YD; Lee WL; Teh LK; Ong CE & Ismail R (2005). Genetic polymorphism of CYP2C8 in three Malaysian ethnics: CYP2C8*2 and CYP2C8*3 are found in Malaysian Indians. *J Clin Pharm Ther.*, 30(5):487-490.

Naisbitt DJ; Ruscoe JE; Williams D; O'Neill PM; Pirmohamed M & Park BK (1997). Disposition of amodiaquine and related antimalarial agents in human neutrophils: implications for drug design. *J Pharmacol Exp Ther.*, 280(2):884-893.

Nakajima M; Fujiki Y; Noda K; Ohtsuka H; Ohkuni H; Kyo S; Inoue M; Kuroiwa Y; & Yokoi T (2003). Genetic polymorphisms of CYP2C8 in Japanese population. *Drug Metab Dispos.*, 31(6):687-690.

Nankabirwa J, Cundill B, Clarke S, Kabatereine N, Rosenthal PJ, Dorsey G, Brooker S, Staedke SG (2010). Efficacy, safety, and tolerability of three regimens for prevention of malaria: a randomized, placebo-controlled trial in Ugandan schoolchildren. *PLoS One*, 5(10):e13438.

Nebert DW; Dalton TP; Okey AB & Gonzalez FJ (2004). Role of aryl hydrocarbon receptor-mediated induction of the CYP1 enzymes in environmental toxicity and cancer. *J Biol Chem.*, 279(23): 23847-23850.

Neftel KA; Woodtly W; Schmid M; Frick PG & Fehr J (1986). Amodiaquine induced agranulocytosis and liver damage. *Br Med J.*, 292(6522): 721-723.

Nosten F; ter Kuile F; Chongsuphajaisiddhi T; Luxemburger C; Webster HK; Edstein M; Phaipun L; Thew KL & White NJ (1991). Mefloquine-resistant falciparum malaria on the Thai-Burmese border. *Lancet.*, 337(8750): 1140-1143.

Nosten F; van Vugt M; Price R; Luxemburger C; Thway KL; Brockman A; McGready R; ter Kuile F; Looareesuwan S & White NJ (2000). Effects of artesunate-mefloquine combination on incidence of Plasmodium falciparum malaria and mefloquine resistance in western Thailand: a prospective study. *Lancet.*, 356(9226):297-302.

Okobia M; Bunker C; Zmuda J; Kammerer C; Vogel V; Uche E; Anyanwu S; Ezeome E; Ferrell R & Kuller L. (2005) Cytochrome P4501A1 genetic polymorphisms and breast cancer risk in Nigerian women. *Breast Cancer Res Treat.*, 94(3):285-293.

Olliaro P; Nevill C; LeBras J; Ringwald P; Mussano P; Garner P & Brasseur P (1996). Systematic review of amodiaquine treatment in uncomplicated malaria. *Lancet.*, 348(9036):1196 1201.

Olliaro P, Mussano P (2003). Amodiaquine for treating malaria. *Cochrane Database Syst Rev.*, (2):CD000016.

Paine MF; Schmiedlin-Ren P & Watkins PB (1999). Cytochrome P-450 1A1 expression in human small bowel: interindividual variation and inhibition by ketoconazole. *Drug Metab Dispos.*, 27(3):360-364.

Paine MF; Hart HL; Ludington SS; Haining RL; Rettie AE & Zeldin DC (2006). The human intestinal cytochrome P450 "pie". *Drug Metab Dispos.*, 34(5):880-886.

Parikh S; Ouedraogo JB; Goldstein JA; Rosenthal PJ & Kroetz DL (2007). Amodiaquine metabolism is impaired by common polymorphisms in CYP2C8: implications for malaria treatment in Africa. *Clin Pharmacol Ther.*, 82(2):197-203.

Peters W (1970). *Chemotherapy and drug resistance in malaria.* Academic press; London, UK.

Phillips-Howard PA, West LJ (1990). Serious adverse drug reactions to pyrimethamine-sulphadoxine, pyrimethamine-dapsone and to amodiaquine in Britain. *J R Soc Med.*, 83(2):82-85.

Pisani P; Srivatanakul P; Randerson-Moor J; Vipasrinimit S; Lalitwongsa S; Unpunyo P; Bashir S & Bishop DT (2006). GSTM1 and CYP1A1 polymorphisms; tobacco; air pollution; and lung cancer: a study in rural Thailand. *Cancer Epidemiol Biomarkers Prev.*, 15(4): 667-674.

Rouveix B; Coulombel L; Aymard JP; Chau F & Abel L (1989). Amodiaquine-induced immune agranulocytosis. *Br J Haematol.*, 71(1):7-11.

Röwer S; Bienzle U; Weise A; Lambertz U; Forst T; Otchwemah RN; Pfützner A & Mockenhaupt FP (2005). Short communication: high prevalence of the cytochrome P450 2C8*2 mutation in Northern Ghana. *Trop Med Int Health.*, 10(12):1271-1273.

Saito T; Egashira M; Kiyotani K; Fujieda M; Yamazaki H; Kiyohara C; Kunitoh H & Kamataki T (2003). Novel nonsynonymous polymorphisms of the CYP1A1 gene in Japanese. *Drug Metab Pharmacokinet.*, 18(3):218-221.

Shah PP; Singh AP; Singh M; Mathur N; Mishra BN; Pant MC & Parmar D (2008). Association of functionally important polymorphisms in cytochrome P4501B1 with lung cancer. *Mutat Res.*;, 643(1-2): 4-10.

Shillcutt S; Morel C; Goodman C; Coleman P; Bell D; Whitty CJ & Mills A (2008). Cost-effectiveness of malaria diagnostic methods in sub-Saharan Africa in an era of combination therapy. *Bull World Health Organ.*, 86(2): 101-110.

Singh R; Ting JG; Pan Y; Teh LK; Ismail R & Ong CE (2008). Functional role of Ile264 in CYP2C8: mutations affect haem incorporation and catalytic activity. *Drug Metab Pharmacokinet.*, 23(3): 165-74 (2008).

Smart J & Daly AK (2000). Variation in induced CYP1A1 levels: relationship to CYP1A1; Ah receptor and GSTM1 polymorphisms. *Pharmacogenetics.*; 10(1):11-24.

Solus JF; Arietta BJ; Harris JR; Sexton DP; Steward JQ; McMunn C; Ihrie P; Mehall JM; Edwards TL & Dawson EP (2004). Genetic variation in eleven phase I drug metabolism genes in an ethnically diverse population. *Pharmacogenomics*, 5(7): 895-931.

Soyama A; Saito Y; Hanioka N; Murayama N; Nakajima O; Katori N; Ishida S; Sai K; Ozawa S & Sawada JI (2001). Non-synonymous single nucleotide alterations found in the CYP2C8 gene result in reduced *in vitro* paclitaxel metabolism. *Biol Pharm Bull.*, 24(12): 1427-1430 (2001).

Soyama A; Saito Y; Komamura K; Ueno K; Kamakura S; Ozawa S & Sawada J (2002). Five novel single nucleotide polymorphisms in the CYP2C8 gene; one of which induces a frame-shift. *Drug Metab Pharmacokinet.*, 17(4): 374-377.

Soyama A; Hanioka N; Saito Y; Murayama N; Ando M; Ozawa S & Sawada J (2002). Amiodarone N deethylation by CYP2C8 and its variants; CYP2C8*3 and CYP2C8 P404A. *Pharmacol Toxicol.*, 91(4): 174-178.

Spurr NK; Gough AC; Stevenson K & Wolf CR (1987). Msp-1 polymorphism detected with a cDNA probe for the P-450 I family on chromosome 15. *Nucleic Acids Res.*, 15(14): 5901.

Sreeja L; Syamala V; Hariharan S; Madhavan J; Devan SC & Ankathil R (2005). Possible risk modification by CYP1A1; GSTM1 and GSTT1 gene polymorphisms in lung cancer susceptibility in a South Indian population. *J Hum Genet.*, 50(12):618-627.

Staedke SG, Kamya MR, Dorsey G, Gasasira A, Ndeezi G, Charlebois ED, Rosenthal PJ (2001). Amodiaquine, sulfadoxine/pyrimethamine, and combination therapy for treatment of uncomplicated falciparum malaria in Kampala, Uganda: a randomised trial. *Lancet.*, 358(9279):368-74.

Stoilov I; Akarsu AN; Alozie I; Child A; Barsoum-Homsy M; Turacli ME; Or M; Lewis RA; Ozdemir N; Brice G; Aktan SG; Chevrette L; Coca-Prados M & Sarfarazi M (1998). Sequence analysis and homology modeling suggest that primary congenital glaucoma on 2p21 results from mutations disrupting either the hinge region or the conserved core structures of cytochrome P4501B1. *Am J Hum Genet.*, 62(3): 573-584.

Struik SS, Riley EM (2004). Does malaria suffer from lack of memory?, *Immunol Rev.* 201:268-290.

Suarez-Kurtz G; Genro JP; de Moraes MO; Ojopi EB; Pena SD; Perini JA; Ribeiro-Dos-Santos A; Romano-Silva MA; Santana I & Struchiner CJ (2010). Global pharmacogenomics: Impact of population diversity on the distribution of polymorphisms in the CYP2C cluster among Brazilians. *Pharmacogenomics J.*, 10(6): 1-10.

Suneetha KJ; Nancy KN; Rajalekshmy KR; Rama R; Sagar TG & Rajkumar T (2011). Role of glutathione-s-transferase and CYP1A1*2A polymorphisms in the therapy outcome of south Indian acute lymphoblastic leukemia patients. *Indian J Med Paediatr Oncol..*, 32(1): 25-29.

Tingle MD; Jewell H; Maggs JL; O'Neill PM & Park BK (1995). The bioactivation of amodiaquine by human polymorphonuclear leucocytes *in vitro*: chemical mechanisms and the effects of fluorine substitution. *Biochem Pharmacol.*, 50(7): 1113-1139.

Ursing J, Kofoed PE, Rodrigues A, Bergqvist Y, Rombo L (2009). Chloroquine is grossly overdosed and overused but well tolerated in Guinea-bissau. *Antimicrob Agents Chemother.*, 53(1):180-185.

Ursing J, Kofoed PE, Rodrigues A, Blessborn D, Thoft-Nielsen R, Björkman A, Rombo L (2011). Similar efficacy and tolerability of double-dose chloroquine and artemether-lumefantrine for treatment of Plasmodium falciparum infection in Guinea-Bissau: a randomized trial. *J Infect Dis.*, 203(1):109-116

Van Duursen MB; Sanderson JT & van den Berg M (2005). Cytochrome P450 1A1 and 1B1 in human blood lymphocytes are not suitable as biomarkers of exposure to dioxin-like compounds: polymorphisms and interindividual variation in expression and inducibility. *Toxicol Sci.*, 85(1): 703-712.

Walsky RL & Obach RS (2004). Validated assays for human cytochrome P450 activities. *Drug Metab Dispos.*, 32(6): 647-660.

Wang Q; Li H; Tao P; Wang YP; Yuan P; Yang CX; Li JY; Yang F; Lee H; & Huang Y (2011). Soy Isoflavones; CYP1A1; CYP1B1; and COMT Polymorphisms; and Breast Cancer: A Case-Control Study in Southwestern China. *DNA Cell Biol.*, 30(8): 585-595.

White NJ (1997). Assessment of the pharmacodynamic properties of antimalarial drugs *in vivo*. *Antimicrob Agents Chemother* , 41(7): 1413-1422.

Willey JC; Coy EL; Frampton MW; Torres A; Apostolakos MJ; Hoehn G; Schuermann WH; Thilly WG; Olson DE; Hammersley JR; Crespi CL & Utell MJ (1997). Quantitative RT-PCR measurement of cytochromes p450 1A1; 1B1; and 2B7; microsomal epoxide hydrolase; and NADPH oxidoreductase expression in lung cells of smokers and nonsmokers. *Am J Respir Cell Mol Biol.*, 17(1): 114-124.

Winstanley P; Edwards G; Orme M & Breckenridge A (1987). The disposition of amodiaquine in man after oral administration. *Br J Clin Pharmacol.*, 23(1): 1-7.

Winstanley PA; Simooya O; Kofi-Ekue JM; Walker O; Salako LA; Edwards G; Orme ML & Breckenridge AM (1990). The disposition of amodiaquine in Zambians and Nigerians with malaria. *Br J Clin Pharmacol.*, 29(6): 695-701.

WHO (1990). Practical chemotherapy of malaria. Report of a WHO Scientific Group.;– Technical Report Series n0 805, Geneva, Switzerland.

WHO (2010); World Malaria Report 2010; WHO; Geneva, Switzerland

Young MD; & Moore DV (1961). Chloroquine resistance in Plasmodium falciparum. *Am J Trop Med Hyg.*, 10: 317-320.

Zhang J; Deng J; Zhang C; Lu Y; Liu L; Wu Q; Shao Y; Zhang J; Yang H; Yu B; & Wan J (2010). Association of GSTT1; GSTM1 and CYP1A1 polymorphisms with susceptibility to systemic lupus erythematosus in the Chinese population. *Clin Chim Acta.*, 411(11-12): 878-881.

11

Pharmacogenetics and Obstetric Anesthesia and Analgesia

C. Ortner, C. Ciliberto and R. Landau
University of Washington, Seattle, WA,
USA

1. Introduction

Approximately 50 years ago, pharmacogenetics emerged as a new field of medicine that may explain human drug action. Anesthesia, in particular, played a key role in these early investigations. An understanding of how an individual's genetic footprint influences drug metabolism and effectiveness may allow tailored prescriptions, improving outcomes and safety; and such concepts, which form the backbone of personalized medicine, have raised a lot of hope. The ultimate goal of pharmacogenetics research is to offer 'tailored personalized medicine' with a view to improving the efficacy of medication as well as patient safety by helping predict risks of adverse outcomes.

In this Chapter, we first present a selection of historical landmarks related to anesthesia as a catalyst for the development of pharmacogenetics, we then cite practical examples of relevant candidates genes and common polymorphisms that are known to alter the response to medication prescribed in the perioperative and peripartum period as well as clinical outcomes in the parturient. To conclude, we hope to present current views and potential exciting perspectives that may arise from the application of pharmacogenetics to the daily practice of obstetric anesthesia and pain medicine.

2. The history of pharmacogenetics related to anesthesia

Medical genetics began with the 20th century rediscovery of Gregor Mendel's original 19th century work on plant genetics [1]. In 1949, the landmark paper in *Science* by Linus Pauling and colleagues linked sickle cell anemia to a derangement in a specific protein [2], and was the first proof that a genetic change alters the structure and function of a protein and results in a human disease. This set the stage for the birth of pharmacogenetics, a field first described by Arno Motulsky in 1957 [3], named by Friedrich Vogel in 1959 [4], and established by Werner Kalow in 1962 [5]. These scientists defined pharmacogenetics as the study of the variability in drug response due to genetic variability. In the early 1950s, prolonged apnea after succinylcholine was one of the drug responses that provided a starting point from which the new field of pharmacogenetics would launch. In 1956, *The Lancet* published a paper that was the first to suggest a genetic basis for prolonged apnea after succinylcholine [6]. Werner Kalow reported soon after the occurrence of prolonged postoperative muscle relaxation following the administration of succinylcholine for endotracheal intubation, and described how an inherited variation of drug metabolism involving the enzyme butyrylcholinesterase affects the response to succinylcholine [7]. Malignant hyperthermia after succinylcholine or inhaled volatile anaesthetics is another example of an adverse reaction important to the history of pharmacogenetics. To date, 30 causative mutations have been identified on the ryanodine receptor gene (RYR1) that are associated with malignant hyperthermia [8,9]. Guidelines proposed by the European Malignant Hyperthermia Group were the first to describe comprehensive genetic screening for a pharmacogenetic test in the field of anesthesia [10].

3. The pharmacogenetics research network

Since the first reports ten years ago describing initial findings from the Human Genome Project [11,12], and its completion in 2003 [13], promises that these discoveries would translate into tangible clinical tests that may change drug prescriptions have been somewhat unfulfilled. Working towards this translation, the pharmacogenetics research network has established a pharmacogenomics knowledge base (PharmGKB) with the goal to collect, encode, and disseminate knowledge about the impact of human genetic variations on drug response, curate primary genotype and phenotype data, annotate gene variants and gene-drug-disease relationships via literature review, and summarize important pharmacogenetic genes and drug pathways (http://www.pharmgkb.org) (Figure 1).

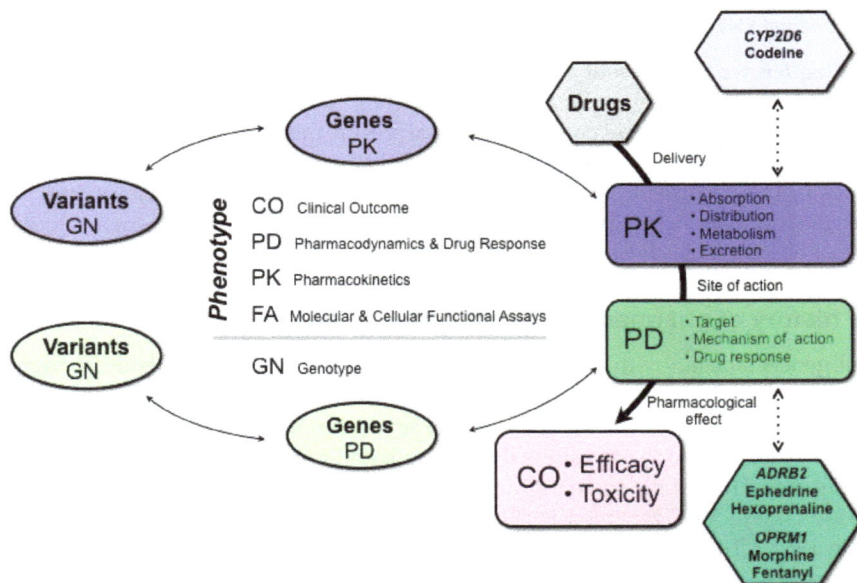

Fig. 1. Pharmacogenomics (PGx) information flow
Adapted from the NIH Pharmacogenomics Research Network – Pharmacogenomics Knowledge Base (http://www.pharmgkb.org)

4. The relevance for obstetric anesthesia and analgesia

Numerous clinical trials and reviews have surfaced in recent years describing genetic associations with clinical outcomes in the field of anesthesia, peri-operative outcomes and pain medicine [14-28]. An overview of all the drugs utilized in the peri-operative and peripartum period is beyond the scope of this review. For this Chapter, we selected several clinical examples for which gentoype/phenotype effects have been evaluated and present their relevance for clinical practice.

4.1 The β_2-adrenergic receptor genotype

Several single nucleotide polymorphisms (SNPs) that have been described in the gene encoding the human β_2-adrenergic receptor (β_2AR) affect the function of the receptor *in vitro*. Substitution of glycine for arginine at position 16 (Arg16Gly) has been associated with enhanced agonist-induced desensitization, while substitution of glutamic acid for glutamine at position 27 (Gln27Glu) has been associated with resistance to desensitization [29]. Significant differences in the response of individuals to β_2AR therapeutic manipulation related to the particular genotype/haplotype of the β_2AR have been demonstrated. The β_2AR is of particular interest for obstetric anesthesia, since drugs that are given to ensure hemodynamic stability at the time of delivery, as well as drugs to promote uterine quiescence (tocolysis) act via β_2-agonism.

4.1.1 Vasopressor requirement during spinal anesthesia for Cesarean delivery

Numerous clinical trials have evaluated the response to vasopressors to prevent and or treat hypotension during spinal anesthesia for elective Cesarean delivery [30]. For decades, ephedrine has been considered the safest and probably the sole acceptable strategy, based on classic studies in sheep that suggested deleterious effects of pure α-adrenergic agonists on uteroplacental blood flow. Ephedrine has been widely used in a variety of regimens (different bolus doses, infusions and in combination with phenylephrine) although no consensus has ever been achieved as to which of these modes of administration provides the most reliable and effective response. Ephedrine is a sympathomimetic amine, the principal mechanism of its action relies on its direct and indirect actions on the adrenergic receptor system (both an α- and β-adrenergic agonist).

A pharmacogenetic study in an obstetric population showed that the incidence and severity of maternal hypotension after spinal anesthesia for Cesarean delivery and the response to treatment is clearly affected by β_2AR genotype/haplotype [31]. Women Gly16 homozygous and carrying one or two Glu at position 27 (heterozygous or homozygous for the minor Glu27 allele) were found to require significantly *less* vasopressors (ephedrine) for treatment of hypotension during spinal anesthesia. The two haplotypes that seem to 'protect' women from requiring higher doses of ephedrine are relatively common in Caucasians, and in this study 20% of the women carried either one of these haplotypes. This pharmacogenetic effect may explain in part why the numerous studies trying to prevent or treat hypotension during spinal anesthesia for Cesarean section failed to define one single optimal strategy (fluid loading, ephedrine or phenylephrine) that would 'fit all'.

Since the incidence of spinal hypotension and vasopressor use is reduced in preeclampsia [32,33], it has been further hypothesized that haplotypes of β_2AR gene influence hemodynamics during spinal anesthesia for Cesarean delivery in women diagnosed with severe pre-eclampsia. In a prospective case-control study, we compared the incidence of hypotension and vasopressor requirements in a predominantly African-American cohort [34]. Despite a trend towards fewer pre-eclamptic women requiring vasopressors, the total vasopressor dose was *higher* in those in whom treatment was indicated. However, no woman in the pre-eclamptic group carried the Gly16Gly/Glu27Glu haplotype, and since this was one of the two haplotypes that predicted less vasopressor requirement in normotensive women [31], this might provide an explanation for these unexpected results. Whether these findings are specific to African-American women remains to be determined in larger studies in other ethnic groups. These findings illustrate the importance of ethnicity when assessing genetic associations, and similar interactions between ethnicity and genetics have been suggested for other SNPs presented in this review (μ-OR). In the long term, if these findings are confirmed, clinical implications could involve using haplotype of β_2AR to predict spinal hypotension and to guide hemodynamic management in women with compromised cardiovascular function and altered uteroplacental perfusion.

4.1.2 Ephedrine-induced neonatal acidosis

Meanwhile, the direct effects of ephedrine on the fetus have been revisited recently [35]. Evidence that ephedrine crosses the placenta to a greater extent and undergoes less early metabolism and redistribution than phenylephrine (a direct α-adrenergic agonist) causing direct fetal metabolic acidosis has made ephedrine less desirable as a first-line treatment [36]. The proposed mechanism is that direct fetal β-adrenergic stimulation increases anaerobic glycolysis and causes a hypermetabolic state. The hypothesis that neonatal *ADRB2* genotype may directly influence the degree of neonatal acidemia in response to ephedrine given to the mother prior to delivery has just recently been explored. The most clinically relevant and intriguing finding of a study conducted in Asian woemen was that umbilical artery (UA) pH was overall higher and UA lactate was lower in neonates that were Arg16 homozygous as compared to neonates with the two other genotypes of *ADRB2* [37]. Furthermore, among babies born to mothers receiving ephedrine, ephedrine dose was associated with neonatal acidemia (decreased UA pH) only in neonates carrying a Gly16 allele, but not in neonates who were Arg16 homozygous. Since there was no significant difference in ephedrine concentration as determined by maternal and umbilical cord assays among genetic groups, any difference in metabolic markers are unlikely to have resulted from differential transplacental transfer of drug or a pharmacokinetic effect. Arg16 homozygous neonates seem to be protected from the risk of developing acidemia when exposed to ephedrine, irrespective of the dose given to the mother (Figure 2). These findings provide interesting insight on fetal acidosis and metabolic responses in neonates born to mothers who have received β-agonists (ephedrine and/or other β-stimulants prescribed for tocolysis or bronchodilation) prior to delivery.

4.1.3 Tocolytics for management of preterm labor and delivery

Stimulation of the β_2AR results in uterine smooth muscle relaxation, and thus the β_2AR has long been a therapeutic target for the treatment of preterm labor. β_2-agonist therapy, in common with virtually all tocolytics, has not been consistently successful at stopping preterm labor or prolonging pregnancy, in part due to the multifactorial nature of preterm labor, and possibly because of a wide variability in therapeutic response within the population. The mechanisms involved in regulation of myometrial smooth muscle contraction and relaxation in preterm labor or even at term are not yet fully elucidated. Genetic variability of *ADRB2* has been evaluated in several studies in the context preterm labor and delivery. Arg16 homozygosity of *ADRB2* appears to confer a protective effect against preterm delivery while the minor allele at position 27 (Glu) increases the risk for preterm delivery [38-40]. Furthermore, a pharmacogenetic effect, with a better response to β₂agonist therapy (hexoprenaline) for tocolysis in women Arg16 homozygous with idiopathic preterm labor between 24 and 34 weeks gestation has been demonstrated [41]. This had a significant impact on neonatal outcomes, with higher birth weights and less neonatal intensive care unit (NICU) admissions for respiratory or other complications due to prematurity in babies born to mothers with that genotype. Meanwhile, a variety of genomic studies have examined the influence of genetic variants on the incidence of preterm labor [42], and proteomic studies to validate biomarkers that could identify women at risk for preterm delivery and serve as predictive tools are ongoing [43,44].

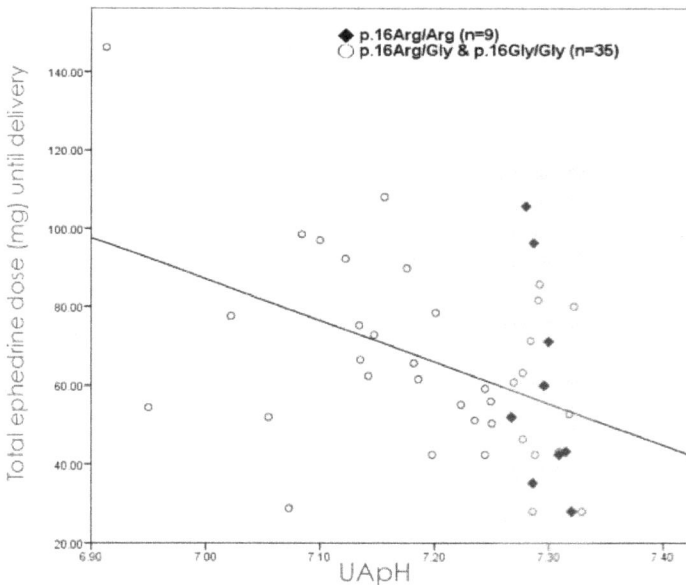

None of the Arg16 homozygous neonates had a pH < 7.28

Fig. 2. Ephedrine-induced neonatal acidosis according to p.16Arg/Gly of *ADRB2*
From Landau R, Liu SK, Blouin JL, Smiley RM, Ngan Kee WD: The Effect of Maternal and Fetal β₂-Adrenoceptor and Nitric Oxide Synthase Genotype on Vasopressor Requirement and Fetal Acid-Base Status During Spinal Anesthesia for Cesarean Delivery. Anesth Analg 2011; 112: 1432-7

4.1.4 Course of labor and delivery

Recent studies have confirmed that *ADRB2* haplotype is important not only in the context of preterm onset of labor and delivery, but also on the course of labor and delivery in the term parturient. In a recent observational study in North-American women enrolled between 34-40 weeks gestation, the progress of active labor was found to be slower in women homozygous for Arg16 [45]. In women at term, the rate of cervical dilatation and duration of labor was shown to be slower in women carrying the wild-allele (Gln) at position 27 [46]. Taken together, both studies confirm that uterine quiescence during pregnancy and progression of cervical dilatation during labor are strongly associated with *ADRB2* haplotype.

5. Analgesia and pain-related candidate genes

Interindividual variability in pain perception and sensitivity to analgesic therapy with a large unpredictability in efficacy, side effects and tolerance profiles to opioids is well described. Genomic and pharmacogenetic research has considered numerous candidate genes as suitable targets for the study of pain and or analgesia [47]. Among the numerous genes and specific polymorphisms that have been considered important in opioid response, the A118G polymorphism of the μ–opioid receptor gene (*OPRM1*), a common variant of the catechol-O-methyltransferase gene (Val158Met of *COMT*), several genetic variants of the ATP-binding cassette, sub- family B gene (*ABCB1*) and genetic variants of the cytochrome P450 family of enzymes have been extensively reviewed [22,24,48]. In addition, a genetic database of *knock-out* mice allowing the study of genetic variations in the context of specific pain phenotypes was made public [49].

Recently an extremely rare phenotype characterized by a total absence of pain perception ('congenital indifference to pain') with no associated neuropathy has been associated with the mutations in the gene SCN9A, encoding the α-subunit of the voltage-gated sodium channel, $Na_v1.7$ [50-52]. Individuals with loss-of-function mutations of the $Na_v1.7$ lack protective mechanisms that allow tissue damage detection and suffer severe injuries because they do not learn pain-avoiding behaviors. This discovery opens new directions for development of novel generations of drugs with blocking $Na_v1.7$ proprieties, which should provide more selective and safe analgesia. Meanwhile, we are still in the era of opioid therapy, and the analgesic effect may be influenced by alterations in the metabolism of analgesic drugs (cytochrome P450), variants coding for the μ-opioid receptor (μOR) as well as other targets.

5.1 Cytochrome P450 and the codeine story

Cytochrome P450 (CYP450) is a super-family of liver enzymes that catalyze phase 1 drug metabolism. The D6 isozyme of the CYP2 family is particularly affected by genetic variability and currently has 80 identified CYP2D6 alleles (http://www.cypalleles.ki.se/), resulting in a variable enzymatic activity ranging from 1 to 200%. As a result, each individual can be classified as having an "ultra-rapid metabolism" (UM), an "extensive metabolism" (EM), an "intermediate metabolism" (IM) or a "poor metabolism" (PM) and microarray technology is available to classify individuals according to their metabolic phenotype. Furthermore, it is important to note that the distribution of CYP2D6 phenotypes varies with race, since mutated alleles differ among racial and ethnic groups. Of note, approximately 7 to 10% of Caucasians have no CYP2D6 activity (poor metabolism) because of deletions, frameshift, or splice-site mutations of the gene. On the other end of the spectrum, 1 to 3% of Middle Europeans and up to 29% of Ethiopians have duplications of the *CYP2D6* gene and are classified as ultra-rapid metabolizers [53]. Ultra-rapid metabolizers have up to 50% higher plasma concentrations compared to extensive metabolizers [54].

Codeine is a pro-drug and needs to be converted into morphine to elicit its analgesic effect; therefore 'poor metabolizers' do not achieve analgesia with codeine while they may encounter side effects such as nausea and vomiting. Codeine is converted to morphine through O-demethylation catalyzed by CYP2D6, and accounts for 10% of codeine clearance. The conversion of codeine into norcodeine by CYP3A4 and into codeine-6-glucuronide by glucuronidation represents approximately 80% of codeine clearance. Morphine is further metabolized into morphine-6-glucuronide (M6G) and morphine-3-glucuronide (M3G), and morphine and M6G have opioid activity. While codeine is undoubtedly not a wonder analgesic, it was initially prescribed because of the belief that being a weak opioid, it is safe. There was a recent FDA warning on codeine use in nursing mothers following the death of a breastfed 13-day-old neonate thought to have suffered a morphine overdose because his mother was taking codeine [55]. Toxic blood levels of morphine or its active metabolite morphine-6-glucuronide (M6G) may arise in mothers and neonates that are CYP2D6 ultra-rapid or extensive metabolizers. The infant in this case report was categorized as a CYP2D6 extensive metabolizer (extensively metabolizing the pro-drug codeine to morphine) and had a blood concentration of morphine at 70ng/mL; neonates breastfed by mothers receiving codeine typically have concentrations of 0-2.2ng/mL. The mother was categorized as a CYP2D6 ultra-metabolizer and her breast milk had a morphine concentration of 87ng/mL – the typical range being 1.9-20.5ng/mL at doses of 60mg codeine every 6 hours. Therefore, the infant had two reasons for having supranormal morphine levels. In light of these findings, it has been suggested that codeine be avoided in breastfeeding mothers with a CYP2D6 extensive or ultra-rapid metabolism genotype. Reports followed that studied the rates of codeine and morphine clearance in breastfeeding mothers and their relation to CYP2D6 genotypes [56-58]. Other life-threatening adverse events have been reported in individuals who are CYP2D6 ultra-rapid metabolizers [59,60].

Since 2007, the FDA requires manufacturers of prescription codeine products to state in the "Precautions" section of the drug label the known risks of prescribing codeine to breastfeeding mothers [61]. An FDA-approved genetic test (AmpliChip CYP450: Roche Diagnostics, Palo Alto, CA, USA) is commercially available to test genetic variants of CYP2D6 [62].

Overall, the level of evidence linking gene variation (CYP2D6) to phenotype (increased biotransformation of codeine into morphine) is strong, however there is no randomized clinical trial assessing the benefits of genetic testing prior to codeine therapy at large. Currently, the only recommendation for risk aversion is a cautionary insert to avoid codeine in breastfeeding mothers (or to apply genetic testing in mothers/neonates if codeine is prescribed).

5.2 The μ-opioid receptor genotype

The μ-opioid receptor gene (OPRM1) is probably the most well studied gene in the context of post-operative and labor analgesia [63]. The most common polymorphism of OPRM1 is a single nucleotide substitution at position 118, with an adenine substitution by a guanine (A118G) reported to occur with an allelic frequency of 10–30% among Caucasians [64], a higher prevalence among Asians [65] and a lower one in African-Americans [66]. Clinicians are well aware of the large and unpredictable inter-individual variability in response to opioids [67]. A recent meta-analysis of all pain studies evaluating the impact of A118G polymorphism of OPRM1 on the response to opioids did not identify a strong association between this polymorphism and the response to opioids [63]. It is likely that the heterogeneity of the clinical situations (experimental pain, acute pain, labor pain, post-operative pain, chronic pain) and diversity of evaluated drugs and dosages precluded from any significant findings.

5.2.1 Response to intrathecal and systemic morphine for post-Cesarean analgesia

The response to an intrathecal solution containing morphine and fentanyl for post-Cesarean analgesia according to *OPRM1* genotype was evaluated in a North-American cohort [68]. There was no difference in the duration of spinal morphine analgesia or need for analgesic supplementation over 72 hours in women carrying the minor allele (G118). The time for first opioid rescue analgesia was on average 22 hours regardless of genotype. The incidence of nausea was similar between groups, however pruritus was less frequent during the first 24 hours in women carrying the minor allele (G118).

In two studies from Singapore in women undergoing Cesarean deliveries under spinal anesthesia (with morphine), women with the minor allele allele exhibited *increased* consumption of iv PCA morphine 24 hours post-delivery [69,70]. Women were given upon arrival in the post-anesthesia care unit (PACU) a morphine iv PCA pump and no other analgesics were prescribed. In the first study on 588 Chinese Singaporean, 24 hours post-operative morphine iv PCA consumption was lowest in women homozygous for the wild-type allele (A118) [69]. Distribution of morphine use over time (doses were recorded in 4 hour time intervals) demonstrated that most of morphine use occurred in the PACU during the first 4 hour after spinal anesthesia. It is possible that this early iv morphine use reflects lack of analgesia upon arrival in the PACU. Consequently, initial differences in iv morphine use may be due to differences in pain perception rather than impaired spinal morphine analgesia in women carrying the minor allele (G118), while differences of morphine use at 24 hour reflect either differences in intrathecal morphine duration and/or efficacy or more likely differences in iv morphine efficacy. The overall incidence of nausea was low; nonetheless it was higher in women homozygous for the wild-type allele (A118).

In the second publication, 994 women from the three main ethnic groups in Singapore were evaluated (n=617 Chinese, n=241 Malays and n=136 Indians) [70]. The authors reported a large inter-individual range with 65 women not using any morphine, 129 using only one dose, while another 122 administered 2 doses. Total iv morphine use over the first 24 hours was significantly higher in women homozygote for the minor allele (G118), and incidence of nausea was again lower in this genotypic group. In a multiple regression analysis, the most important factor contributing to morphine usage was maximum pain score, followed by ethnicity and A118G polymorphism. After correction for genotype, ethnicity was still a significant contributing factor, with Indian women reporting higher pain scores and using higher doses of iv morphine.

This apparent discrepancy between the North-American study reporting no effect of *OPRM1* A118G polymorphism on intrathecal morphine analgesia and the Singaporean results may be explained by differences in ethnicity, study design and primary outcomes. In the Singaporean studies, the intrathecal solution did not include fentanyl therefore it is possible that onset of intrathecal analgesia occurred after women arrived in the PACU. Since women were given iv PCA morphine as the initial rescue analgesic (rather than ibuprofen as in the North-American study), such study design was more likely to evaluate the effect of A118G polymorphism on iv morphine analgesic rather than intrathecal analgesic response.

Another obvious explanation may be that *OPRM1* genotype interacts differently with opioid analgesia in different ethnic groups.

Study	Subjects (N)	Study cohort	Route of administration	Measured outcomes	Observed associations
Landau (34)	223	Nulliparous women in early labor	Spinal (up-down sequential and randomized doses)	ED50 (median effective dose providing 60min of early labor analgesia)	G118 carriers requested analgesia at later stage (greater cervical dilatation) and required *less* spinal fentanyl
Wong (35)	147	Nulliparous women in early labor	Spinal (25mcg)	Duration of effective analgesia in early labor	No difference in duration of analgesia between genotypes
Fukuda (36)	280 (183 women)	Healthy Japanese, orodental surgery	• Pre-op IV test: (2mcg/kg) • Post-op iv PCA (40mcg/10min)	• Cold-pressor test before vs after iv dose • 24h post-op iv PCA consumption	• Pre-iv test: decreased sensitivity in A118 • Post-iv test: enhanced analgesic effect in A118 • Reduced fentanyl sensitivity in women vs men • No difference in VAS scores and 24h post-op fentanyl consumption between genotypes
Wu (37)	189 (97 women)	Han Chinese, laparoscopic abdominal surgery	• Pre-op IV (5mcg/kg) • Intra-op IV (1mcg/kg/30min) • Post-op IV (1mcg/kg)	• Post-op pain scores (15, 30, 45, 60min) • Time to awakening • Respiratory depression • PaCO2	• Lower pain scores in A118 (at 15 and 30min) • Longer time for awakening in A118 • Higher PaCO2 in A118 subjects
Zhang (38)	174	Han Chinese, hysterectomy	• Pre-extubation (1mcg/kg) • Post-op IV PCA (continuous 5mcg/h bolus 20mcg/5min)	• Pre-op electrical pain threshold • 24h post-op VAS scores • 24h post-op IV PCA consumption	• No difference in pain threshold • Lower electrical pain tolerance threshold in G118 carriers (gene-dose dependant effect) • No difference of initial post-op or averaged 24h pain scores • Higher consumption of post-op fentanyl in G118 homozygotes • Trend for higher incidence PONV in A118 subjects

Table 1. Recent studies evaluating *OPRM1* A118G SNP and fentanyl analgesic effect
From Landau R, Kraft JC: Pharmacogenetics in obstetric anesthesia. Curr Opin Anaesthesiol 2010; 23: 323-9

5.2.2 Response to intrathecal fentanyl for labor analgesia

Using the up-down sequential allocation model to identify differences in analgesic requirement according to *OPRM1* genotype in a Swiss cohort of nulliparous women requesting neuraxial analgesia early in labor, women carrying the minor allele (G118) required substantially lower doses of intrathecal fentanyl [71]. The ED50 (median effective dose providing labor pain relief defined on a 0-10 verbal numerical pain scale as being < 1 for at least 60 minutes) of intrathecal fentanyl given as part of a combined-spinal epidural (CSE) was 1.5 fold higher in A118 homozygotes versus that in women carrying at least one minor allele (G118). Moreover, this finding was replicated using random-dose allocation (doses ranging from 2.5-35µg), with a 2.1-fold difference between genetic groups. Of note, cervical dilatation at the time of analgesia request was significantly *less* in women homozygote for wild-type allele (A118) than in women carrying one or two minor alleles (G118). This is of interest because women received the CSE analgesic when they requested pain relief at the time they experienced painful contractions. It has previously been demonstrated that epidural analgesic requirements increase with progress of labor and cervical dilatation, therefore women carrying the variant G118 allele should have greater analgesic requirements due to the greater cervical dilatation at which they requested analgesia; our finding that these women require *less* fentanyl may actually underestimate the true effect of genotype. Since provision of optimal labor analgesia remains an ongoing challenge for obstetric anesthesiologists, the variability in ED50 according to genotype is clearly relevant from a clinical standpoint. These findings suggest genotyping may help improve the administration of labor analgesia with 30% of Caucasian women (and probably a vast majority of Asian women) potentially requiring lower doses of intrathecal fentanyl for effective analgesia during labor and delivery.

In a North-American cohort, the effect of the A118G polymorphism on the duration of intrathecal fentanyl analgesia in early labor and found no difference between genotypes [68]. The severity of nausea, pruritus or incidence of vomiting was also not different between genetic groups. While the A118G polymorphism may influence intrathecal fentanyl potency, there may be no pharmacokinetic effect altering duration of analgesic action.

Overall, the level of evidence linking gene variation to morphine or fentanyl response is moderate, probably due to the inherent complexity of studying pain (different nociceptive modalities, gender differences, limitations in extrapolating data from animal models to the response in humans, interethnic and environmental differences) in addition to the obvious polygenic nature of pain and analgesic response. The design and execution of large clinical studies analyzing multiple haplotypes simultaneously remains to be the true challenge to date. Meanwhile, a genome-wide study in the context of acute post-operative pain was published [21], the possible impact of epigenetics-based strategies for pain therapy is proposed [72] and researchers are actively working on gene therapies for chronic pain [73-75]. It will also be of interest to see the new insights and developments brought by more research on the SCN9A gene, a gene involved in channelopathies that result in the inability to experience pain, and potential targeted therapies [76].

6. The future of personalized medicine

Perhaps the most exciting yet challenging development of personalized medicine emerged with the highly sophisticated technology that now allows whole genome sequencing at a cost that is no longer prohibitive. Therefore, extensive considerations are needed to decide how to best utilize whole genome sequencing data in clinical practice [77]. Among these challenges, patients will need to receive complex and detailed genetic counseling before they can decide whether they wish to undergo such genetic risk assessment, and effective ways to convey meaningful information to patients about the many implications of their whole-genome sequences need to be developed. In addition, interpretation should take into account the limits of the sequencing method used. Databases with easily accessible and well validated information about the associations between genomic sequences and diseases needs to be created, maintained, and frequently updated to incorporate new information about disease risks, and changes in assessment will have to be communicated to patients.

A fascinating report on the first integrated analysis of a complete human genome in the clinical context of a 40 year old male who presented with a family history of coronary artery disease and sudden death addressed these issues [78]. Disease and risk analysis of the genome for this individual study was focused on variants associated with genes for known Mendelian disease, novel mutations, variants known to have a pharmacogenetic effect, and SNPs previously associated with complex disease. The subject was found to have an increased genetic risk for myocardial infarction, type II diabetes and certain cancers. With this report, the authors developed tools to integrate the subject's clinical characteristics, his family history and the results from whole genome sequencing including 2.6 million SNPs and 752 copy number variations to assist clinical decision-making. Large-scale implementation of such sophisticated methodology will require multidisciplinary approaches that include medical and genetic professionals, ethicists and regulatory agencies.

7. Conclusions

There is no doubt that genetic variants affect drug responses to an extent that can have relevant implications beyond just the efficacy of a prescribed drug. For the clinician, and in particular for the anesthesiologist providing anesthesia and post-operative pain management, there are to date no guidelines or recommendations that suggest any pharmacogenetic testing prior to administering any anesthesia-related drug. Consequently, it is still too early to foresee immediate implications of pharmacogenetics in general and pharmacogenetic diagnostic tests specifically, but one can hope that future discoveries in the field of genomics will soon aid anesthesiologists and other clinicians in predicting efficacy or toxicity for some drugs.

8. References

[1] Weber WW: Pharmacogenetics. New York, Oxford University Press, 1997

[2] Pauling L, Itano HA, et al.: Sickle cell anemia, a molecular disease. Science 1949; 109: 443

[3] Motulsky AG: Drug reactions enzymes, and biochemical genetics. J Am Med Assoc 1957; 165: 835-7

[4] Vogel F: Moderne Probem der Humangenetik. Ergeb. Inn. Med. U. Kinderheilk. 1959; 12: 52-125

[5] Kalow W: Pharmacogenetics; heredity and the response to drugs. Philadelphia,, W.B. Saunders Co., 1962

[6] Lehmann H, Ryan E: The familial incidence of low pseudocholinesterase level. Lancet 1956; 271: 124

[7] Kalow W, Gunn DR: The relation between dose of succinylcholine and duration of apnea in man. J Pharmacol Exp Ther 1957; 120: 203-14

[8] Davis PJ, Brandom BW: The association of malignant hyperthermia and unusual disease: when you're hot you're hot or maybe not. Anesth Analg 2009; 109: 1001-3

[9] Maintained as an up-to-date list by the European Malignant Hyperthermia Group at http://www.emhg.org/index.pdp?option=com_ryr1&Itemid=66:

[10] Urwyler A, Deufel T, McCarthy T, West S: Guidelines for molecular genetic detection of susceptibility to malignant hyperthermia. Br J Anaesth 2001; 86: 283-7

[11] The human genome. Science genome map. Science 2001; 291: 1218

[12] Venter JC, Adams MD, Myers EW, Li PW, Mural RJ, Sutton GG, Smith HO, Yandell M, Evans CA, Holt RA, Gocayne JD, Amanatides P, Ballew RM, Huson DH, Wortman JR, Zhang Q, Kodira CD, Zheng XH, Chen L, Skupski M, Subramanian G, Thomas PD, Zhang J, Gabor Miklos GL, Nelson C, Broder S, Clark AG, Nadeau J, McKusick VA, Zinder N, Levine AJ, Roberts RJ, Simon M, Slayman C, Hunkapiller M, Bolanos R, Delcher A, Dew I, Fasulo D, Flanigan M, Florea L, Halpern A, Hannenhalli S, Kravitz S, Levy S, Mobarry C, Reinert K, Remington K, Abu-Threideh J, Beasley E, Biddick K, Bonazzi V, Brandon R, Cargill M, Chandramouliswaran I, Charlab R, Chaturvedi K, Deng Z, Di Francesco V, Dunn P, Eilbeck K, Evangelista C, Gabrielian AE, Gan W, Ge W, Gong F, Gu Z, Guan P, Heiman TJ, Higgins ME, Ji RR, Ke Z, Ketchum KA, Lai Z, Lei Y, Li Z, Li J, Liang Y, Lin X, Lu F, Merkulov GV, Milshina N, Moore HM, Naik AK, Narayan VA, Neelam B, Nusskern D, Rusch DB, Salzberg S, Shao W, Shue B, Sun J, Wang Z, Wang A, Wang X, Wang J, Wei M, Wides R, Xiao C, Yan C, et al.: The sequence of the human genome. Science 2001; 291: 1304-51

[13] Collins FS, Morgan M, Patrinos A: The Human Genome Project: lessons from large-scale biology. Science 2003; 300: 286-90

[14] Allen PD: Anesthesia and the human genome project: the quest for accurate prediction of drug responses. Anesthesiology 2005; 102: 494-5

[15] Ama T, Bounmythavong S, Blaze J, Weismann M, Marienau MS, Nicholson WT: Implications of pharmacogenomics for anesthesia providers. AANA J 2010; 78: 393-9

[16] Avram MJ, Gupta DK, Atkinson AJ, Jr.: Anesthesia: a discipline that incorporates clinical pharmacology across the DDRU continuum. Clin Pharmacol Ther 2008; 84: 3-6

[17] Bukaveckas BL, Valdes R, Jr., Linder MW: Pharmacogenetics as related to the practice of cardiothoracic and vascular anesthesia. J Cardiothorac Vasc Anesth 2004; 18: 353-65

[18] Galinkin JL, Demmer L, Yaster M: Genetics for the pediatric anesthesiologist: a primer on congenital malformations, pharmacogenetics, and proteomics. Anesth Analg 2010; 111: 1264-74

[19] Galley HF, Mahdy A, Lowes DA: Pharmacogenetics and anesthesiologists. Pharmacogenomics 2005; 6: 849-56

[20] Iohom G, Fitzgerald D, Cunningham AJ: Principles of pharmacogenetics--implications for the anaesthetist. Br J Anaesth 2004; 93: 440-50

[21] Kim H, Clark D, Dionne RA: Genetic contributions to clinical pain and analgesia: avoiding pitfalls in genetic research. J Pain 2009; 10: 663-93

[22] Kosarac B, Fox AA, Collard CD: Effect of genetic factors on opioid action. Curr Opin Anaesthesiol 2009; 22: 476-82

[23] Landau R: Pharmacogenetic influences in obstetric anaesthesia. Best Pract Res Clin Obstet Gynaecol 2010; 24: 277-87

[24] Landau R, Kraft JC: Pharmacogenetics in obstetric anesthesia. Curr Opin Anaesthesiol 2010; 23: 323-9

[25] Palmer SN, Giesecke NM, Body SC, Shernan SK, Fox AA, Collard CD: Pharmacogenetics of anesthetic and analgesic agents. Anesthesiology 2005; 102: 663-71

[26] Schwinn DA, Podgoreanu M: Pharmacogenomics and end-organ susceptibility to injury in the perioperative period. Best Pract Res Clin Anaesthesiol 2008; 22: 23-37

[27] Searle R, Hopkins PM: Pharmacogenomic variability and anaesthesia. Br J Anaesth 2009; 103: 14-25

[28] Sweeney BP: Pharmacogenomics and anaesthesia: explaining the variability in response to opiates. Eur J Anaesthesiol 2007; 24: 209-12

[29] Liggett SB: Polymorphisms of the beta2-adrenergic receptor. N Engl J Med 2002; 346: 536-8

[30] Ngan Kee WD, Khaw KS: Vasopressors in obstetrics: what should we be using? Curr Opin Anaesthesiol 2006; 19: 238-43

[31] Smiley RM, Blouin JL, Negron M, Landau R: beta2-Adrenoceptor Genotype Affects Vasopressor Requirements during Spinal Anesthesia for Cesarean Delivery. Anesthesiology 2006; 104: 644-650

[32] Aya AG, Mangin R, Vialles N, Ferrer JM, Robert C, Ripart J, de La Coussaye JE: Patients with severe preeclampsia experience less hypotension during spinal anesthesia for elective cesarean delivery than healthy parturients: a prospective cohort comparison. Anesth Analg 2003; 97: 867-72

[33] Aya AG, Vialles N, Tanoubi I, Mangin R, Ferrer JM, Robert C, Ripart J, de La Coussaye JE: Spinal anesthesia-induced hypotension: a risk comparison between patients with severe preeclampsia and healthy women undergoing preterm cesarean delivery. Anesth Analg 2005; 101: 869-75

[34] Ramanathan J, Ramsay R, Blouin J, Richebe P, Landau R: β_2Adrenoceptor Haplotypes and Vasopressor Response during Spinal Anesthesia for CS in Preeclampsia. ASA Abstract 2009; A860

[35] Cooper DW, Carpenter M, Mowbray P, Desira WR, Ryall DM, Kokri MS: Fetal and maternal effects of phenylephrine and ephedrine during spinal anesthesia for cesarean delivery. Anesthesiology 2002; 97: 1582-90

[36] Ngan Kee WD, Khaw KS, Tan PE, Ng FF, Karmakar MK: Placental transfer and fetal metabolic effects of phenylephrine and ephedrine during spinal anesthesia for cesarean delivery. Anesthesiology 2009; 111: 506-12

[37] Landau R, Liu SK, Blouin JL, Smiley RM, Ngan Kee WD: The Effect of Maternal and Fetal β_2-Adrenoceptor and Nitric Oxide Synthase Genotype on Vasopressor Requirement and Fetal Acid-Base Status During Spinal Anesthesia for Cesarean Delivery. Anesth Analg 2011; 112: 1432-7

[38] Landau R, Xie HG, Dishy V, Stein CM, Wood AJ, Emala CW, Smiley RM: β_2-Adrenergic receptor genotype and preterm delivery. Am J Obstet Gynecol 2002; 187: 1294-8

[39] Ozkur M, Dogulu F, Ozkur A, Gokmen B, Inaloz SS, Aynacioglu AS: Association of the Gln27Glu polymorphism of the β_2-adrenergic receptor with preterm labor. Int J Gynaecol Obstet 2002; 77: 209-15

[40] Doh K, Sziller I, Vardhana S, Kovacs E, Papp Z, Witkin SS: β_2-adrenergic receptor gene polymorphisms and pregnancy outcome. J Perinat Med 2004; 32: 413-7

[41] Landau R, Morales MA, Antonarakis SE, Blouin JL, Smiley RM: Arg16 homozygosity of the β_2-adrenergic receptor improves the outcome after β_2-agonist tocolysis for preterm labor. Clin Pharmacol Ther 2005; 78: 656-63

[42] Esplin MS, Varner MW: Genetic factors in preterm birth--the future. BJOG 2005; 112 Suppl 1: 97-102

[43] Romero R, Espinoza J, Rogers WT, Moser A, Nien JK, Kusanovic JP, Gotsch F, Erez O, Gomez R, Edwin S, Hassan SS: Proteomic analysis of amniotic fluid to identify women with preterm labor and intra-amniotic inflammation/infection: the use of a novel computational method to analyze mass spectrometric profiling. J Matern Fetal Neonatal Med 2008; 21: 367-88

[44] Buhimschi CS, Rosenberg VA, Dulay AT, Thung S, Sfakianaki AK, Bahtiyar MO, Buhimschi IA: Multidimensional system biology: genetic markers and proteomic biomarkers of adverse pregnancy outcome in preterm birth. Am J Perinatol 2008; 25: 175-87

[45] Miller RS, Smiley RM, Daniel D, Weng C, Emala CW, Blouin JL, Flood PD: β_2-adrenoceptor genotype and progress in term and late preterm active labor. Am J Obstet Gynecol 2011

[46] Reitman E, Conell-Price J, Evansmith J, Olson L, Drosinos S, Jasper N, Randolph P, Smiley RM, Shafer S, Flood P: β_2-adrenergic receptor genotype and other variables that contribute to labor pain and progress. Anesthesiology 2011; 114: 927-39

[47] Foulkes T, Wood JN: Pain genes. PLoS Genet 2008; 4: e1000086

[48] Stamer UM, Zhang L, Stuber F: Personalized therapy in pain management: where do we stand? Pharmacogenomics 2010; 11: 843-64

[49] Lacroix-Fralish ML, Ledoux JB, Mogil JS: The Pain Genes Database: An interactive web browser of pain-related transgenic knockout studies. Pain 2007; 131: 3 e1-4

[50] Cox JJ, Reimann F, Nicholas AK, Thornton G, Roberts E, Springell K, Karbani G, Jafri H, Mannan J, Raashid Y, Al-Gazali L, Hamamy H, Valente EM, Gorman S, Williams R, McHale DP, Wood JN, Gribble FM, Woods CG: An SCN9A channelopathy causes congenital inability to experience pain. Nature 2006; 444: 894-8

[51] Goldberg YP, MacFarlane J, MacDonald ML, Thompson J, Dube MP, Mattice M, Fraser R, Young C, Hossain S, Pape T, Payne B, Radomski C, Donaldson G, Ives E, Cox J, Younghusband HB, Green R, Duff A, Boltshauser E, Grinspan GA, Dimon JH, Sibley BG, Andria G, Toscano E, Kerdraon J, Bowsher D, Pimstone SN, Samuels ME, Sherrington R, Hayden MR: Loss-of-function mutations in the Nav1.7 gene underlie congenital indifference to pain in multiple human populations. Clin Genet 2007; 71: 311-9

[52] Nilsen KB, Nicholas AK, Woods CG, Mellgren SI, Nebuchennykh M, Aasly J: Two novel SCN9A mutations causing insensitivity to pain. Pain 2009; 143: 155-8

[53] Cascorbi I: Pharmacogenetics of cytochrome p4502D6: genetic background and clinical implication. Eur J Clin Invest 2003; 33 Suppl 2: 17-22

[54] Kirchheiner J, Schmidt H, Tzvetkov M, Keulen JT, Lotsch J, Roots I, Brockmoller J: Pharmacokinetics of codeine and its metabolite morphine in ultra-rapid metabolizers due to CYP2D6 duplication. Pharmacogenomics J 2007; 7: 257-65

[55] Koren G, Cairns J, Chitayat D, Gaedigk A, Leeder SJ: Pharmacogenetics of morphine poisoning in a breastfed neonate of a codeine-prescribed mother. Lancet 2006; 368: 704

[56] Ferner RE: Did the drug cause death? Codeine and breastfeeding. Lancet 2008; 372: 606-8

[57] Madadi P, Ross CJ, Hayden MR, Carleton BC, Gaedigk A, Leeder JS, Koren G: Pharmacogenetics of neonatal opioid toxicity following maternal use of codeine during breastfeeding: a case-control study. Clin Pharmacol Ther 2009; 85: 31-5

[58] Willmann S, Edginton AN, Coboeken K, Ahr G, Lippert J: Risk to the breast-fed neonate from codeine treatment to the mother: a quantitative mechanistic modeling study. Clin Pharmacol Ther 2009; 86: 634-43

[59] Ciszkowski C, Madadi P, Phillips MS, Lauwers AE, Koren G: Codeine, ultrarapid-metabolism genotype, and postoperative death. N Engl J Med 2009; 361: 827-8

[60] Gasche Y, Daali Y, Fathi M, Chiappe A, Cottini S, Dayer P, Desmeules J: Codeine intoxication associated with ultrarapid CYP2D6 metabolism. N Engl J Med 2004; 351: 2827-31

[61] US-FDA: Information for Healthcare Professionals: Use of Codeine Products in Nursing Mothers - 17 August 2007. http://www.fda.gov/drugs/drugsafety/postmarketdrugsafetyinformationforpati entsandproviders/ucm124889.htm. [Accessed: 2/11/2011].

[62] de Leon J, Susce MT, Murray-Carmichael E: The AmpliChip CYP450 genotyping test: Integrating a new clinical tool. Mol Diagn Ther 2006; 10: 135-51

[63] Walter C, Lotsch J: Meta-analysis of the relevance of the OPRM1 118A>G genetic variant for pain treatment. Pain 2009; 146: 270-5

[64] Landau R, Cahana A, Smiley RM, Antonarakis SE, Blouin JL: Genetic variability of mu-opioid receptor in an obstetric population. Anesthesiology 2004; 100: 1030-3

[65] Tan EC, Tan CH, Karupathivan U, Yap EP: Mu opioid receptor gene polymorphisms and heroin dependence in Asian populations. Neuroreport 2003; 14: 569-72

[66] Crowley JJ, Oslin DW, Patkar AA, Gottheil E, DeMaria PA, Jr., O'Brien CP, Berrettini WH, Grice DE: A genetic association study of the mu opioid receptor and severe opioid dependence. Psychiatr Genet 2003; 13: 169-73

[67] Nielsen CS, Staud R, Price DD: Individual differences in pain sensitivity: measurement, causation, and consequences. J Pain 2009; 10: 231-7

[68] Wong C, McCarthy R, Blouin JL, Landau R: Observational study of the effect of mu-opioid receptor genetic polymorphism on intrathecal opioid labor analgesia and post-cesarean delivery analgesia. Int J Obstet Anesth 2010; in press

[69] Sia AT, Lim Y, Lim EC, Goh RW, Law HY, Landau R, Teo YY, Tan EC: A118G single nucleotide polymorphism of human mu-opioid receptor gene influences pain perception and patient-controlled intravenous morphine consumption after intrathecal morphine for postcesarean analgesia. Anesthesiology 2008; 109: 520-6

[70] Tan EC, Lim EC, Teo YY, Lim Y, Law HY, Sia AT: Ethnicity and OPRM variant independently predict pain perception and patient-controlled analgesia usage for post-operative pain. Mol Pain 2009; 5: 32

[71] Landau R, Kern C, Columb MO, Smiley RM, Blouin JL: Genetic variability of the mu-opioid receptor influences intrathecal fentanyl analgesia requirements in laboring women. Pain 2008; 139: 5-14

[72] Doehring A, Geisslinger G, Lotsch J: Epigenetics in pain and analgesia: an imminent research field. Eur J Pain 2011; 15: 11-6

[73] Mata M, Fink DJ: Gene therapy for pain. Anesthesiology 2007; 106: 1079-80

[74] Mata M, Hao S, Fink DJ: Applications of gene therapy to the treatment of chronic pain. Curr Gene Ther 2008; 8: 42-8

[75] Wolfe D, Wechuck J, Krisky D, Mata M, Fink DJ: A clinical trial of gene therapy for chronic pain. Pain Med 2009; 10: 1325-30

[76] Lotsch J, Geisslinger G: Pharmacogenetics of new analgesics. Br J Pharmacol 2010

[77] Ormond KE, Wheeler MT, Hudgins L, Klein TE, Butte AJ, Altman RB, Ashley EA, Greely HT: Challenges in the clinical application of whole genome sequencing. Lancet 2010; 375: 1749-51

[78] Ashley EA, Butte AJ, Wheeler MT, Chen R, Klein TE, Dewey FE, Dudley JT, Ormond KE, Pavlovic A, Morgan AA, Pushkarev D, Neff NF, Hudgins L, Gong L, Hodges LM, Berlin DS, Thorn CF, Sangkuhl K, Hebert JM, Woon M, Sagreiya H, Whaley R, Knowles JW, Chou MF, Thakuria JV, Rosenbaum AM, Zaranek AW, Church GM, Greely HT, Quake SR, Altman RB: Clinical assessment incorporating a personal genome. Lancet 2010; 375: 1525-35

12

Pharmacogenetics of Asthma

Andrzej Mariusz Fal and Marta Rosiek-Biegus
Wroclaw Medical University, Wroclaw,
Poland

1. Introduction

Pharmacogenetics uses genetic information to help adjusting treatment for individual patients. It improves efficacy of therapy and enables avoiding side effects basing on genetic knowledge. Different asthmatic patients with similar disease severity, who are treated with the same medication, may respond to the therapy differently. After excluding non-genetic causes of such variability (like patient's compliance, environmental and psychological factors), the most possible reason for the variability appears to be a different genetic structure. Changes in gene structure resulting in inter-individual dissimilarities, occur mostly as single nucleotide polymorphism (SNP). Different strategies play a role in searching and identifying SNPs, that influence pathogenesis of asthma and its response to treatment, (Kazani et al., 2010). One of the strategies involved is candidate gene studying, that focuses on finding genes responsible for therapy effectiveness as well as asthma development and its clinical severity (Moffatt & Cookson, 1997). Pharmacogenetics of asthma concentrates on genes coding: drug binding receptors, enzymes (important both in drug metabolism and metabolic cycles, eg. arachidonic acid cascade), chemokines, cytokines or growth factors relevant to asthma pathogenesis and pathophysiology. Genes need to be studied for known SNPs and new variants as well. When an SNP is found a thorough check for possible correlation between this polymorphism and disease phenotype or treatment response is needed. An expanded strategy for searching candidate genes involves screening of genes encoding proteins (enzymes) active in metabolic cycles important for drug response or key disease pathologies. In asthmatic patients this last method is often used to examine the leukotriene pathway in order to elucidate different patient reactions to leukotriene modifiers. Other options are genome-wide association studies that analyze genetic markers across the entire genome that may be connected with the phenotype. The identification of such a marker generated investigation of surrounding genes for SNPs related to the phenotype (Kazani et al., 2010). This procedure needs numerous and phenotypically well characterised populations and enables examination of the most frequent SNPs. There are some fields of medicine where pharmacogenetics is already in clinical use but in asthma treatment further investigation is still needed. This chapter reviews recent knowledge of pharmacogenetics of drugs commonly used in asthma treatment. We focus on bronchodilators, iCS (inhaled corticosteroids) and leukotriene modifiers.

2. Pharmacogenetics of antiasthmatic medications

2.1 Pharmacogenetics of β2-agonists

β2-adrenoreceptor (β2-ADR) agonists are fundamental relief medications and among the most important chronic treatments in asthma. These drugs exert their action by activation of β2-adrenoreceptors located among others on smooth muscle cells. This results in smooth muscle relaxation, airway dilatation and improved airflow. Depending on the duration of their action β2-agonistss are divided into two groups: short acting (SABA) and long acting β2-agonists (LABA). SABA are used exclusively as rescue medicines. They quickly reduce asthma symptoms: wheezing, shortness of breath and coughing. While LABA when used on a daily basis in combination with iCS help to improve asthma control. The side effects are common for both groups and these are: tachycardia, muscle tremble, mild hypokalaemia.

The β2-adrenoreceptor is a member of the 7-transmembrane domain G-protein coupled receptor family. It consists of seven transmembrane spanning domains, 3 extracellular and 3 intracellular (Fig. 1) (Dixon et al., 1986). Stimulation of β2-adrenoreceptor is G-protein dependent and results in activation of the second messenger, the adenylate cyclase. This in turn leads to an increase of cAMP level and smooth muscle relaxation. Another mechanism resulting from β2-adrenoreceptor stimulation is potassium channels opening by cAMP or directly by G-protein (Kowalski & Woszczek, 2002).

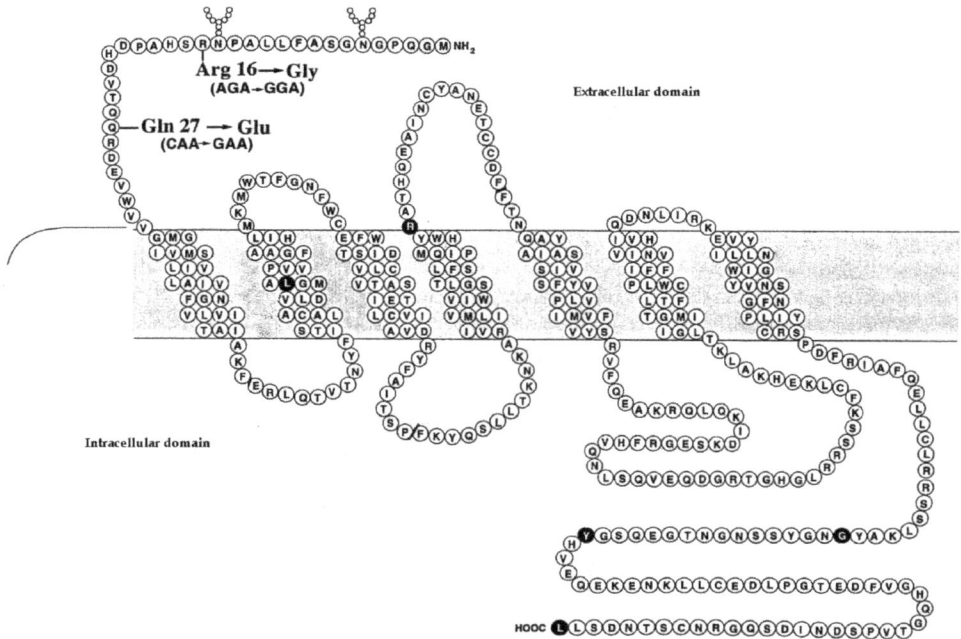

Fig. 1. Most common clinically relevant polymorphisms of the β2-adrenoreceptor (Ligget, 1997-changed). Black - nucleic acid deviations from wild type not resulting in nucleotide changes.

2.1.1 Polymorphisms of the β2-adrenergic receptor

Examination of the intronless β2-adrenoreceptor gene, which is located on chromosome 5q31.32 (Kobilka et al., 1987), revealed over 80 SPNs (Weiss et al., 2006). Two of these polymorphisms: Arg→Gly16 (46A→G) and Gln→Glu27 (79C→G) are the most frequent ones (see Figure 1.) (Green et al.,1994, 1995; Lee et al., 2004). Their occurrence results in receptor function change, different ligand binding and impaired signal transmission. The occurrence of the Gly16 gene variant is higher than that of the wild-type Arg16 and ranges between 67% in British asthmatics and 72% in British and American healthy subjects (Liggett, 1997; Tan et al., 1997; Lipworth et al., 1999). It has been estimated that the homozygous genotype Arg16 appears in 16% Caucasians and 25% Afro-Americans. Studies of Xie (Xie, et al., 2001) and co-workers revealed further differences between β2-adrenoreceptor polymorphisms and ethnic groups. In a study, that examined 415 healthy subjects, Glu27 allele were the most frequent in Caucasian-Americans (34.8%). Other groups had much lower occurrence of this allele: Afro-Americans (20.7%) and Chinese (7.2%). Individuals with homozygous Glu27 genotype were mostly Caucasian-Americans (15.4%). This genotype occured only in 4.9% African-Americans and was not observed in Chinese subjects (Xie, et al., 2001). Both Gly16 and Glu27 polymorphisms are involved in higher agonist promoted receptor down-regulation, moreover, Glu27 is related with a stronger desensitization of the receptor (Green et al., 1994, 1995). Another defined polymorphism: Thr→Ile164 is associated with diminished affinity of β2-agonist to the receptor, decreased adenylate cyclase binding and 50% shorter lasting salmeterol (one of the long acting beta2 agonists) effect (Green et al., 2001).

2.1.1.1 Correlation between β2-adrenoreceptor gene polymorphism and short acting β-agonists action

Short acting β-agonists are drugs commonly used in asthma treatment, especially in asthma exacerbations or as regular rescue medications. However, they are not recommended as regular antiasthmatic drugs. Several studies demonstrated higher FEV1 increase (forced expiratory volume in the first second, a spirometric parameter used to determine the level of airways narrowing) increase after SABA (salbutamol) administration in homozygous Arg16 individuals as compared to heterozygous and homozygous Gly16 patients with polynosis (Martinez et al., 1997; Woszczek et al., 2005). Different results were obtained during asthma exacerbation. Patients who were homozygous Arg16 had impaired SABA response compared to homozygous Gly16 individuals (Carroll et al., 2009). Systematic administration of SABA to Arg16 asthmatics caused deterioration of lung function (as evaluated with PEF - peak expiratory flow, another parameter used to monitor airway narrowing), that did not stop even with treatment discontinuation. In contrast patients homozygous for Gly16 demonstrated improved lung function (evaluated by PEF measurement as well) (Israel, 2000, 2004). Based on these studies it has been postulated that Arg16 homozygotes may be at higher risk during long-term SABA therapy. According to the 2010 updated GINA guidelines (Global Initiative for Asthma [GINA], 2010) regular long-term SABA treatment is not recommended for any individual. But due to relatively low differences in PEF-worsening between the two groups more research is needed to fully elucidate this problem.

2.1.1.2 Correlation between β2-adrenoreceptor gene polymorphisms and long acting β-agonists action

Long acting β2-agonists as opposed to SABA are drugs commonly used in long-term asthma therapy. There are several population studies suggesting increased risk of therapy with long acting β2-agonists in patients with the Arg16 homozygous genotype. However, no genotype is currently considered a direct contraindication for LABA treatment. Some patients treated with salmeterol, experienced rare but severe asthma exacerbations (Nelson et al., 2006). Further investigation suggested a dependence between Arg16 genotype and faster decline of lung parameters (FEV1) after LABA application (Nelson et al., 2006; Wechsler et al., 2006; Lee et al., 2004; Palmer et al., 2006). A good example is a study of Wechsler and co-workers comparing salmeterol response in individuals with asthma homozygous for arginine (Arg16) with glycine homozygous (Gly16) group of patients. Patients were divided in two groups . The first group was treated with salmeterol without iCS and the second continued iCS therapy while randomized for salmeterol. In both groups Arg16 patients didn't draw benefit from salmeterol therapy comparing to Gly16 patients, which resulted in lower morning PEF, increased symptom scores and albuterol rescue use especially in trial without iCS. Present asthma treatment guidelines allow use of LABA only together with iCS since it has been demonstrated that iCS ameliorate the LABA effect. It is possible that in the future patients with Arg16Arg genotype will constitute a group requiring different treatment guidelines, but up to date therapeutic indications are uniform irrespective of the patient's genotype.

2.1.1.3 Correlation between β2-adrenoreceptor gene polymorphisms and asthma exacerbations

It has been proven that exacerbations of asthma during short acting β-agonist therapy is related to β2-adrenoreceptor gene polymorphisms (Taylor et al., 2000). Recent studies reveal, that children and adolescent asthmatics with the Arg16 genotype suffer from asthma exacerbations more frequently than the Gly16 subpopulation (OR 2.05, 95% CI 1.19 to 3.53, p=0.010). This genotype-exacerbation correlation significantly increases after salmeterol treatment (OR 3.40, 95% CI 1.19 to 9.40, p=0.022) (Palmer et al., 2006). Other studies confirm the conclusion that risk of asthma exacerbation in the Arg16 group rises with higher doses and more frequent use of β2-agonists. Individuals with the Arg16 genotype receiving short- or long-acting β2-agonists on everyday basis had significantly higher risk of asthma exacerbation (OR 1.64, 95% CI 1.22 to 2.20, p=0.001) than patients with the Arg16 genotype taking β2-agonist less than once daily (Basu et al., 2009). According to the LARGE study patients with the Gly16 genotype have diminished bronchial hyperresponsiveness to matacholine after adding inhaled corticosteroids (at an average dose 480µg of beclomethasone daily) to salmeterol treatment (Wechsler et al., 2009). Arg16 genotype Afro-Americans have a lower chance for lung function improvement after co-administration of LABA and inhaled corticosteroids what may be related to more frequent prevalence of Arg16 polymorphism in this population (25%). This can also explain ethnic differences in asthma manifestation – more frequent severe asthma occurrence in Afro-Americans. According to Liggett (Liggett, SB., 2000) β2-adrenoreceptors in Gly16 subjects are down regulated at baseline by exposure to endogenous cathecholamines what explains why reaction to exogenous β2-agonists is more evident in Arg16Arg individuals. At the same time however, Arg16 patients seem to have higher risk of asthma exacerbation especially during β2-agonist therapy. Despite these differences present guidelines [GINA, BTS (British Thoracic Society)] do not recommend checking the patients' genotype before starting therapy. In our opinion LABA-treatment failure should be a recommendation for β2-adrenoreceptor genotype verification. This may increase both treatment effectiveness and safety. More research in this field is needed, however.

2.2 Pharmacogenetics of leukotriene modifiers

Leukotrienes are a family of polyunsaturated eicosatetraenoic acids that are derived from arachidonic acid in an enzymatic pathway called arachidonic acid cascade (see Figure 2.). In this pathway 5-lipoxygenase plays probably the most important role (Dixon et al., 1990). 5-lipoxygenase (5-LOX) catalyzes the conversion of arachidonic acid to leukotriene-A4 (LTA4) (Silverman & Drazen, 1999). All leukotrienes include cysteine and are called cysteinyl leukotrienes (with the exception of LTB4). Cysteinyl leukotrienes bind to CysLT1 receptor causing among others airway smooth muscle contraction, eosinophilic influx and mucus hypersecretion. Another important enzyme in the leukotriene pathway is LTC4 synthase, which is responsible for LTA4 to LTC4 conversion. Leukotrienes have been shown to be potent pro-inflammatory mediators in asthma pathology (Chanarin & Johnston, 1994). They are produced and released by several types of inflammatory cells including eosinophils, neutrophils and mast cells.

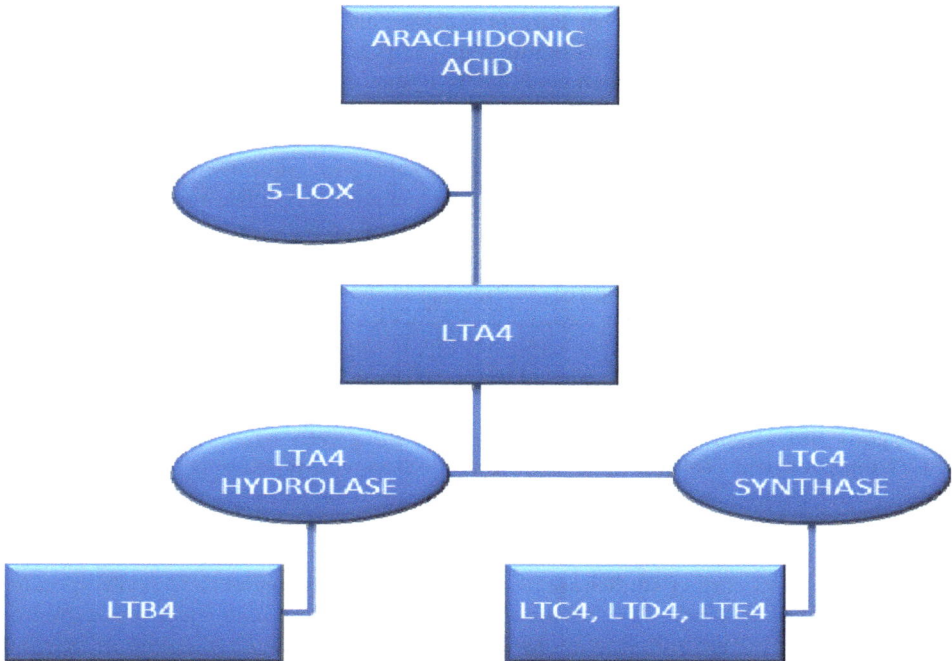

Fig. 2. The lipoxygenase pathway of leukotriene synthesis

Leukotriene modifiers are an important group of drugs in asthma treatment as well as in other diseases including allergic rhinitis. Based on their mode of action they can be divided into two groups: first – cysteine leukotrienes receptor antagonists (montelukast, zafirlukast, pranlukast and tomelukast), second - 5-lipoxygenase inhibitors (zileuton). These drugs show strong anti-inflammatory activity, ameliorate asthma clinical course and improve disease control with minimal or no side effects. Currently, they are listed in GINA 2010 (GINA, 2010) guidelines for asthma treatment as number two anti-inflammatory treatment (number one are still inhaled steroids), even though not all asthmatic patients benefit substantially from anti-leukotriene therapy. Based on the knowledge on leukotriene synthesis pathway, studies of genotype dependent therapeutic reactions have used strategies of candidate gene screening and examination of SNPs in genes encoding different proteins (enzymes) of the arachidonic acid cascade. To date, most investigations of the genetic factors which may affect therapy with anti-leukotriene drugs have focused on the 5-LOX enzyme and the LTC4 synthase. Possible genetic alterations of cysteine leukotriene receptors have also been investigated. The following paragraphs discuss the most important pharmacogenetic studies presenting major polymorphisms relevant in asthma and allergy as well as their impact on drug action.

2.2.1 Polymorphisms of the 5-lipoxygenase gene

The 5-LOX gene (ALOX5) is located on chromosome 10q11.12, contains 14 exons and its activity is associated with a number of repetitions of Sp1/Erg1 binding motifs in the promoter region (Hoshiko et al., 1990; Funk et al., 1989; Silverman et al., 1998). The promoter region containing five tandem motifs binding Sp1/Erg1 transcription factors (GGGCGG) is known as wild-type allele (Silverman et al., 1998). Polymorphisms of this region result from additions or deletions of binding motifs and are called non-wild-type alleles (In et al., 1997; Silverman et al., 1998). A polymorphism with one additional Sp1/Erg1 binding motif has been found in 35% of both asthmatic and non-asthmatic population (Fenech, A & Hall, IP., 2002). Further, 3% of the subjects without any copy of a wild-type allele are expected to have lower ALOX-5 gene transcription, which leads to reduced enzyme production and finally to lower LTA4 levels (Drazen et al., 1999; Kalayci et al., 2003). In consequence, the low level of cysteinyl leukotriene does not intensify allergic inflammation in asthma, but patients who do not have a wild-type allele, experience only 1% FEV1 improvement after 5-LOX inhibitor treatment comparing to wild-type patients (FEV1 improves up to 15-20%) and are considered non-responders for this type of therapy (Drazen et al., 1999). The same concerns to montelukast treatment (antagonist of cysteine leukotriene receptors): wild-type homozygous and heterozygous patients present benefit greatly from treatment (measured as FEV1 improvement (Telleria et al., 2008)), while non-wild-type are considered relative-non-responders. Other studies demonstrated however, that subjects with non-wild-type allele(s) treated with montelukast had reduced (73%) risk of asthma exacerbation (Lima et al., 2006). Because the role of leukotriene modifiers in asthma control increased significantly in the past five years, further studies are necessary to define responders and non-responders phenotypes. Defining standards of responding to leukotriene modifier therapy is extremely important at least in two subpopulations: in non-wild-type individuals, who in previous tudies have not experienced treatment benefit and in patient with steroid resistance or at least with partially impaired response to iCS.

2.2.2 Polymorphisms of the leukotriene C4 synthase gene (LTC4S)

LTC4 synthase (LTC4S) belongs to S-glutathione synthases family and is responsible for leukotriene A4 and glutathione bonding. This reaction results in leukotriene C4 synthesis. LTC4 is a potent contractor of bronchial smooth muscles. The gene for LTC4 synthase is located on chromosome 5q35. In the promoter region of this gene several polymorphism have been described. One of the most important is substitution of nucleotide A by C in position 444 (-444A→C). The -444A→C SNP results in increased LTC4S gene transcription and therefore higher LTC4 level in eosinophils (Sampson et al., 2000; Sanak et al., 2000). This variant occurs more often in patients suffering from aspirin induced asthma (in patients with aspirin idiosyncrasy in general) (Sanak et al., 1997). Presence of the C nucleotide is also related to better response to cysteine leukotriene receptor 1 (LTRA1) blockers. During montelukast therapy 80% reduction of asthma exacerbation risk was observed in heterozygous individuals with C allele when compared to AA homozygous (Lima et al., 2006). Similar results were reported from a study in Japan, where patients with moderate, well controlled asthma, treated with inhaled corticosteroids, received pranlukast as an add-on treatment. Again, individuals with the C allele had more pronounced FEV1 improvement than AA homozygous patients (FEV1 improvement in C allele group 5.3% vs. in AA group 2.4%). Heterozygous population also showed higher values of bronchial dilatation after salbutamol usage (Asano et al., 2002).

2.2.3 Polymorphisms of the cysteine leukotriene receptors 1 and 2 genes (CYSTLTR1, CYSTLTR2)

The human CYSLT1 and CYSLT2 receptors have been characterized as G-protein coupled receptors (Lynch et al., 1999; Heise et al., 2000). The gene coding for the CYSLT1 receptor is located on chromosome X and the CYSLT2 receptor gene maps to chromosome 13q14 (Lynch et al., 1999; Heise et al., 2000). Polymorphisms of these genes are studied in relation to the probability of asthma development. Previous data suggest however, that polymorphisms of CYSTLTR1 and CYSTLTR2 genes play a minor role in the determination of asthma severity and clinical symptoms' expression (alike other genes encoding proteins related to leukotriene pathway) (Tantisira & Drazen, 2009). As for now there are no unequivocal results concerning polymorphisms of the CYSLT receptor genes in relation to anti-leukotriene treatment effects.

Although zileuton does not directly act through the CYSLT1 receptor, the possible correlation between this medication and CYSLT1R polymorphisms was also investigated. These studies, including genotype analysis of over five hundred patients treated with zileuton did not show any significant correlation between CYSLT1R gene polymorphisms and clinical response to therapy (Tantisira et al., 2009).

2.2.4 Polymorphisms of the ABCC1 gene

The ABCC1 gene (ATP-binding cassette, subfamily C, member 1) encodes MRP1 (Multiple Drug Resistance Protein 1) that takes a part in transmembrane LTC4 transport. This gene is located on chromosome 16p13.12 and demonstrates significant heterogeneity (Saito et al., 2002; van der Deen et al., 2005). One of the polymorphisms of this gene, that was thought to be correlated to drug response, namely rs119774, described by Lima et al. was related to a significant FEV1 improvement in subjects receiving montelukast for 6 months (Lima et al., 2006). Heterozygous patients had a 24% FEV1 rise as compared to only a 2% improvement in homozygous individuals (Lima et al., 2006). Since there are no further studies of this correlation available data are insufficient to have any treatment implications. Again, further studies would help to elucidate whether the two phenotypes differ enough to justify different treatment regimens.

2.2.5 Polymorphism of LTA4 hydrolase gene

Hydrolase LTA4 is an enzyme that converts LTA4 to LTB4. The gene encoding this protein is located on chromosome 12q22. One of the known polymorphisms for this gene (rs2660845) involves a nucleotide change A->G at intron. Patients, whose genotypes contain at least one G allele (heterozygous), when treated with montelukast, have 4-5 higher risk of asthma exacerbation when compared to AA homozygous subjects (Lima et al., 2006). The pathogenetic mechanism of this phenomenon remains unclear. It has been hypothesized that this SNP causes a decreased enzyme activity that results in diminished LTB4 synthesis, therefore stimulating the LTC4-synthase pathway and leading to cysteine leukotriene synthesis (Lima et al., 2006) (Fig. 2).

There are big individual differences in response to leukotriene modifiers. All polymorphisms listed in paragraph 2.2 contribute to these differences. It remains extremely important to determine which patient subpopulation benefit most from the treatment.

2.2.6 Polymorphisms of the SLCO2B1 gene

The gene SLCO2B1 (solute carrier organic anion transporter family - 2B1) encodes the protein 2B1, that plays an important role in the active transport of organic anions through the intestinal wall. Protein 2B1 is thought to be a key transporter of montelukast through the intestinal wall. A recently described, common, SLCO2B1 polymorphism, namely rs12422149 935G→A (Arg312Gln), appears to relate to changes in montelukast pharmacokinetics. Specifically, individuals with this SNP have a significantly lower serum drug concentration (Mougey et al., 2009). So far, there are no data on other possible SLCO2B1 gene polymorphisms that could affect montelukast transport or serum level.

Gene	Chromosomal location	Polymorphisms with potential pharmacogenetic consequences during leukotriene modifier therapy
ALOX5	10q11.12	Promoter Sp1/Egr1binding motif (G+C rich sequence, i.e. – GGGCGG-) different than 5 sequence repeats, -212 to -88 bp
LTC4S	5q35	Promoter -444A→C
CYSLTR1	Xq13.2-q21.1	927C→T
ABCC1	16p13.12	rs119774, G→A intron
LTA4H	12q22	rs2660845, A→G intron
SLCO2B1	11q13	rs12422149 935G→A

Table 1. Genes polymorphisms with potential pharmacogenetic consequences for leukotriene modifier therapy

Leukotriene modifiers are widely used in asthma treatment and they are orally administered which improves patients compliance and therefore efficacy. However, genes linked to their metabolism, drug-receptor interactions etc. have not intensively investigated. In our opinion, cytochrome P450, that metabolises both groups of leukotriene modifiers (especially CYP1A2 and CYP3A4), is a promising target. Studies investigating genetic variants of cytochrome P450 enzymes in relation to leukotriene modifiers response are necessary to establish possible dosing variations.

2.3 Pharmacogenetics of inhaled corticosteroids (iCS)

Corticosteroids are the most important and the most effective medication in asthma therapy. They are powerful anti-inflammatory agents in asthma management, mostly being "anti-eosinophilic". Although many asthmatics derive therapeutic benefit from inhaled corticosteroids, many fail to respond or at least need to be treated with much higher doses. Despite iCS being considered a safe treatment, side effects of increased dosage may be clinically significant and include: adrenal suppression, osteoporosis, skin changes, cataract, and growth retardation in children. There at least two different mechanisms of CS resistance, but both are still under investigation.

Candidate gene studies were used to determine the pharmacogenetics of response to inhaled corticosteroids.

2.3.1 Glucocorticoid receptor

Corticosteroids exert their action by binding to the glucocorticoid intracellular receptor (GR), a nuclear receptor. The GR gene is located on the long arm of chromosome 5 (5q31-32). Members of the superfamily of nuclear receptors share a structural pattern containing a short central DNA-binding domain, a variable N-terminal domain as well as a C-terminal, which is the steroid hormone binding part, and a transcription regulator (Beato et al., 1996; Gronemeyer, 1992). There are two different GR isoforms known: one consisting of 777 (called GRα) and the other of 742 amino acids called GRβ. These isoforms are created during alternative splicing of the GR pre-mRNA (Bamberger et al., 1996). GRβ varies from the other isoform only in the length of C-terminal domain, which is shorter by five amino acids. This results in reduced glucocorticoid binding affinity of the GRβ receptor. Both receptors are expressed in all human cells, but GRβ plays a regulatory role and its concentration is much lower than that of GRα. Although there is no evidence to support that this polymorphism is responsible for reduced responsiveness to GC in clinical practice, this concept has been widely discussed and related studies are currently carried out (Brogan et al., 1999; Gagliardo et al., 2000; Malmstrom et al., 1999). In the cytoplasm, the glucocorticoid receptor is linked with several regulatory proteins, with the heat shock protein (hsp90), p59 immunophilin and p23 phosphoprotein being the most important (Smith & Toft, 1993). GR and hsp90 coupling enables ligand (CS) binding to the receptor and facilitates correct receptor "maturation" after synthesis (Smith & Toft, 1993). After CS binding the complex GR/hsp90 is disunited and activated GR/CS translocates to the nucleus and binds to DNA via the central domain consisting of two "zinc fingers"(Mitchell & Tjian, 1989). On the DNA side the fragment interacting with GR is called GRE (glucocorticoid response elements). This is one of the two mechanisms for CS to stimulate or inhibit transcription and therefore mRNA synthesis. The other mechanism involves intra-cytoplasmic interaction of GR/CS with transcription factors, resulting in the blockage of their activity and consequently hampering transcription of several inflammatory agents as cytokines and chemokines, simplifying synthesis of anti-inflammatory agents (Barnes, 1996).

The importance of iCS in asthma treatment made the glucocorticoid receptors gene polymorphisms the obvious target of pharmacogenetic studies. However, despite the large number of researchers involved and the considerable funds devoted by both academic and industrial teams, only few polymorphisms have been discovered until now: Val→Asp641, that results in a three-fold lower binding affinity for dexamethasone, Val→Ile729 - with four-fold decrease in dexamethasone activity and Asn→Ser363 that results in higher activity to exogenous corticosteroids (Hurley et al., 1991; Malchof et al., 1993; Huizenga et al., 1998). From published studies we know, that patients with GR gene polymorphisms Val→Asp641 and Val→Ile729 may be predisposed to a relatively decreased response to CS therapy (Koper et al., 1997; Lane et al., 1994). A three marker long haplotype G-A-T (frequency 23% in general population; G allele - BclI SNP, A allele - intron B 33389, T allele - intron B 33388) was described in 2004 by Stevens and coworkers. It is associated with enhanced GC sensitivity measured as low postdexamethasone cortisol (frequency 41%). Subjects homozygous for G-A-T had over twofold FEV1 improvement after CS treatment compared to heterozygous or non-G-A-T haplotypes (Tantisira et al., 2004).

However, all these studies have not demonstrated a correlation between GR polymorphisms and corticosteroid resistance in asthma. Corticosteroid resistance does not seem to be dependent on a single GR gene polymorphism.

2.3.2 Polymorphisms of the CRHR1 gene (corticotropin releasing hormone receptor type 1)

In contrast to the GR gene polymorphism studies, CRHR1 investigations seem to yield more promising results. The CRHR1 gene is the major receptor for corticotropin that in turn is the key regulator of corticosteroids synthesis and catecholamine production. The gene for CRHR1 is located on chromosome 17q12-22, in the genomic region linked to asthma in a genome-wide-screen (Zandi et al., 2001). Most important data came from studies by Tantisira et al (Tantisira et al., 2004) that analyzed 14 genes connected with biological pathways of corticosteroids in three large groups of patients. Study participants were recruited from several other clinical trials studying the use of inhaled corticosteroids in asthma. The first group consisted of 470 adult individuals and was encoded AD (Adult Study), the second included 336 adult patients - ACRN (Asthma Clinical Research Network), and the third one included 311 children from CAMP (Childhood Asthma Management Program). This project revealed a significant correlation between lung function improvement after inhaled corticosteroid therapy and SNPs (rs1876828, rs242939 and rs242941) and haplotype occurrence within the CRHR1 gene, especially rs242941 (G→T, intron located) polymorphism, in all populations. In the AD population homozygous individuals with this polymorphism had average FEV1 improvement, higher than homozygous patients lacking this SNP. Similar results were obtained for the paediatric population that was studied. These data can contribute to our understanding of the diverse patient reactions to iCS treatment but further investigation is still necessary.

2.3.3 Polymorphisms of the TBX21 gene (T-box expressed in T cells)

Another gene modulating inhaled corticosteroids action is TBX21 that encodes T-bet transcription factor (Tantisira et al., 2004). It plays an important role in balancing lymphocyte subpopulations, enhancing Th1 and inhibiting Th2 clone formation. TBX21 knockout mice develop bronchial hyperresponsiveness, enhanced airway eosinophilia and faster airway remodelling (Finotto et al., 2002) proving that TBX21 is crucial for asthma protection.

So far one clinically important SNP, His→Glu33 (H33Q), was found within this gene's area in mice. Cellular models suggest that the H33Q allele can activate Th1 cytokine production (including interferon γ – INFγ) that in turn decreases Th2 cytokine synthesis providing a stable protection against asthma and allergy development. Surprisingly enough, it has been demonstrated that corticosteroids are able to inhibit T-bet induction (Refojo et al., 2003) resulting in Th2 domination. These findings still require a direct in vivo confirmation.

Studies in children (CAMP population) showed 4.5% occurrence in general population of homozygous Glu33 individuals. The presence of even one copy of this allele in subjects treated with iCS was associated with a significant decrease in airway hyperresponsiveness (measured as PC20) as compared to His33His homozygous subjects and individuals not iCS-treated (Tantisira et al., 2004).

2.3.4 Polymorphisms of the FCER2 gene (Fc fragment of IgE, low affinity II, receptor for (CD23))

The FCER2 gene encodes a protein, which is the low-affinity receptor for IgE and a key molecule for B-cell activation and growth. FCER2 gene polymorphism was predicted to bronchial hypperresponsiveness and IgE-mediated allergic diseases. Within this gene three SNPs have been described, all connected to higher risk of severe asthma and asthma exacerbations in spite of inhaled corticosteroids therapy. The polymorphism 2206T→C occurs relatively often (allelic frequency 0.26 in Caucasians and 0.44 in black population) and was carefully analyzed for potential association to inhaled corticosteroids therapy response (Tantisira et al., 2007). The presence of the C allele increases three- to four-fold the risk of severe asthma exacerbations. This effect was confirmed both in Afro-American and Caucasian individuals being under iCS therapy.

2.3.5 Polymorphism of AC9 gene (cyclase adenylate 9)

Although adenylate cyclase is activated via the β2-adrenoreceptor it may also influence inhaled corticosteroids reaction. Individuals carrying the polymorphism Ile→Met 772 demonstrate increased bronchial dilatation after SABA when treated with corticosteroids compared to wild-type individuals (isoleucine in 772 position) (Tantisira et al., 2005). This substitution results in a loss of function. Met772 has lower basic as well as beta2-mediated adenylyl cyclase activities compared to Ile772.

Gene	Chromosomal location	Polymorphism with potential pharmacogenetic consequences during iCS therapy
CRHR1	17q12-22	rs242941 (G→T, intron)
TBX21	17q21.32	His→Glu33 (H33Q)
FCER2	19p13.3	2206T→C
AC9	16p13.3-13.2	Ile→Met 772

Table 2. List of gene polymorphism examples that could have pharmacogenetic consequences during corticosteroids therapy

2.4 Pharmacogenetics of anticholinergic treatment

2.4.1 Polymorphisms of the muscarinic receptor

Anticholinergics are used mainly in chronic obstructive pulmonary disease (COPD) but sometimes also in asthma as second line bronchodilators. Anticholinergics are antagonists of muscarinic receptors: M1, M2 and M3. SNPs have been found in coding regions of M2 and M3 receptors (Fenech, 2001). The expression of M2 and M3 receptors is dependent on transcription regulation in the gene promoter region and polymorphisms have been demonstrated in both promoter regions (Fenech, 2004; Donfack, 2003). Furthermore different expression of M2 receptor may be related to various number of dinucleotide CA repetitions in gene promoter region. None of these changes has been investigated in relation to bronchodilation in asthma or COPD yet.

3. Conclusions

Genome analysis, candidate gene studies and SNP investigation represent a new approach to pharmacological treatment in all chronic diseases. Genetically defined differences combined with clinical phenotyping lead to treatment personalization. At this point "personalization" means selecting different treatment regimens for different groups of patients. The more knowledge on pharmacogenetics and general genetics we have, the smaller these groups are likely to be.

iCS remain the mainstream therapy in asthma. Despite intensive research in this field there is only one biological treatment available for asthma and allergy (anti-IgE monoclonal antibody). Several other have been suggested and underwent pre-clinical or clinical tests, but to prove either their effectiveness and safety.

All the studies presented in this chapter have aimed at the identification and characterization of subgroups of asthmatic patients that will derive optimal therapy benefit while minimizing or eliminating drug side effects. The ultimate goal in the pharmacogenetics of antiasthmatic medication is to enable the optimization of individual therapies from the very start, maximizing efficacy without exposing patients to side effects. That would also significantly improve patient's treatment compliance. The amount of clear data from pharmacogenetics of antiasthmatic drugs is still limited due, among others, to the vast number of genotype variants in different populations.

Combined research of the past decade seem to suggests that either asthma has several phenotypes distinct in terms of inflammatory mechanisms (eosinophilic versus neutrophilic, IL-17 dependent vs non-dependent etc.) or "asthma" is rather a group of respiratory diseases with similar symptomatology than a uniform disease. Computerized multivariate analysis has to be employed in the process of defining clinically relevant disease phenotypes of asthma before effective pharmacogenetic research can be undertaken.

4. References

Asano, K.; Shiomi, T.; Hasegawa, N.; Nakamura, H.; Kudo, H. & Matsuzaki, T. (2004) *Leukotriene C4 synthase gene A(-444)C polymorphism and clinical response to a CYS-LT(1) antagonist, pranlukast, in Japanese patients with moderate asthma.* Pharmacogenetics, 12:565-70.

Bamberger, CM.; Schulte, HM. & Chrousos, GP. (1996). *Molecular determinants of glucocorticoid receptor function and tissue sensitivity to glucocorticoids.* Endocrine Reviews, 17:245–61.

Barnes, PJ. (1996). *Mechanisms of action of glucocorticoids in asthma.* American journal of respiratory and critical care medicine, 154: S21–S26.

Basu, K.; Palmer, CN.; Tavendale, R.; Lipworth, BJ. & Mukhopadhyay, S. (2009). *Adrenergic beta(2)-receptor genotype predisposes to exacerbations in steroid-treated asthmatic patients taking frequent albuterol or salmeterol.* Journal of Allergy and Clinical Immunology, 124:1188-94.

Beato, M.; Chavez, S. & Truss, S. (1996). *Transcriptional regulation by steroid hormones.* Steroids, 61:240–51.

Brogan, IJ.; Murray, IA.; Cerillo, G.; Needham, M.; White, A. & Davis, JR.(1999) *Interaction of glucocorticoid receptor isoforms with transcription factors AP-1 and NF-kappaB: lack of effect of glucocorticoid receptor beta.* Molecular and Cellular Endocrinology, 157, 95–104.

Carroll, CL.; Stoltz, P.; Schramm, CM. & Zucker, AR. (2009). *Beta2-adrenergic receptor polymorphisms affect response to treatment in children with severe asthma exacerbations.* Chest, 135:1186-92.

Chanarin, N. & Johnston, SL.(1994). *Leukotrienes as a target in asthma therapy.* Drugs, 47: 12–24.

Dixon, RA.; Diehl, RE. & Opas, E. (1990). *Requirement of a 5-lipoxygenase-activating protein for leukotriene synthesis.* Nature, 343: 282–284.

Dixon, RA.; Kobilka, BK.; Strader, DJ.;, Benovic, JL.; Dohlman, HG.& Frielle, T. (1986). *Cloning of the gene and cDNA for mammalian beta-adrenergic receptor and homology with rhodopsin.* Nature, 321:75-9.

Donfack, J.; Kogut, P.; Forsythe, S.; Solway, J.; Solway, J. & Ober, C. (2003). *Sequence variation in the promoter region of the cholinergic receptor muscarinic 3 gene and asthma and atopy.* Journal of Allergy and Clinnical Immunology, 111: 527-532.

Drazen, JM.; Yandava, CN.; Dube, L.; Szczerback, N.; Hippensteel, R.; Pillari, A. & Israel, E. (1999). *Pharmacogenetic association between ALOX5 promoter genotype and the response to anti-asthma treatment.* Nature Genetics, 22, 168–170.

Fenech, AG. & Hall, IP. (2002). *Pharmacogenetics of asthma.* Journal of Clinical Pharmacology, 53, 3-15.

Fenech, AG., Ebejer MJ.; Felice, AE.; Ellul-Micallef, R. & Hall, IP. (2001). *Mutation screening of the muscarinic M2 and M3 receptor genes in normal and asthmatic subjects.* British Journal of Pharmacology, 133: 43-48.

Fenech, AG.; Billington, CK. & Swan, C. (2004). *Novel polymorphisms influencing transcription of the human CHRM2 gene in airway smooth muscle.* American Journal of Respiratory Cell and Molecular Biology, 30: 678-686.

Finotto, S.; Neurath, MF.; Glickman, JN.; Qin, S.; Lehr, HA.; Green, FH. & Ackerman, K. (2002). *Development of spontaneous airway changes consistent with human asthma in mice lacking T-bet.* Science, 295, 336–368.

Funk, CD.; Hoshiko, S.; Matsumoto, T.; Radmark, O. & Samuelsson, B. (1989). *Characterization of the human 5-lipoxygenase gene.* Proceedings of the National Academy of Sciences, 86: 2587–2591.

Gagliardo, R.; Chanez, P.; Vignola, AM.; Bousquet, J.; Vachier, I.; Godard, P. & Bonsignore, G. (2000) *Glucocorticoid receptor alpha and beta in glucocorticoid dependent asthma.* American Journal of Respiratory and Critical Care Medicine, 162, 7–13.

GINA (Global Initiative for Asthma, updated 2010)

Green, SA.; Rathz, DA.; Schuster, AJ. & Liggett, SB. (2001). *The Ile164 beta(2)-adrenoceptor polymorphism alters salmeterol exosite binding and conventional agonist coupling to G(s).* European Journal of Pharmacology, 421:141-7.

Green, SA.; Turki, J.; Bejarano, P.; Hall, IP. & Liggett, SB. (1995) *Influence of beta 2-adrenergic receptor genotypes on signal transduction in human airway smooth muscle cells.* American Journal of Respiratory Cell and Molecular Biology, 13, 25–33.

Green, SA.; Turki, J.; Innis, M. & Liggett, SB. (1994). *Amino-terminal polymorphisms of the human beta 2-adrenergic receptor impart distinct agonist-promoted regulatory properties.* Biochemistry, 33, 9414–9419.

Gronemeyer, H. (1992). *Control of transcription activation by steroid hormone receptors.* FASEB Journal, 6:2524–9.

Heise, CE.; O'Dowd, BF. & Figueroa, DJ. (2000). *Characterization of the human cysteinyl leukotriene 2 receptor.* Journal of Biological Chemistry, 275: 30531–30536.

Hoshiko, S.; Radmark, O. & Samuelsson, B. (1990). Characterization *of the human 5-lipoxygenase gene promoter.* Proceedings of the National Academy of Sciences, 87: 9073–9077.

Huizenga, NA.; De Koper, JW. & Lange, P. (1998). *A polymorphism in the glucocorticoid receptor gene may be associated with and increased sensitivity to glucocorticoids in vivo.* The Journal of Clinical Endocrinology and Metabolism, 83: 144–151.

Hurley, DM.; Accili, D. & Stratakis, CA. (1991). *Point mutation causing a single amino acid substitution in the hormone binding domain of the glucocorticoid receptor in familial glucocorticoid resistance.* Journal of Clinical Investigation, 87: 680–686.

In, KH.; Asano, K.; Beier, D.; Grobholz, J.; Finn, PW.; Silverman, EK. & Silverman, ES. (1997). *Naturally occurring mutations in the human 5-lipoxygenase gene promoter that modify transcription factor binding and reporter gene transcription.* Journal of Clinical Investigation, 99, 1130–1137.

Israel, E.; Chinchilli, VM.; Ford, JG.; Boushey, HA.; Cherniack, R. & Craig, TJ. (2004). *Use of regularly scheduled albuterol treatment in asthma: genotype-stratified, randomised, placebo-controlled cross-over trial.* Lancet, 364:1505-12.

Israel, E.; Drazen, JM.; Liggett, SB.; Boushey, HA.; Cherniack, RM. & Chinchilli, VM. (2000). *The effect of polymorphisms of the beta(2)-adrenergic receptor on the response to regular use of albuterol in asthma.* American Journal of Respiratory and Critical Care Medicine, 162:75-80.

Kalayci, O.; Wechsler, M.; Galper, B.; Hong, C.; Israel, E.; Drazen, JM. & Lilly, CM. (2003). *LTC4 production by eosinophils in asthmatic subjects with alternative forms of ALOX-5 core promoter.* Advances in Experimental Medicine and Biology, 525, 11–14.

Kazani, S.; Wechsler, ME. & Israel, E. (2010). *The role of pharmacogenomics in improving the management of asthma.* Journal of Allergy and Clinical Immunology, 125: 295-302.

Klotsman, M.; York, TP.; Pillai, SG.; Vargas-Irwin, C.; Sharma, SS.; van den Oord, EJ. & Anderson, WH. (2007). *Pharmacogenetics of the 5-lipoxygenase biosynthetic pathway and variable clinical response to montelukast.* Pharmacogenetics and Genomics, 17:189-96.

Kobilka, BK.; Dixon, RA. & Frielle, T. (1987). *cDNA for the human β2-adrenergic receptor: a protein with multiple membrane-spanning domains and encoded by a gene whose chromosomal location is shared with that of the receptor for platelet-derived growth factor.* Proceedings of the National Academy of Sciences, 84: 46–50.

Koper, JW.; De Stolk, RP. & Lange, P. (1997). *Lack of association between five polymorphisms in the human glucocorticoid receptor gene and glucocorticoid resistance.* Human Genetics, 99: 663–668.

Kowalski, ML. & Woszczek, G. (2002). *Pharmacogenetics of β2-adrenoreceptor and asthmatic phenotypes.* New trends in Allergy V. Springer-Verlag. Berlin Heidelberg, Germany; 13-20.

Lane, SJ.; Arm, JP.; Staynov, DZ. & Lee, TH. (1994). *Chemical mutational analysis of the human glucocorticoid receptor cDNA in glucocorticoid-resistant bronchial asthma.* American Journal of Respiratory Cell and Molecular Biology, 11: 42–48.

Lee, DK.; Currie, GP.; Hall, IP.; Lima, JJ. & Lipworth, BJ. (2004). *The arginine-16 beta2-adrenoceptor polymorphism predisposes to bronchoprotective subsensitivity in patients treated with formoterol and salmeterol.* British Journal of Clinical Pharmacology, 57:68-75.

Liggett, SB. (1997). *Polymorphisms of the β2-adrenergic receptor and asthma.* American Journal of Respiratory and Critical Care Medicine, 156: S156–S162.

Lima, JJ.; Zhang, S.; Grant, A.; Shao, L.; Tantisira, KG. & Allayee, H.(2006). *Influence of leukotriene pathway polymorphisms on response to montelukast in asthma.* American Journal of Respiratory and Critical Care Medicine, 173:379-85.

Lipworth, BJ.; Hall, IP.; Tan, S.; Aziz, I. & Coutie, W. (1999). *Effects of genetic polymorphism on ex vivo and in vivo function of β2-adrenoceptors in asthmatic patients.* Chest, 115: 324–328.

Lynch, KR.; O'Neill, GP. & Liu, Q.(1999). *Characterization of the human cysteinyl leukotriene CysLT1 receptor.* Nature, 399: 789–793.

Malchoff, DM. Brufsky, A. & Reardon, G. (1993). *A mutation of the glucocorticoid receptor in primary cortisol resistance.* Journal of Clinical Investigation, 91: 1918–1925.

Malmstrom, K.; Rodriguez-Gomez, G.; Guerra, J.; Villaran, C.; Pineiro, A.; Wei, LX. & Seidenberg, BC. (1999). *Oral montelukast, inhaled beclomethasone, and placebo for chronic asthma. A randomized, controlled trial.* Montelukast/Beclomethasone Study Group. Annals of Internal Medicine, 130, 487–495.

Martinez, FD.; Graves, PE.; Baldini, M.; Solomon, S. & Erickson, R. *Association between genetic polymorphisms of the beta 2-adrenoceptor and response to albuterol in children with and without a history of wheezing.* Journal of Clinical Investigation, 100:3184-8.

Mitchell, PJ. & Tjian, R.(1989). *Transcriptional regulation in mammalian cells by sequence-specific DNA binding proteins.* Science,245:371-8.

Moffatt, MF. & Cookson, WO. (1997). *Linkage and candidate gene studies in asthma.* American Journal of Respiratory and Critical Care Medicine, 156: S110–S112.

Mougey, EB.; Feng, H.; Castro, M.; Irvin, CG. & Lima, JJ. (2009). *Absorption of montelukast is transporter mediated: a common variant of OATP2B1 is associated with reduced plasma concentrations and poor response.* Pharmacogenetics and Genomics, 19:129-38.

Nelson, HS.; Weiss, ST.; Bleecker, ER.; Yancey, SW. & Dorinsky, PM. (2006). *The Salmeterol Multicenter Asthma Research Trial: a comparison of usual pharmacotherapy for asthma or usual pharmacotherapy plus salmeterol.* Chest, 129:15-26.

Palmer, CN.; Lipworth, BJ.; Lee, S.; Ismail, T.; Macgregor, DF. & Mukhopadhyay, S. (2006). *Arginine- 16 {beta}2 adrenoceptor genotype predisposes to exacerbations in young asthmatics taking regular salmeterol.* Thorax, 61:940-4.

Refojo, D.; Liberman, AC.; Giacomini, D.; Carbia Nagashima, A.; Graciarena, M.; Echenique, C. & Paez Pereda, M. (2003). *Integrating systemic information at the molecular level: cross-talk between steroid receptors and cytokine signaling on different target cells.* Annals of the New York Academy of Science, 992, 196–204.

Saito, S.; Iida, A.; Sekine, A.; Miura, Y.; Ogawa, C.; Kawauchi, S.; Higuchi, S. & Nakamura, Y. (2002). *Identification of 779 genetic variations in eight genes encoding members of the ATP-binding cassette, subfamily C (ABCC/MRP/CFTR).* Journal of Human Genetics, 47:147-171.

Sampson, AP.; Siddiqui, S.; Buchanan, D.; Howarth, PH.; Holgate, ST.& Holloway, JW. (2000). *Variant LTC(4) synthase allele modifies cysteinyl leukotriene synthesis in eosinophils and predicts clinical response to zafirlukast.* Thorax, 55(suppl 2): S28-31.

Sanak, M.; Pierzchalska, M.; Bazan-Socha, S. & Szczeklik, A. (2000). *Enhanced expression of the leukotriene C4 synthase due to overactive transcription of an allelic variant associated with aspirin-intolerant asthma.* American Journal of Respiratory Cell and Molecular Biology, 23:290-6.

Sanak, M.; Simon, HU. & Szczeklik, A. (1997). *Leukotriene C4 synthase promoter polymorphism and risk of aspirin-induced asthma.* Lancet, 350:1599-600.

Silverman, ES. & Drazen, JM. (1999). *The biology of 5-lipoxygenase: function, structure, and regulatory mechanisms.* Proceedings of the Association of American Physicians, 111, 525–536.

Silverman, ES.; In, KH.; Yandava, C. & Drazen, JM. (1998). *Pharmacogenetics of the 5-lipoxygenase pathway in asthma.* Clinical and Experimental Allergy, Suppl 5, 164–170.

Smith, DF. & Toft, DO. (1993). *Steroid receptors and their associated proteins.* Molecular Endocrinology, 7:4–11.

Stevens A.; Ray DW.; Zeggini E.; John E.; Richard HL.; Griffith CEM.; Donn R (2004) *Glucocorticoid sensitivity is determined by a specific glucocorticoid receptor haplotype.* The Journal of Clinical Endocrinology & Metabolism 89:892–897

Tan, S.; Hall, IP.; Dewar, J.; Dow, E. & Lipworth, B. (1997). *Association between β2-adrenoceptor polymorphism and susceptibility to bronchodilator desensitisation in moderately severe stable asthmatics.* Lancet, 350: 995–999.

Tantisira, KG. & Drazen, JM. (2009). *Genetics and pharmacogenetics of the leukotriene pathway.* Journal of Allergy and Clinical Immunology, 124:422-7.

Tantisira, KG.; Hwang, ES. & Raby, BA. (2004). *TBX21: a functional variant predicts improvement in asthma with the use of inhaled corticosteroids.* Proceedings of the National Academy of Sciences, 101:18099–18104.

Tantisira, KG.; Lake, S. & Silverman, ES. (2004) *Corticosteroid pharmacogenetics: association of sequence variants in CRHR1 with improved lung function in asthmatics treated with inhaled corticosteroids.* Human Molecular Genetics, 13:1353–1359.

Tantisira, KG.; Lima, J.; Sylvia, J.; Klanderman, B. & Weiss, ST. (2009). *5-lipoxygenase pharmacogenetics in asthma: overlap with Cys-leukotriene receptor antagonist loci.* Pharmacogenetics and Genomics, 19:244-7.

Tantisira, KG.; Silverman, ES.; Mariani, TJ.; Xu, J.; Richter, BG. &, Klanderman, BJ. (2007). *FCER2: a pharmacogenetic basis for severe exacerbations in children with asthma.* Journal of Allergy Clinical Immunology, 120:1285-91.

Tantisira, KG.; Small, KM.; Litonjua, AA.; Weiss, ST. & Liggett, SB. (2005). *Molecular properties and pharmacogenetics of a polymorphism of adenylyl cyclase type 9 in asthma: interaction between beta-agonist and corticosteroid pathways.* Human Molecular Genetics, 14:1671-7.

Taylor, DR.; Drazen, JM.; Herbison, GP.; Yandava, CN.; Hancox, RJ. & Town, GI. (2000). *Asthma exacerbations during long term beta agonist use: influence of beta(2)adrenoceptor polymorphism.* Thorax, 55:762-7.

Telleria, JJ.; Blanco-Quiros, A.; Varillas, D.; Armentia, A.; Fernandez-Carvajal, I.; Jesus Alonso, M. & Diez, I. (2008). *ALOX5 promoter genotype and response to montelukast in moderate persistent asthma.* Respiratory Medicine,102:857-61.

van der Deen, M.; de Vries, EG.; Timens, W.; Scheper, RJ.; Timmer-Bosscha, H.& Postma, DS. (2005). *ATP-binding cassette (ABC) transporters in normal and pathological lung.* Respiratory Research, 6:59

Wechsler, ME.; Kunselman, SJ.; Chinchilli, VM.; Bleeker, E.; Boushey, HA. & Calhounb, WJ. (2009). *Effect of beta2-adrenergic receptor polymorphism on response to longacting beta2 agonist in asthma (LARGE trial): a genotype-stratified, randomised, placebo-controlled, crossover trial.* Lancet, 374:1754-64.

Wechsler, ME.; Lehman, E.; Lazarus, SC.; Lemanske, RF.; Boushey, HA. & Deykin, A. (2006). *beta-Adrenergic receptor polymorphisms and response to salmeterol.* American Journal of Respiratory and Critical Care Medicine, 173:519-26.

Weiss, ST.; Litonjua, AA.; Lange, C.; Lazarus, R.; Liggett, SB. & Bleecker, ER. (2006). *Overview of the pharmacogenetics of asthma treatment.* Pharmacogenomics Journal, 6: 311-26.

Woszczek, G.; Borowiec, M.; Ptasinska, A.; Kosinski, S.; Pawliczak, R. & Kowalski, ML. (2005). *Beta2-ADR haplotypes/polymorphisms associate with bronchodilator response and total IgE in grass allergy.* Allergy, 60:1412-7.

Xie HG.; Stein, CM.; Kim, RB.; Xiao, ZS.; He, N., Zhou, HH.; Gainer, JV., Brown, NJ.; Haines, JL. & Wood, AJ.. (2001). *Frequency of functionally important beta-2 adrenoceptor polymorphisms varies markedly among African-American, Caucasian and Chinese individuals.* Pharmacogenetics, 11(2):185.

Zandi, PP.; Klein, AP.; Addington, AM.; Hetmanski, JB.; Roberts, L. & Peila, R. (2001). *Multilocus linkage analysis of the German asthma data. Genetics Epidemiology,* 21: S210–S215.

Part 5

Future Prospects

13

Beyond Pharmacogenetics

Roberto Canaparo
University of Torino
Italy

1. Introduction

It has been observed that similar medication is subject to a considerable efficacy heterogeneity and toxicity across the human population and numerous studies, over the last 30 years, have indicated that individual genetic make-up might well be the major determinants of this variability in drug action (Nebert et al., 2008).

The intellectual foundation of the hypothesis that variation among individuals in drug response might be due to subtle genetic differences with little or no obvious phenotypes, except in response to the relevant drug, was first articulated by Arno Motulsky (Motulsky, 1957). Although the notion that certain individuals inherited a predisposition, such as to alcaptonuria or other conditions, may most likely be attributed to the British physician Archibald Garrod (Garrod, 1975). Garrod observed that parental consanguinity was more common than usual among parents of children with alcaptonuria and, with particular foresight, he developed the concept of "Chemical Individuality in Man". He proposed that drugs undergo biotransformation by specific pathways similarly to endogenous substrates and defects in such pathways, that occur with inborn metabolic errors, that could alter drug concentrations and, therefore, their effects (Meyer, 2004). It was then William Bateson (Meyer, 2004), a biologist ahead of his time, who interpreted Garrod's reports as a recessive inheritance when he popularized Mendelian genetics in Britain. Bateson discovered genetic linkage and introduced the term "genetics" at some time between 1902 and 1913.

The concept of familial clustering of unusual xenobiotic responses was reinforced during the 1940s, when a high incidence of haemolysis was observed among individuals with glucose-6-phosphate dehydrogenase deficiency when exposed to antimalarial drugs (Beutler et al., 1955a, 1955b). In the 50s, Evans et al. identified N-acetylation as a major route of isoniazid elimination (Evans et al., 1960). Although individuals varied substantially in terms of the extent to which a single dose of the drug was acetylated, less variability was observed between monozygotic twins than dizygotic twins (Roden & George Jr, 2002). This observation led to further studies that defined the clinical consequences and genetic basis underlying the fast and slow acetylator phenotypes. Shortly thereafter, Friedrich Vogel first coined the term "Pharmacogenetics", defining it as the "study of the role of genetics in drug response" (Nebert et al., 2008). More generally, the late 20th century witnessed developments in the understanding of the molecular basis of drug disposition, action and the mechanisms that determine the observed variability in drug action.

Along with the increased understanding of the molecular, cellular and genetic determinants of drug action, has come the appreciation that variants in many genes might contribute to variability in drug action.

Single Nucleotide Polymorphisms (SNPs) have been long recognized as the main source of genetic and phenotypic human variation and numerous recent studies have tried to demonstrate that SNPs make a major genetic contribution to the variability in drug effects (Evans & McLeod, 2003; Gardiner & Begg, 2006). However, the complete mapping of all human genes, arrived through the Human Genome Project, along with the advent of more powerful molecular technologies and other studies showing a poor correlation between SNPs in candidate genes and phenotypes, modifying this perception (Nebert & Vesell, 2004). Therefore, this chapter focuses on the development of Pharmacogenetics from SNPs to the new area of Genomics, or Pharmacogenomics, in an attempt to better understand and predict variations in drug response phenotypes.

2. From pharmacogenetics to pharmacogenomics

An SNP is a DNA sequence variation which occurs when a single nucleotide (A, T, C, or G) in the genome, or other shared sequences, differs between members of a biological species, or paired chromosomes in an individual. For example, a SNP might change the DNA sequence AAGGCTAA to ATGGCTAA (Fig.1).

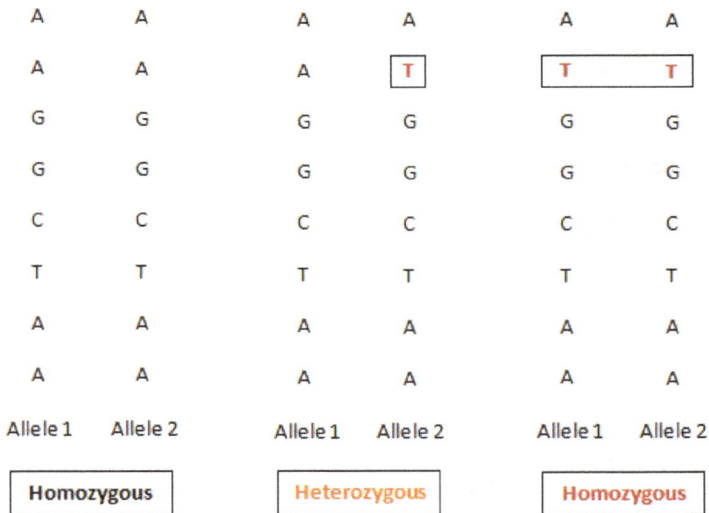

Fig. 1. Single Nucleotide Polymorphism

For a variation to be considered a SNP, it must occur in at least 1% of the population. Single Nucleotide Polymorphisms, representing about 90% of all human genetic variations, occur every 100 to 300 bases along the 3-billion-base human genome. Consequently, it has been estimated that there are at least 10 million SNPs within the human population (Kruglyak & Nickerson, 2001). They can be in coding regions (where they may be either synonymous, or non-synonymous) or, more commonly, in non-coding regions and frequently vary according to ethnicity (Sachidanandam et al., 2001). It is in these heritable variations among individuals that the principles of Pharmacogenetics are found. However, other types of genetic variations, such as small insertions (usually <1 kb), deletions, inversions, variable numbers of tandem repeats (minisatellite), short tandem repeats (microsatellite), copy number variations (Nakamura, 2009) and combinations of these changes, can also contribute to variability in drug response, even if to a less extent than do SNPs. Therefore, the selection of a non-synonymous SNPs, or other genetic variations in coding regions, in hypothesis driven pharmacogenetic association studies, is based on their functionality, where the genetic variant leads to, or is predicted to lead to, alterations in protein function and hence drug response variability.

There are at least four examples where this approach has been correlated with significant changes in drug effects (Evans & McLeod, 2003; Gardiner & Begg, 2006). One of the best examples of SNPs relating to the outcome of therapy is the polymorphism of the gene thiopurine S-methyltransferase (*TPMT*) (Yates et al., 1997). Thiopurine S-methyltransferase is a cytosolic drug-metabolizing enzyme that catalyzes the S-methylation of 6-mercaptopurine (6-MP) and azathioprine. Weinshilboum et al. demonstrated a very clear tri-modal frequency of TPMT activity in red blood cells from 298 unrelated control adults (Weinshilboum & Sladek, 1980). One in 300 subjects lacked TPMT activity and 11% had intermediate levels. Family studies have demonstrated that the frequency distribution is due to inheritance (Weinshilboum & Sladek, 1980). While phenotypic studies have shown a clear tri-modal distribution, the genetic basis of phenotypic variation is a more complex question (Evans & Krynetsky, 2003).

To date, about seventeen variant *TPMT* alleles have been identified, although 3 variant alleles account for the majority (>95%) of persons with intermediate (1 variant allele), or low (2 variant alleles) TPMT activity (Krynetski et al., 1995; Yates et al., 1997). Subsequent clinical studies demonstrated that *TPMT* polymorphism is able to predict 6-MP toxicity and consequences of therapy (Lennard et al., 1990; Relling et al., 1999).

Another good example of SNPs influencing therapeutic efficacy is the polymorphism of genes belonging to the superfamily of cytochrome P450 enzymes (CYP450) (Wilkinson, 2005). *CYP2D6* polymorphism is clinically important mainly due to the greater likelihood of adverse reactions (ADRs) amongst individuals, because they can be associated with poor metabolism of certain drugs, resulting in high plasma concentrations and increased likelihood of ADRs. For example, patients carrying some of the *CYP2D6* variants identified (http://www.imm.ki.se/cypalleles), have a greater risk of adverse effects from metoprolol, venlafaxine and tricyclic antidepressants, or have impaired ability to metabolically activate prodrugs like codeine and the selective oestrogen receptor modulator (SERM), tamoxifen, to form active drug metabolites (Bertilsson et al., 2002; Jin et al., 2005; Lessard et al., 1999; Mortimer et al., 1990; Sindrup & Brøsen, 1995; Stearns et al., 2003; Wuttke et al., 2002).

CYP2C19 is important in the metabolism of proton-pump inhibitors (omeprazole, lansoprazole, rabeprazole and pantoprazole), fluoxetine, sertaline and nelfinavir. Although there are several inactive genetic variants, two (*CYP2C19*2* and *CYP2C19*3*) account for more than 95% of cases of poor metabolism of these drugs (Wedlund, 2000). Marked differences in the plasma levels of protein-pump inhibitors occur between genotypes and phenotypes and are reflected in drug-induced changes in gastric pH (Furuta et al., 1999).

CYP2C9 is an enzyme involved in the hydroxylation of the S form of the anti-epileptic agent phenytoin and the anticoagulant warfarin. Many *CYP2C9* variant alleles have now been reported (http://www.imm.ki.se/cypalleles) and decreased activity has been confirmed in cases with *CYP2C9*3*, by an expression system using COS cells and yeast and an *in vivo* test on healthy volunteers and patients with a known genetic polymorphism (Takahashi et al., 1998b, 2000).

Indeed, there was a 50% decrease in oral clearance capacity of (S)-warfarin in individuals with heterozygous polymorphism for *CYP2C9*3* (*CYP2C9*1/*3*), dropping to less than 10% in homozygous individuals for *CYP2C9*3* (Takahashi et al., 1998a).

These successful pharmacogenetic studies, together with the glucuronidation of an anticancer drug, irinotecan, by a member of the UDP-glucuronosyltransferase (UGT) enzyme family (Gagné et al., 2002), showing gene-drug interactions, represented a predominantly monogenic, high-penetrance trait where the functional consequence of a major gene was recognized. However, these associations were not replicated by other investigators (Hu & Ziv, 2008) and might lead to false-positive findings (Serpe et al., 2009). Indeed, even with the very strong single-gene high-penetrance disorder *TPMT*, a study correlating thiopurine related ADRs with *TPMT* genotype, noted that 78% of ADRs were not associated with *TPMT* gene polymorphism and were attributable to factors other than this drug-metabolizing enzyme (van Aken et al., 2003).

Although the presence of non-synonymous SNPs in a candidate gene may be suspected to cause variance in drug response, this cannot account for all SNPs able to cause drug response variance or susceptibility in drug response variance. Other functional SNPs implicated in variance in drug response or susceptibility variance in drug response include SNPs located in promoter, introns, splice sites and intragenic regions. Furthermore, it has been postulated that even synonymous or silent SNPs are implicated in functional consequence via hypothesized mechanisms (Kimchi-Sarfaty et al., 2007).

A more comprehensive approach is the genome-wide method (GWA) using SNP arrays (Grant & Hakonarson, 2008). With this strategy we move from studies involving the effects of single genes on drug disposition and response, to studies where the effects of several genes up to whole genome are investigated. In other words we move from Pharmacogenetics to Pharmacogenomics.

A clear advantage of this method is that it is hypothesis-free and that this may reveal unexpected SNPs related to drug response. Hence this method does not rely on current knowledge of the metabolism and mechanism of action to drug response. Recent genome-wide association studies have presented novel associations between SNPs and drug response. Studies on drug response have detected significant genome-wide associations for interferon-α, clopidogrel response and anticoagulant dose requirement (Cooper et al., 2008; Shuldiner et al., 2009; Takeuchi et al., 2009; Tanaka et al., 2009; Teichert et al., 2009). As to ADRs, significant associations have been reported for statin-induced myopathy and flucloxacillin induced liver injury (Daly et al., 2009; Link et al., 2008). Most of these studies reported novel findings and made important contributions to the field, some even with the potential to influence clinical practice.

Since it has been estimated that the human genome contains more than 10 million SNPs, comprehensive genome-wide SNP pharmacogenomic association studies would require too many SNPs. Various strategies may be adopted to overcome these challenges: one could be to improve high-throughput sequencing technologies capable of sequencing a full human genome in the most cost-effective way, another to combine the candidate gene approach with the genome wide SNP association studies strategy (Kooloos et al., 2009), or to apply genome-wide haplotype pharmacogenomic association studies (Srinivasan et al., 2009).

Haplotypes are a combination of alleles at different markers along the same chromosome that are inherited as a unit. Unlike a genotype, the identity of a single polymorphic location on both chromosomal alleles, a haplotype is the specific combination of nucleotides present at all of the polymorphic locations within a single chromosomal allele. All the genetic variations in a population, or species, can be described as the sum of all haplotypes present among the individuals of that population, or species. Nucleotide differences between these haplotypes are responsible for heterozygous genotypes and provide information useful in ascertaining the identity and/or structure of a haplotype. Consequently, haplotyping nucleotide polymorphisms requires two steps: firstly, the identification of the polymorphisms and, secondly, the determination of which polymorphisms are allelic to one another (Fig.2).

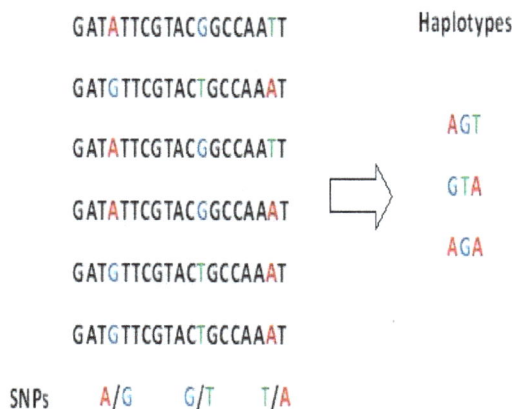

Fig. 2. Haplotypes: a set of closely linked genetic markers (SNPs) present on one chromosome which tend to be inherited together

Although the primary tool used in pharmacogenetic association studies has traditionally been the genotyping of SNPs, recent evidence indicates that determining haplotypes may be more informative than genotyping single variants (Evans & McLeod, 2003). Indeed, in this context, a study evaluated whether the response to inhaled β_2-agonist therapy for asthma was best predicted by individual non-synonymous SNPs, or 13 SNPs within the β_2-adrenoceptor gene (*ADRB2*) (Drysdale et al., 2000). It reported that these 13 SNPs were organized into only 12 of the possible 8,192 SNP haplotype combinations. Although haplotype analyses did define a patient group with a significantly superior response to β_2-agonist therapy, only 5/12 appeared with more than a 10% frequency in the multiethnic cohort studies. Therefore, there has been a great deal of interest in defining the haplotype structure of the human genome (e.g. the human "HapMap" project). The HapMap project (The International HapMap Project, 2003) focuses on SNPs that are relatively common among human populations; assessing these SNPs at an appropriate density (i.e. number and position across the human genome) will provide new insights into the polymorphic nature of the human genome.

As common SNPs are phylogenetically older than rare SNPs, they have arisen from recombination events of ancestral haplotypes (Wall & Pritchard, 2003). Therefore, focusing on these common SNPs will allow for the reconstruction of these ancestral haplotypes, tracing human evolutionary history. More importantly, the use of common SNPs to map the human haplotype structure will identify the haplotypes that make up the majority (perhaps up to 90%) of human variations and will be the most informative source for GWA pharmacogenomic studies. Recent evidence suggests that genotyping just 6 to 8 "haplotype tag" SNPs per 10–100 kb of genomic DNA may provide enough information to determine an individual's haplotype for that region (Gabriel et al., 2002; Wall & Pritchard, 2003). This suggests that genotyping these haplotype tag SNPs will be the method of choice for the haplotyping of individual patients for common variations in genome-wide haplotype pharmacogenomic association studies. According to these new strategies, there is an ever increasing use of genome-wide association studies in the field of Pharmacogenomics, with several studies appearing between 2010 and 2011 (Daly, 2010). However, it has become apparent that there may be allelic epigenetic modifications at some genes that cause these alleles to exhibit different expression patterns (Fournier et al., 2002). Indeed, in the future it may be important to refine our concept of haplotypes and, therefore, GWA, beyond DNA sequence variations, to include other information, such as allelic epigenetic factors, which are inherited through mitosis and meiosis with the DNA itself and serve to extend the information content of the human genome (Jenuwein & Allis, 2001).

3. Pharmacoepigenetics and pharmacoepigenomics

Epigenetics is usually defined as the study of mitotically heritable changes in gene expression that are not attributable to nucleic acid sequence alterations. Therefore epigenetics refers to the regulation of various genomic functions controlled by stable, but potentially reversible changes in DNA methylation and chromatin structure (Henikoff & Matzke, 1997). Epigenomics refers to the study of epigenetics on a genome-wide basis (Peedicayil, 2008).

There are two major mechanisms of epigenetic regulation, methylation of cytosines in the DNA sequence and modification of the histone proteins that the DNA is wrapped around. The coordination of both mechanisms results in dramatic changes in the remodelling of chromatin and altered gene transcription (Flanagan & Petronis, 2005). One of the most recent important observations is the increasing evidence that epigenetic factors play an important role in the etiopathogenesis of human diseases and the discovery that epigenetic risk factors open new opportunities for diagnostic, prognostic and therapeutic approaches in human biology. Indeed, epigenetic factors contribute to numerous genomic functions, from the regulation of gene activity to genome stability and segregation of chromosomes, such as: genomic imprinting, X chromosome inactivation and suppression of parasitic DNA elements (Urnov & Wolffe, 2001). Moreover, epigenetic variation across individuals is much richer in comparison to DNA sequence variation and identical DNA sequences in unrelated individuals exhibit significant epigenetic variation. Therefore, such epigenetic differences may have an impact on gene expression that translates into differential density of receptors, or varied numbers of molecules of an enzyme, factors that might contribute to the pharmacokinetic and pharmacodynamic drug variability. The main goals of Pharmacoepigenomics and Pharmacoepigenetics are to predict drug response and/or adverse reactions, based on the epigenetic individuality of an organism.

3.1 The effect of methylation/deacetylation on drug response

There are almost 300 genes involved in the absorption, distribution, metabolism, and excretion (ADME) of pharmaceutical compounds in humans. It has been demonstrated that DNA methylation, or histone modifications, potentially participate in the regulation of almost 60 human ADME genes (Kacevska et al., 2011). A correlation between the epigenetic state of the gene and a possible influence on drug therapy outcome has been experimentally established only for a few ADME genes. Nevertheless, there is credible evidence that epigenetic factors influence ADME gene expression, which, in turn, leads to changes in the metabolism and distribution of drugs. For example, about 30% of the lungs of heavy smokers and 70% of light smokers' lungs have a CYP1A1 expression, with complete, or partial methylation of the *CYP1A1* gene (Anttila et al., 2003). An increase in the methylation level was observed as early as 1-7 days after individuals had stopped smoking, possibly explaining the smoking-related increase in CYPA1A expression (Anttila et al., 2003). Moreover, hypomethylation at sites coinciding with the transcription activator binding sites, such as Arnt and Sp1, leads to overexpression of CYP1B1 in prostate cancer and correlates to the progression of malignancy (Tokizane et al., 2005).

Similarly, CYP1A2, an enzyme abundant in the liver, is involved in the metabolism of many drugs (Zhou et al., 2010). Known SNPs account only partially for the wide interindividual differences observed for CYP1A2 (Jiang et al., 2006). Therefore, it has been implied that an epigenetic component in CYP1A2 regulation is responsible for the variability in CYP1A2 expression and the methylation status of a CpG island in exon 2, consisting of 17 CpG dinucleotides, has been shown to correlate with interindividual differences in CYP1A2 mRNA levels (Ghotbi et al., 2009). It has also been demonstrated that the methylation status of even a single CpG located far upstream from the transcriptional start site (−2579 bp) could contribute to differential CYP1A2 expression. Such interindividual variations might affect the pharmacokinetic and pharmacodynamic metabolization of the drug through CYP1A2, potentially failing the drug treatment or leading to ADRs. Among the members of the CYP2 family, the *CYP2A6, CYP2C9, CYP2D6, CYP2J2, CYP2R1, CYP2S1* and *CYP2W1* genes contain putative important CpG islands, suggesting a potential role for DNA methylation in their regulation (Ingelman-Sundberg et al., 2007).

As to phase II drug metabolism, glutathione-S-transferase genes, it has been shown that the extent of promoter methylation is dependent on the haplotype of the glutathione-S-transferase P1 (*GSTP1*) gene in breast cancer patients (Rønneberg et al., 2008). Moreover, hypermethylation of *GSTP1* is a common molecular alteration in human prostate cancer (Woodson et al., 2008). Irinotecan is a first-line treatment for metastatic colorectal cancer. Its active metabolite is inactivated through glucuronidation mediated by the UGT1A1 enzyme. The level of UGT1A1 expression is highly variable among primary colon tumours, thereby contributing to their differential sensitivity to irinotecan treatment. UGT1A1 expression in colon tumours correlates with the methylation of its promoter and the outcome of cancer chemotherapy (Gagnon et al., 2006).

The *SLC19A1* gene encodes the reduced folate carrier. This enzyme is responsible for cellular uptake of reduced folates and of antifolate drugs, including methotrexate, the most effective drug against primary central nervous system lymphoma. The level of reduced folate carrier differs significantly among lymphoma samples and is associated with methylation of the *SLC19A1* promoter. It has been hypothesized that an increase in SLC19A1 methylation can contribute to methotrexate resistance in tumour cells (Ferreri et al., 2004).

The promoter of the *ABCB1* gene that encodes the P-gp transporter is found hypomethylated in cancer cell lines, manifesting a multidrug-resistance phenotype compared to drug-sensitive cell lines (Baker & El-Osta, 2004). These differences in methylation are also associated with histone modifications. Such epigenetic mechanisms have been shown to be responsible for the increased tolerance shown by certain types of cancer cells to anticancer drugs, such as doxorubicin, paclitaxel and vincristine. Hypomethylation of *ABCB1* can also be induced by exposure of drug-sensitive cells to chemotherapeutic drugs (Baker et al., 2005). Once established, this epigenetic mark can then stably perpetuate through mitotic divisions of cells, manifesting as acquired multidrug resistance.

In addition to these ADME genes, epigenetic influence has also been documented for the α-1 adrenergic receptors (α1-ARs). The three subtypes of α1-AR (α_{1a}AR, α_{1b}AR, and α_{1d}AR) display tissue-specific expression patterns and undergo subtype switching in response to many pathological stimuli. Basal expression of the α_{1d}AR (*ADRA1D*) subtype is dependent on the binding of Sp1 in the two proximal promoter GC boxes of the gene and this binding was shown to be dependent on the methylation status of the promoter region (Michelotti et al., 2007). The expression of the chemokine receptor CXCR4, involved in leukocyte trafficking, seems to be epigenetically regulated, as reported in human pancreatic cancer, where aberrant methylation influences CXCR4 expression (Sato et al., 2005). This finding may pave the way for the development of anticancer drugs that target the CXCR4 receptor, which is overexpressed in various cancers. Moreover, the CXCR4 receptor ligand CXCL12, which has also been shown to be regulated by DNA methylation, has a role in tumour invasion and metastasis and may offer another target for anticancer drugs (Kubarek & Jagodzinski, 2007). The *MGMT* gene, which encodes the DNA repair enzyme O6-methylguanine-DNA methyltransferase, plays a prominent role in the repair of DNA lesions caused by alkylating agents. The extent of methylation of the *MGMT* promoter has been shown to correlate with the responsiveness of gliomas to alkylating drugs, such as carmustine and temozolomide (Paz et al., 2004). Lastly, although the oestrogen receptor is also regulated epigenetically, both by DNA methylation and histone modifications (Bovenzi & Momparler, 2001) in cancer, a non-cancer-related event (ischemia) has also been shown to affect the methylation and expression status of the oestrogen receptor in an animal model (Westberry et al., 2008), demonstrating the wide range of genes that may contribute to drug response variations by means of epigenetic regulation.

As reported for the oestrogen receptor, also histone modifications play an important role in the control of genes encoding drug targets and proteins involved in drug ADME. However, it must not be forgotten that DNA methylation and histone modification are interconnected events. Let's go back then to CYP1A1, this enzyme has been shown to be also under histone modification control, particularly methylation of lysine 4, a H3 histone (3meK4H3) (Okino et al., 2006). Again, in phase I drug metabolism, an increase in CYP2A6 mRNA and protein levels was observed in human hepatocytes in response to dexamethasone. This was shown to be mediated by the hepatic nuclear factor 4α and the glucocorticoid receptor (GR). The binding of the hepatic nuclear factor 4α to the hepatic nuclear factor 4α response element was promoted by the increased acetylation of histone H4, also in response to dexamethasone (Onica et al., 2008). This modification relaxes the chromatin, thereby allowing the binding of DNA-binding proteins. As a response to cisplatin treatment of HeLa cells, specific phosphorylation of Ser-10 at histone H3 is mediated by the p38 mitogen-activated protein kinase pathway. Likewise, cisplatin induces phosphorylation of H3 at Ser-28 and acetylation of histone H4 (Wang & Lippard, 2004). These findings provide a link between the drug response and chromosomal structural alterations through histone modifications.

3.2 The effect of drugs on methylation/deacetylation

Several chemicals are able to affect the epigenome, either as agents used in clinical practice, or causing ADRs. A range of first-generation compounds that target the epigenome, including DNA methyltransferases (DNMTs) and histone deacetylase inhibitors, have met with success in the treatment of haematological disorders. The earliest of these, 5-azacytidine and azacytidine, are chemical analogs of the nucleoside cytidine and its deoxy derivative, 5-aza-2'-deoxycytidine (decitabine). Through incorporation into DNA (during replication) and RNA (during transcription), they inhibit methyltransferases and lead to demethylation of the sequence (Christman, 2002). Other drugs that affect the epigenome have also emerged, such as zebularine, a cytidine analog that inhibits DNA methylation (Bradbury, 2004). Second-generation drugs that target epigenetic enzymes with more tightly defined modes of action are, at time of writing, still in the investigation phase. Some such drugs include MG98, an antisense oligonucleotide that targets the 3'-untranslated region of the maintenance methyltransferase DNMT1, inhibiting it (Goffin & Eisenhauer, 2002); RG108, a small molecule that effectively blocks DNMTs, particularly DNMT1 and inhibits their activity (Suzuki et al., 2010), and psammaplin, a natural product derived from the sea sponge Pseudoceratina purpurea that inhibits DNMTs as well as histone deacetylases (McCulloch et al., 2009). Increasing attention is being paid not only to research on drugs that modify the DNA methylation landscape, but also to developing drugs that affect histone modifications. Histone deacetylase inhibitors have been object of research in anticancer drug development, as they present a potential strategy to reverse aberrant epigenetic changes associated with cancer (Dannenberg & Edenberg, 2006). However, there is also an increasing awareness that commonly used drugs can affect epigenome and cause ADRs. Among the better-documented examples are valproic acid (VPA), hydralazine, and procainamide. Although VPA is an established antiepileptic and mood-stabilizing drug, clinically used since the 1960s, only recently it has been found that VPA is a direct inhibitor of histone deacetylase (Phiel et al., 2001). Furthermore, the resultant increase in histone acetylation caused by VPA was shown to be interrelated with changes in genomic DNA methylation (Milutinovic et al., 2007). Animal and cell culture studies have implicated the epigenetic mode of action of VPA in a wide range of gene expression changes associated with VPA-induced side-effects, such as teratogenicity and cognitive disorders (Fukuchi et al., 2009;

Nagai et al., 2008; Tung & Winn, 2010). Procainamide, an antiarrythmic sodium channel blocker and hydralazine, a vasodilator used to treat hypertension, did not have well-characterized mechanisms of action when they were first introduced. Mechanistic studies have now shown that procainamide directly inhibits methyltransferases activity, specifically DNMT1 (Lee et al., 2005), whereas hydralazine mainly inhibits DNMT expression (Arce et al., 2006). Consequently, the extensive hypomethylation induced by these drugs alters appropriate protein expression in T cells and triggers a lupus-like autoimmune disease (Chang & Gershwin, 2010; Yung et al., 1996).

The notion that some drug-induced epigenetic marks may have a transgenerational impact is even more alarming. It has been suggested that drugs, such as thalidomide, a sedative–hypnotic and immunomodulatory agent and the synthetic oestrogen diethylstilbestrol may induce transgenerational epigenetic alterations that result in persistent pathological changes in subsequent generations (Holliday, 1998; Newbold et al., 2006). However, given the inadequacy of experimental tools and approaches, solid evidence for true transgenerational epigenetic impact has not been clearly established, although it is an attractive hypothesis to explain such observations.

Other drugs, such as isotretinoin, methylphenidate, tamoxifen, methotrexate and even families of drugs, such as conventional neuroleptics, selective serotonin reuptake inhibitor antidepressant, β-blockers, and chloroquine and fluoroquinolone antibiotics, have all been suggested to affect the epigenome (Csoka & Szyf, 2009). Such conclusions have been based mainly on observations of altered DNA methylation patterns, chromatin remodeling, or substantial changes in gene and protein expression that persist even after therapy has ceased. However, the exact mechanisms through which these drugs influence the epigenome and the consequences of the drug-induced epigenetic reprogramming have not been sufficiently investigated

4. Pharmacogenomics of microRNA

Although sequencing the whole genome and identifying genetic variations, such as SNPs, small insertions, deletions, inversions, variable numbers of tandem repeat (minisatellite), short tandem repeat (microsatellite), and copy number variations (Nakamura, 2009), are important for the understanding of human biology, having information on only these genomic aspects is limiting when attempting to explain interindividual differences in drug response and ADRs. Consequently, researchers have suggested that knowledge and understanding of functional genomics related to gene expression, such as transcriptional and translational processes, be included. One of the first steps to be taken towards understanding the difference in gene expression to identify the variability in drug response is investigating the role of nuclear receptors, or transcription factors, such as the arylhydrocarbon receptor (AhR), peroxisoma proliferator activated receptor (PPAR), pregnane X receptor (PXR) and constitutive androstane receptor (CAR), in the transcription control of genes encoding drug transporters, enzymes and drug targets (Lehmann et al., 1998; Smirlis et al., 2001; Synold et al., 2001; Xie et al., 2000a, 2000b). However the discovery of the world of small regulatory RNAs, or microRNA (miRNA), which are coded in our genomes and implicated in post-transcriptional control, has been more promising. Some researchers classify microRNA regulation as an epigenetic phenomenon (Peedicayil, 2008) but, even if it is closely related to epigenetic phenomena, microRNAs are not themselves epigenetic factors (Chuang & Jones, 2007).

MiRNAs are small, single stranded, 21–23 nucleotide-long, independent functional units of noncoding RNA (Lagos-Quintana et al., 2001; Lau et al., 2001; Lee & Ambros, 2001) which bind to the target transcript in the 3'-untraslated region (3'-UTR) to inhibit the translation of proteins and destabilize their target mRNAs (Baek et al., 2008, Selbach et al., 2008). MiRNAs regulate specific genes broadly involved in multiple pathways, like cell death, cell proliferation, stress resistance and fat metabolism (Ambros, 2003, Lim et al., 2003a, 2003b).

Work on miRNA knock-down and miRNA transfections has recently shown that approximately one third of the miRNA targets are translationally repressed in a cell display mRNA destabilization (Baek et al., 2008, Selbach et al., 2008). Consequently, miRNAs fine-tune protein output in the cell by translationally repressing and destabilizing the target mRNA (Baek et al., 2008; Mishra et al., 2007; Selbach et al., 2008). Other evidence suggests that a gain, or loss in miRNA function is associated to disease progression and prognosis (Lu et al., 2005; Mishra et al., 2007), as several studies have now established that miRNAs are expressed differently in human cancers than in normal healthy tissue (Calin et al., 2004; He et al., 2007; Lu et al., 2005).

4.1 Effect of polymorphisms in miRNA in drug response and adverse drug reactions

Polymorphisms in the miRNA regulatory pathway (miR-polymorphisms) are a novel class of functional polymorphisms present in the human genome. MiR-polymorphisms reside at, or near to, a miRNA binding site of a functional gene, influencing its expression by interfering with miRNA function (Bertino et al., 2007; Mishra et al., 2007, 2008). Several groups worldwide have acknowledged the role of miR-polymorphisms, suggesting a strong association between miR-polymorphisms and disease progression, as well as with drug response. Indeed, a single miR-polymorphism can potentially affect the expression of multiple genes involved in pathways regulating drug absorption, metabolism, disposition and may affect the overall clinical efficacy of a drug and/or resistance to that drug.

An analysis of the publicly available SNP database revealed the presence of a relatively high level of variations in the 3'-UTRs of miRNA target genes (Saunders et al., 2007) demonstrating that some of these variations may interfere with the function of miRNA and are potential miR-polymorphisms with the capacity to affect the expression of miRNA targets (Barnes et al., 2007; Kertesz et al., 2007; Mishra et al., 2007). MiRNA mutation (miR-mutations) can be defined as a mutation that interferes with miRNA function. MiR-polymorphisms and miR-mutations can be present either in heterozygous, or homozygous forms in a population. These variants in the human genome may take the form of insertions, deletions, amplifications, or chromosomal translocations, resulting in loss, or gain of miRNA site/function (Mishra et al., 2007). Functional miR-polymorphisms, or mutations, may create, or destroy, a miRNA binding site within a target mRNA and affect gene expression by interfering with the function of a miRNA (Bertino et al., 2007; Mishra et al., 2007, 2008).

Recently, the role of miRNA in drug-resistance/sensitivity has been investigated. It was functionally demonstrated that a polymorphism in a miRNA binding site could lead to drug-resistance/drug sensitivity (Bertino et al., 2007; Mishra et al., 2007, 2008). For example, a C>T SNP present in the 3'-UTR of dihydrofolate reductase gene (DHFR) was originally identified in a case–control study of childhood leukaemia patients to occur with 14.2% allelic frequency in the Japanese population (Goto et al., 2001). Later it was demonstrated that the

SNP is present near a miR-24 miRNA-binding site in human DHFR. The C>T SNP near the miRNA-binding site acts as a loss-of-function mutation and interferes with miR-24 function. The loss of miR-24 function results in high steady-state levels of DHFR mRNA and protein levels leading to drug resistance (Mishra et al., 2007). Interestingly, loss of miR-24 function, due to the SNP, led to a twofold increase in the half-life of the mRNA target. This observation not only explained the corresponding increase in DHFR mRNA and protein levels, but also suggested that the target mRNA destabilization could be a principle mechanism of action of a miRNA (Mishra et al., 2007). This finding may also be useful in predicting the clinical outcome of methotrexate treatment in clinical settings. Consequently, various miR-polymorphisms, located in many important genes that are drug targets, may affect drug response in patients and may lead to drug resistance and/or drug sensitivity and even unexpected toxicity.

This new insight has introduced a novel and promising field of research: Pharmacogenomics of miRNA, that holds new possibilities for tailor-made medical therapy. MiRNA pharmacogenomics can be defined as the study of miRNAs and polymorphisms affecting miRNA function in order to predict drug behaviour and improve drug efficiency (Bertino et al., 2007; Mishra et al., 2008). There are several reasons why miRNA pharmacogenomics have strong clinical implications: miRNAs are attractive drug targets, are differentially expressed in abnormal cells in all different diseases versus normal cells and regulate the expression of several important proteins in the cell (Calin et al., 2002; Iorio et al., 2005) supporting the hypothesis that miRNA polymorphisms, located near the miRNA-binding site of important genes involved in the drug pharmacokinetics and pharmacodynmics, have the potential to affect drug behaviour. Therefore, these miR-polymorphisms are potential predictors of drug response in the clinical setting and will hopefully lead to the development of more accurate methods of determining appropriate drug dosages based on a patient's genetic make-up and decrease the likelihood of drug overdose (Bertino et al., 2007)

4.2 MiRNA expression and drugs

Even though each miRNA appears to regulate the expression of tens to hundreds of different genes at time of writing, there are only a few examples demonstrating the relevance of miRNA in the regulation of proteins involved in drug metabolism, transporting and targeting. In CYP research, miR-27b expression was found to be lower in breast cancer tissues than in neighbouring healthy tissue (P < 0.0005). This expression profile correlated inversely with CYP1B1 expression and, *in vitro* studies, showed the involvement of miR-27b in the post-transcriptional regulation of CYP1B1 (Tsuchiya et al., 2006). Human CYP2E1 expression, an important CYP450 isoform from a pharmacologically and toxicological point of view, is regulated by miR-378, mainly via translational repression (Mohri et al., 2010). Again, CYP24 by miR-125b post-transcriptionally, which serves as a possible mechanism for the high CYP24 expression in tumour tissues, since CYP24 catalyzes the inactivation of 1α,25-dihydroxyvitamin D3 (calcitriol), which exerts antiproliferative effects (Komagata et al., 2009). Moreover, the transcription factor pregnane X receptor, which regulates the expression of a number of CYP members, including CYP3A4, was shown to be regulated by miR-148a (Takagi et al., 2008). The miR-148a–dependent decreases in pregnane X receptor protein attenuated the induction of CYP3A4 mRNA (P < 0.05) and protein levels (P < 0.010).

As to drug transporters, ABCG2 expression was found to be inhibited by miR-519c in a parental S1 colon cancer cell line. However, this inhibition was lost in the drug-resistant counterpart due to a shorter 3'-UTR in these cells, most likely responsible for the resistance (To et al., 2008). There was a similar effect on drug resistance in the multidrug resistant cell lines (A2780DX5 and KB-V1.27), where miR-27a and miR-451 led to overexpression of P-glycoprotein (P-gp) (Zhu et al., 2008). Again, some researchers reported that miR-451 regulates P-gp expression in doxorubicin-resistant MCF-7 cells (Kovalchuk et al., 2008). There is other evidence on miRNA and anticancer agents, such as tamoxifen (Cittelly et al., 2010), cisplatin (Bian et al., 2011; Imanaka et al., 2011), 5-fluorouracil (Shah et al., 2011; Valeri et al., 2010) and other anticancer drugs (Giovannetti et al., 2011).

Other examples involve the role of miRNA as regulators of nuclear receptors. Peroxisome proliferator-activated receptor gamma (PPARγ) has gained considerable interest as a therapeutic target during chronic inflammatory diseases. Indeed, the pathogenesis of diseases such as multiple sclerosis, or Alzheimer, might be associated with impaired PPARγ expression. Jennewein and colleagues have provided, *in vitro*, evidence of the PPARγ mRNA destabilization through miRNA 27b binding *PPARγ* 3'-UTR, which is induced by inflammatory response (Jennewein et al., 2010). Hepatocyte nuclear factor (HNF) 4α is a key transcription factor regulating endo/xenobiotic-metabolizing enzymes and transporters and this nuclear factor was down-regulated, *in vitro*, by miR-24 and miR-34a, affecting the metabolism and cellular biology (Takagi et al., 2010). Glucocorticoids (GCs) exert profound effects on a variety of physiological processes, including adaptation to stress, metabolism, immunity, and neuronal development. Vreugdenhil et al. tested the hypothesis that miRNA might control GR activity by reducing GR protein levels in neuronal tissues and found that miRNA 18 and 124a not only reduced GR-mediated events, but also decreased GR protein levels, providing a better understanding of the etiology of stress-related diseases as well as the efficacy of GC therapy (Vreugdenhil et al., 2009). When considered as a whole, these results indicate a possibility of intervening in the drug response mechanisms by modulating miRNA expression but many hurdles must be overcome before finding methodologies or agents (anti-miRNA) capable of efficiently modulating miRNA expression (Thai et al., 2010).

5. Complementary approaches

Even if the process of understanding the mechanisms responsible for variable responses to the powerful therapeutic agents have been accelerated by these new approaches, the identification of a particular phenotype unequivocally from an equivocal genotype still remains a challenge. Nebert et al. report several reasons why no example can be cited in which a single genotype is always associated with a phenotype in all individuals within all human populations (Nebert & Vesell, 2004). Indeed, there is always a reason why a genomic event, or another phenomenon might override a single DNA variant site somewhere in a gene (Nebert & Vesell, 2004). Therefore, studies on drug response are expanding beyond genomics to new horizons encompassing trascriptomics, metabonomics, proteomics and mathematical models, to become a systems-based discipline, or system biology approach. Even if much still remains to be done in the field of genomics to better understand the exact role of the genotype in the development of the phenotype e.g. through gene-gene interactions resulting from particular stimuli that affect a complex circuitry of pathways, ending in a response by the cell, or organism, these new fields are very promising to understand and predict variation in drug response phenotype. Trascriptomics refers to the study of gene transcripts (Kiechle & Holland-Staley, 2003), generally analyzed by cDNA expression microarrays. Such cDNA expression studies have led to a number of exciting breakthroughs in basic science. For example, microarray analysis of certain tumours has been successful in correlating particular expression patterns with patient prognosis (Macgregor, 2003). Microarrays of cDNA expression have also been used effectively as predictors of success for hormone responsiveness, hormone non-responsiveness, clinical outcomes and anticancer chemotherapeutic drugs (Domchek & Weber, 2002; Liu & Karuturi, 2004), even if other phenotypes may also be directly related to drug response. One of those phenotypes is the level of metabolites, not drug metabolites, but rather all small molecules that can be accurately assayed in the organism. These thousands of small molecules i.e. the metabolome, may also be altered by drug exposure and, consequently, able to predict variation in drug response. Metabonomics or metabolomics refers to the study of metabolite profiling, or metabolome i.e. the repertoire of small molecules present in cell, tissues, organs and biological fluids (Dettmer & Hammock, 2004; Lindon et al., 2004; Maddox et al., 2006; Plumb et al., 2003; Reo, 2002; Schmidt, 2004a, 2004b; van der Greef et al., 2007). The metabonome represents a real time integrated response to all endogenous and all exogenous stimuli (drugs, chemical exposures, occupation, lifestyle, nutrition, age, gender). Therefore, metabonomics might provide a sensitive means to follow an individual patient's phenotype as a function of all these stimuli. Recently, metabonomics has achieved major new advances due to novel, highly sensitive techniques for the measurement of urinary metabolite profiles. The analytical data in these studies are derived from electrospray mass spectrometry coupled to gas chromatography, liquid chromatography, or mass spectrometry time-of-flight (Plumb et al., 2002). The metabolites measured include, not only those from drugs, but hundreds of small-molecular weight compounds present in synthetic and degradation pathways.

Animal model studies, using the metabonomic approach have been reported to perform a study of drug-induced hepatotoxicity. Hepatotoxicity is a common and potentially serious adverse reaction to drugs, such as acetaminophen (Fontana & Quallich, 2001; Watkins et al., 2006). In this metabolomic study, male Sprague-Dawley rats were treated with acetaminophen and both pre and post-drug exposure urine samples were subjected to Nuclear Magnetic Resonance (NMR) analysis. A model was then developed that used pre-drug metabolomic data to predict both ratios of acetaminophen glucuronide conjugate to parent drug and post-acetaminophen hepatotoxicity (Clayton et al., 2006).

Clinical studies using metabonomics are still in the teething stage. For example, one study focused on metabolic profiles of antipsychotic drugs and used a specialized lipidomic platform to measure more than 300 lipid metabolites for the evaluation of global lipid changes in schizophrenia after treatment with three commonly prescribed atypical antipsychotics: olanzapine, risperidone and aripiprazole (Kaddurah-Daouk et al., 2007). A major side-effect associated with the use of these drugs is weight gain. Effects of the three antipsychotic drugs on lipid biochemical pathways were then evaluated by comparing metabolic profiles at baseline with post treatment assays. Phosphotidylethanolamine concentrations were elevated after treatment with all three drugs. Olanzapine and risperidone affected a much broader range of lipid classes than did aripiprazole, with an increase in about 50 lipids after exposure to these drugs, but not after aripiprazole therapy.

Thus, metabonomics might well help the physician to provide each patient with personalized drug therapy and avoid toxicity, consequently minimizing the risk of ADRs. This new form of metabolite profiling would resemble what clinical pharmacology has done previously, with the difference that it would be several orders of magnitude more sensitive in detecting subtle toxicity, or other ADRs, long before these become clinically evident. Changes in an individual's metabolite profile might warrant an aggressive regimen, for example, to prevent, or impede the onset of arthritis, or renal disease, long before clinical symptoms appear. It seems practicable that, in the distant future, metabonomics will go hand in hand with genomics to revolutionize and individualize drug therapy.

Proteomics is the study of all proteins encoded by the genome (Tuma, 2004). Although a recent study (Rual et al., 2004) estimated an average of 2 to 3 human proteins per gene, others have estimated that the true number of proteins per gene might be considerably higher. Even though proteomics has not yet been widely applied to the study of drug response, it is however, both conceivable and feasible, that, in the future, proteomic investigators might identify certain protein profiles, similar to ways in which metabonomics can identify certain metabolite profiles, which might be useful in predicting ADRs long before they become overt.

6. Future challenges

The purpose of this chapter is to provide an overview of the development of Pharmacogenetics and the scientific advances that have contributed to the continuing evolution of this discipline. Therefore, the ultimate approach in this field would be the union of genomic, trascriptomic, metabonomic and proteomic data as well as clinical diagnosis and pharmacological treatment response to build a computational cellular, or organ model. If the model is sufficiently accurate and detailed, it will then be possible, firstly to predict the behaviour of a system given any disturbance within it, secondly, gene regulatory networks could be redesigned to create new system properties. This second possibility could take on an extremely important role in Pharmacogenomic research for the development of new drugs.

However, to fully realize the potential of this approach and new insights, a number of issues and challenges must be met. First and foremost, researchers should continue training on systems biology. This will require developing new global technologies for genomics, trascriptomics, proteomics, metabolomics and phenotyping. It will also involve the development of software able to capture, store, analyze, graphically display, integrate, model and disperse the global data sets of systems biology. We must learn how to determine the nature of proteins and gene regulatory networks and their integrations and how to integrate many types of data as well as analyze and integrate global data sets across the dynamic transitions of development, or physiological responses. We also must deal with the challenge of providing access for the laboratories practicing small science to these global technologies and powerful computational tools. Lastly, access to biological samples from a large number of healthy and diseased subjects must be made available so as to begin the global correlative studies able to establish the foundational framework of predictive medicine and pave the way for moving forward into preventive medicine. There is, however, little doubt that the application of Systems Biology will significantly advance our ability to individualize drug therapy over the next few years.

7. Conclusions

Although Pharmacogenetics and Pharmacogenomics hold out the promise of leading to individualized therapy, to date, relatively few Pharmacogenetic/Pharmacogenomic tests are currently used in the clinical setting and even those that are used are done so less frequently than indicated. Even if there has recently been an increase in the awareness on the part of the Food and Drug Administration of the necessity to integrate genomic data into regulatory review (http://www.fda.gov/cder/genomic/), the goal of individualized prescribing still remains an arduous task. Therefore, Pharmacogenetics and/or Pharmacogenomics requires further research in various areas of science and the development of the capability to integrate them so as to be able to treat each patient as they deserve i.e. as the complex, unique and fascinating individual they really are.

8. Acknowledgements

The author thanks Dr. Loredana Serpe for valuable discussion and helpful suggestions during the preparation of this chapter and Mrs Barbara Wade for her linguistic advice. This work was supported by grant number 2010.3097 from Fondazione CRT, Torino, Italy.

9. References

Ambros V (2003) MicroRNA pathways in flies and worms: growth, death, fat, stress, and timing. Cell 113: 673-676.

Anttila S, Hakkola J, Tuominen P, Elovaara E, Husgafvel-Pursiainen K, Karjalainen A, Hirvonen A, Nurminen T (2003) Methylation of cytochrome P4501A1 promoter in the lung is associated with tobacco smoking. Cancer Res 63: 8623-8628.

Arce C, Segura-Pacheco B, Perez-Cardenas E, Taja-Chayeb L, Candelaria M, Dueñnas-Gonzalez A (2006) Hydralazine target: from blood vessels to the epigenome. J Transl Med 4: 10.

Baek D, Villén J, Shin C, Camargo FD, Gygi SP, Bartel DP (2008) The impact of microRNAs on protein output. Nature 455: 64-71.

Baker EK, El-Osta A (2004) MDR1, chemotherapy and chromatin remodeling. Cancer Biol. Ther 3: 819-824.

Baker EK, Johnstone RW, Zalcberg JR, El-Osta A (2005) Epigenetic changes to the MDR1 locus in response to chemotherapeutic drugs. Oncogene 24: 8061-8075.

Barnes MR, Deharo S, Grocock RJ, Brown JR, Sanseau P (2007) The micro RNA target paradigm: a fundamental and polymorphic control layer of cellular expression. Expert Opin Biol Ther 7: 1387-1399.

Bertilsson L, Dahl M-L, Dalén P, Al-Shurbaji A (2002) Molecular genetics of CYP2D6: clinical relevance with focus on psychotropic drugs. Br J Clin Pharmacol 53: 111-122.

Bertino JR, Banerjee D, Mishra PJ (2007) Pharmacogenomics of microRNA: a miRSNP towards individualized therapy. Pharmacogenomics 8: 1625-1627.

Beutler E, Dern RJ, Alving AS (1955a) The hemolytic effect of primaquine. VI. An in vitro test for sensitivity of erythrocytes to primaquine. J. Lab. Clin. Med 45: 40-50.

Beutler E, Dern RJ, Flanagan CL, Alving AS (1955b) The hemolytic effect of primaquine. VII. Biochemical studies of drug-sensitive erythrocytes. J. Lab. Clin. Med 45: 286-295.

Bian HB, Pan X, Yang JS, Wang ZX, De W (2011) Upregulation of microRNA-451 increases cisplatin sensitivity of non-small cell lung cancer cell line (A549). J. Exp. Clin Cancer Res 30: 20.

Bovenzi V, Momparler RL (2001) Antineoplastic action of 5-aza-2'-deoxycytidine and histone deacetylase inhibitor and their effect on the expression of retinoic acid receptor beta and estrogen receptor alpha genes in breast carcinoma cells. Cancer Chemother. Pharmacol 48: 71-76.

Bradbury J (2004) Zebularine: a candidate for epigenetic cancer therapy. Drug Discov. Today 9: 906-907.

Calin GA, Dumitru CD, Shimizu M, Bichi R, Zupo S, Noch E, Aldler H, Rattan S, Keating M, Rai K, Rassenti L, Kipps T, Negrini M, Bullrich F, Croce CM (2002) Frequent deletions and down-regulation of micro- RNA genes miR15 and miR16 at 13q14 in chronic lymphocytic leukemia. Proc. Natl. Acad. Sci. U.S.A 99: 15524-15529.

Calin GA, Sevignani C, Dumitru CD, Hyslop T, Noch E, Yendamuri S, Shimizu M, Rattan S, Bullrich F, Negrini M, Croce CM (2004) Human microRNA genes are frequently located at fragile sites and genomic regions involved in cancers. Proc. Natl. Acad. Sci. U.S.A 101: 2999-3004.

Chang C, Gershwin ME (2010) Drugs and autoimmunity--a contemporary review and mechanistic approach. J. Autoimmun 34: J266-275.

Christman JK (2002) 5-Azacytidine and 5-aza-2'-deoxycytidine as inhibitors of DNA methylation: mechanistic studies and their implications for cancer therapy. Oncogene 21: 5483-5495.

Chuang JC, Jones PA (2007) Epigenetics and microRNAs. Pediatr. Res 61: 24R-29R.

Cittelly DM, Das PM, Spoelstra NS, Edgerton SM, Richer JK, Thor AD, Jones FE (2010) Downregulation of miR-342 is associated with tamoxifen resistant breast tumors. Mol. Cancer 9: 317.

Clayton TA, Lindon JC, Cloarec O, Antti H, Charuel C, Hanton G, Provost J-P, Le Net J-L, Baker D, Walley RJ, Everett JR, Nicholson JK (2006) Pharmaco-metabonomic phenotyping and personalized drug treatment. Nature 440: 1073-1077.

Cooper GM, Johnson JA, Langaee TY, Feng H, Stanaway IB, Schwarz UI, Ritchie MD, Stein CM, Roden DM, Smith JD, Veenstra DL, Rettie AE, Rieder MJ (2008) A genome-wide scan for common genetic variants with a large influence on warfarin maintenance dose. Blood 112: 1022-1027.

Csoka AB, Szyf M (2009) Epigenetic side-effects of common pharmaceuticals: a potential new field in medicine and pharmacology. Med. Hypotheses 73: 770-780.

Daly AK (2010) Genome-wide association studies in pharmacogenomics. Nat. Rev. Genet 11: 241-246.

Daly AK, Donaldson PT, Bhatnagar P, Shen Y, Pe'er I, Floratos A, Daly MJ, Goldstein DB, John S, Nelson MR, Graham J, Park BK, Dillon JF, Bernal W, Cordell HJ, Pirmohamed M, Aithal GP, Day CP (2009) HLA-B*5701 genotype is a major determinant of drug-induced liver injury due to flucloxacillin. Nat. Genet 41: 816-819.

Dannenberg LO, Edenberg HJ (2006) Epigenetics of gene expression in human hepatoma cells: expression profiling the response to inhibition of DNA methylation and histone deacetylation. BMC Genomics 7: 181.

Dettmer K, Hammock BD (2004) Metabolomics--a new exciting field within the «omics» sciences. Environ. Health Perspect 112: A396-397.

Domchek SM, Weber BL (2002) Recent advances in breast cancer biology. Curr Opin Oncol 14: 589-593.

Drysdale CM, McGraw DW, Stack CB, Stephens JC, Judson RS, Nandabalan K, Arnold K, Ruano G, Liggett SB (2000) Complex promoter and coding region beta 2-adrenergic receptor haplotypes alter receptor expression and predict in vivo responsiveness. Proc. Natl. Acad. Sci. U.S.A 97: 10483-10488.

Evans DA, Manley KA, McKusick VA (1960) Genetic control of isoniazid metabolism in man. Br Med J 2: 485-491.

Evans WE, McLeod HL (2003) Pharmacogenomics--drug disposition, drug targets, and side effects. N. Engl. J. Med 348: 538-549.

Evans WE, Krynetsky E (2003) Drug methylation in cancer therapy: lessons from TPMT polymorphism. Oncogene 22: 7403-7413.

Ferreri AJM, Dell'Oro S, Capello D, Ponzoni M, Iuzzolino P, Rossi D, Pasini F, Ambrosetti A, Orvieto E, Ferrarese F, Arrigoni G, Foppoli M, Reni M, Gaidano G (2004) Aberrant methylation in the promoter region of the reduced folate carrier gene is a potential mechanism of resistance to methotrexate in primary central nervous system lymphomas. Br. J. Haematol 126: 657-664.

Flanagan James, Petronis Arturas (2005) Pharmacoepigenetics. In Pharmacogenomics, Second Edition, 461-491. Informa Healthcare, Giugno 17. Drugs and the Pharmaceutical Sciences.

Fontana RJ, Quallich LG (2001) Acute liver failure. Curr. Opin. Gastroenterol 17: 291-298.

Fournier C, Goto Y, Ballestar E, Delaval K, Hever AM, Esteller M, Feil R (2002) Allele-specific histone lysine methylation marks regulatory regions at imprinted mouse genes. EMBO J 21: 6560-6570.

Fukuchi M, Nii T, Ishimaru N, Minamino A, Hara D, Takasaki I, Tabuchi A, Tsuda M (2009) Valproic acid induces up- or down-regulation of gene expression responsible for the neuronal excitation and inhibition in rat cortical neurons through its epigenetic actions. Neurosci. Res 65: 35-43.

Furuta T, Ohashi K, Kosuge K, Zhao XJ, Takashima M, Kimura M, Nishimoto M, Hanai H, Kaneko E, Ishizaki T (1999) CYP2C19 genotype status and effect of omeprazole on intragastric pH in humans. Clin. Pharmacol. Ther 65: 552-561.

Gabriel SB, Schaffner SF, Nguyen H, Moore JM, Roy J, Blumenstiel B, Higgins J, DeFelice M, Lochner A, Faggart M, Liu-Cordero SN, Rotimi C, Adeyemo A, Cooper R, Ward R, Lander ES, Daly MJ, Altshuler D (2002) The structure of haplotype blocks in the human genome. Science 296: 2225-2229.

Gagné J-F, Montminy V, Belanger P, Journault K, Gaucher G, Guillemette C (2002) Common human UGT1A polymorphisms and the altered metabolism of irinotecan active metabolite 7-ethyl-10-hydroxycamptothecin (SN-38). Mol. Pharmacol 62: 608-617.

Gagnon J-F, Bernard O, Villeneuve L, Têtu B, Guillemette C (2006) Irinotecan inactivation is modulated by epigenetic silencing of UGT1A1 in colon cancer. Clin. Cancer Res 12: 1850-1858.

Gardiner SJ, Begg EJ (2006) Pharmacogenetics, drug-metabolizing enzymes, and clinical practice. Pharmacol. Rev 58: 521-590.

Garrod AE (1975) The Lancet. The incidence of alkaptonuria: a study in chemical individuality. Nutr. Rev 33: 81-83.

Ghotbi R, Gomez A, Milani L, Tybring G, Syvänen A-C, Bertilsson L, Ingelman-Sundberg M, Aklillu E (2009) Allele-specific expression and gene methylation in the control of CYP1A2 mRNA level in human livers. Pharmacogenomics J 9: 208-217.

Giovannetti E, Erozenci A, Smit J, Danesi R, Peters GJ (2011) Molecular mechanisms underlying the role of microRNAs (miRNAs) in anticancer drug resistance and implications for clinical practice. Crit. Rev. Oncol. Hematol xxx:xxx.

Goffin J, Eisenhauer E (2002) DNA methyltransferase inhibitors-state of the art. Ann. Oncol 13: 1699-1716.

Goto Y, Yue L, Yokoi A, Nishimura R, Uehara T, Koizumi S, Saikawa Y (2001) A novel single-nucleotide polymorphism in the 3'-untranslated region of the human dihydrofolate reductase gene with enhanced expression. Clin. Cancer Res 7: 1952-1956.

Grant SFA, Hakonarson H (2008) Microarray technology and applications in the arena of genome-wide association. Clin. Chem 54: 1116-1124.

He L, He X, Lowe SW, Hannon GJ (2007) microRNAs join the p53 network--another piece in the tumour-suppression puzzle. Nat. Rev. Cancer 7: 819-822.

Henikoff S, Matzke MA (1997) Exploring and explaining epigenetic effects. Trends Genet 13: 293-295.

Holliday R (1998) The possibility of epigenetic transmission of defects induced by teratogens. Mutat. Res 422: 203-205.

Hu D, Ziv E (2008) Confounding in genetic association studies and its solutions. Methods Mol. Biol 448: 31-39.

Imanaka Y, Tsuchiya S, Sato F, Shimada Y, Shimizu K, Tsujimoto G (2011) MicroRNA-141 confers resistance to cisplatin-induced apoptosis by targeting YAP1 in human esophageal squamous cell carcinoma. J. Hum. Genet 56: 270-276.

Ingelman-Sundberg M, Sim SC, Gomez A, Rodriguez-Antona C (2007) Influence of cytochrome P450 polymorphisms on drug therapies: pharmacogenetic, pharmacoepigenetic and clinical aspects. Pharmacol. Ther 116: 496-526.

Iorio MV, Ferracin M, Liu C-G, Veronese A, Spizzo R, Sabbioni S, Magri E, Pedriali M, Fabbri M, Campiglio M, Ménard S, Palazzo JP, Rosenberg A, Musiani P, Volinia S, Nenci I, Calin GA, Querzoli P, Negrini M, Croce CM (2005) MicroRNA gene expression deregulation in human breast cancer. Cancer Res 65: 7065-7070.

Jennewein C, von Knethen A, Schmid T, Brüne B (2010) MicroRNA-27b contributes to lipopolysaccharide-mediated peroxisome proliferator-activated receptor gamma (PPARgamma) mRNA destabilization. Cardiovasc. Res 89: 98-108.

Jenuwein T, Allis CD (2001) Translating the histone code. Science 293: 1074-1080.

Jiang Z, Dragin N, Jorge-Nebert LF, Martin MV, Guengerich FP, Aklillu E, Ingelman-Sundberg M, Hammons GJ, Lyn-Cook BD, Kadlubar FF, Saldana SN, Sorter M, Vinks AA, Nassr N, von Richter O, Jin L, Nebert DW (2006) Search for an association between the human CYP1A2 genotype and CYP1A2 metabolic phenotype. Pharmacogenet. Genomics 16: 359-367.

Jin Y, Desta Z, Stearns V, Ward B, Ho H, Lee K-H, Skaar T, Storniolo AM, Li L, Araba A, Blanchard R, Nguyen A, Ullmer L, Hayden J, Lemler S, Weinshilboum RM, Rae JM, Hayes DF, Flockhart DA (2005) CYP2D6 genotype, antidepressant use, and tamoxifen metabolism during adjuvant breast cancer treatment. J. Natl. Cancer Inst 97: 30-39.

Kacevska M, Ivanov M, Ingelman-Sundberg M (2011) Perspectives on Epigenetics and Its Relevance to Adverse Drug Reactions. Clin Pharmacol Ther 89: 902-907.

Kaddurah-Daouk R, McEvoy J, Baillie RA, Lee D, Yao JK, Doraiswamy PM, Krishnan KRR (2007) Metabolomic mapping of atypical antipsychotic effects in schizophrenia. Mol. Psychiatry 12: 934-945.

Kertesz M, Iovino N, Unnerstall U, Gaul U, Segal E (2007) The role of site accessibility in microRNA target recognition. Nat. Genet 39: 1278-1284.

Kiechle FL, Holland-Staley CA (2003) Genomics, transcriptomics, proteomics, and numbers. Arch. Pathol. Lab. Med 127: 1089-1097.

Kimchi-Sarfaty C, Oh JM, Kim I-W, Sauna ZE, Calcagno AM, Ambudkar SV, Gottesman MM (2007) A «silent» polymorphism in the MDR1 gene changes substrate specificity. Science 315: 525-528.

Komagata S, Nakajima M, Takagi S, Mohri T, Taniya T, Yokoi T (2009) Human CYP24 catalyzing the inactivation of calcitriol is post transcriptionally regulated by miR-125b. Mol. Pharmacol 76:702-709.

Kooloos WM, Wessels JAM, van der Straaten T, Huizinga TWJ, Guchelaar H-J (2009) Criteria for the selection of single nucleotide polymorphisms in pathway pharmacogenetics: TNF inhibitors as a case study. Drug Discov. Today 14: 837-844.

Kovalchuk O, Filkowski J, Meservy J, Ilnytskyy Y, Tryndyak VP, Chekhun VF, Pogribny IP (2008) Involvement of microRNA-451 in resistance of the MCF-7 breast cancer cells to chemotherapeutic drug doxorubicin. Mol. Cancer Ther 7: 2152-2159.

Kruglyak L, Nickerson DA (2001) Variation is the spice of life. Nat. Genet 27: 234-236.

Krynetski EY, Schuetz JD, Galpin AJ, Pui CH, Relling MV, Evans WE (1995) A single point mutation leading to loss of catalytic activity in human thiopurine S-methyltransferase. Proc. Natl. Acad. Sci. U.S.A 92: 949-953.

Kubarek Ł, Jagodzinski PP (2007) Epigenetic up-regulation of CXCR4 and CXCL12 expression by 17 beta-estradiol and tamoxifen is associated with formation of DNA methyltransferase 3B4 splice variant in Ishikawa endometrial adenocarcinoma cells. FEBS Lett 581: 1441-1448.

Lagos-Quintana M, Rauhut R, Lendeckel W, Tuschl T (2001) Identification of novel genes coding for small expressed RNAs. Science 294: 853-858.

Lau NC, Lim LP, Weinstein EG, Bartel DP (2001) An abundant class of tiny RNAs with probable regulatory roles in Caenorhabditis elegans. Science 294: 858-862.

Lee BH, Yegnasubramanian S, Lin X, Nelson WG (2005) Procainamide is a specific inhibitor of DNA methyltransferase 1. J. Biol. Chem 280: 40749-40756.

Lee RC, Ambros V (2001) An extensive class of small RNAs in Caenorhabditis elegans. Science 294: 862-864.

Lehmann JM, McKee DD, Watson MA, Willson TM, Moore JT, Kliewer SA (1998) The human orphan nuclear receptor PXR is activated by compounds that regulate CYP3A4 gene expression and cause drug interactions. J. Clin. Invest 102: 1016-1023.

Lennard L, Lilleyman JS, Van Loon J, Weinshilboum RM (1990) Genetic variation in response to 6-mercaptopurine for childhood acute lymphoblastic leukaemia. Lancet 336: 225-229.

Lessard E, Yessine MA, Hamelin BA, O'Hara G, LeBlanc J, Turgeon J (1999) Influence of CYP2D6 activity on the disposition and cardiovascular toxicity of the antidepressant agent venlafaxine in humans. Pharmacogenetics 9: 435-443.

Lim LP, Glasner ME, Yekta S, Burge CB, Bartel DP (2003a) Vertebrate microRNA genes. Science 299: 1540.

Lim LP, Lau NC, Weinstein EG, Abdelhakim A, Yekta S, Rhoades MW, Burge CB, Bartel DP (2003b) The microRNAs of Caenorhabditis elegans. Genes Dev 17: 991-1008.

Lindon JC, Holmes E, Nicholson JK (2004) Metabonomics and its role in drug development and disease diagnosis. Expert Rev. Mol. Diagn 4: 189-199.

Link E, Parish S, Armitage J, Bowman L, Heath S, Matsuda F, Gut I, Lathrop M, Collins R (2008) SLCO1B1 variants and statin-induced myopathy--a genomewide study. N. Engl. J. Med 359: 789-799.

Liu ET, Karuturi KR (2004) Microarrays and clinical investigations. N. Engl. J. Med 350: 1595-1597.

Lu J, Getz G, Miska EA, Alvarez-Saavedra E, Lamb J, Peck D, Sweet-Cordero A, Ebert BL, Mak RH, Ferrando AA, Downing JR, Jacks T, Horvitz HR, Golub TR (2005) MicroRNA expression profiles classify human cancers. Nature 435: 834-838.

Macgregor PF (2003) Gene expression in cancer: the application of microarrays. Expert Rev. Mol. Diagn 3: 185-200.

Maddox JF, Luyendyk JP, Cosma GN, Breau AP, Bible RH Jr, Harrigan GG, Goodacre R, Ganey PE, Cantor GH, Cockerell GL, Roth RA (2006) Metabonomic evaluation of idiosyncrasy-like liver injury in rats cotreated with ranitidine and lipopolysaccharide. Toxicol. Appl. Pharmacol 212: 35-44.

McCulloch MWB, Coombs GS, Banerjee N, Bugni TS, Cannon KM, Harper MK, Veltri CA, Virshup DM, Ireland CM (2009) Psammaplin A as a general activator of cell-based signaling assays via HDAC inhibition and studies on some bromotyrosine derivatives. Bioorg. Med. Chem 17: 2189-2198.

Meyer UA (2004) Pharmacogenetics - five decades of therapeutic lessons from genetic diversity. Nat. Rev. Genet 5: 669-676.

Michelotti GA, Brinkley DM, Morris DP, Smith MP, Louie RJ, Schwinn DA (2007) Epigenetic regulation of human alpha1d-adrenergic receptor gene expression: a role for DNA methylation in Sp1-dependent regulation. FASEB J 21: 1979-1993.

Milutinovic S, D'Alessio AC, Detich N, Szyf M (2007) Valproate induces widespread epigenetic reprogramming which involves demethylation of specific genes. Carcinogenesis 28: 560-571.

Mishra PJ, Humeniuk R, Mishra PJ, Longo-Sorbello GSA, Banerjee D, Bertino JR (2007) A miR-24 microRNA binding-site polymorphism in dihydrofolate reductase gene leads to methotrexate resistance. Proc. Natl. Acad. Sci. U.S.A 104: 13513-13518.

Mishra PJ, Mishra PJ, Banerjee D, Bertino JR (2008) MiRSNPs or MiR-polymorphisms, new players in microRNA mediated regulation of the cell: Introducing microRNA pharmacogenomics. Cell Cycle 7: 853-858.

Mohri T, Nakajima M, Fukami T, Takamiya M, Aoki Y, Yokoi T (2010) Human CYP2E1 is regulated by miR-378. Biochem. Pharmacol 79: 1045-1052.

Mortimer O, Persson K, Ladona MG, Spalding D, Zanger UM, Meyer UA, Rane A (1990) Polymorphic formation of morphine from codeine in poor and extensive metabolizers of dextromethorphan: relationship to the presence of immunoidentified cytochrome P-450IID1. Clin. Pharmacol. Ther 47: 27-35.

Motulsky AG (1957) Drug reactions, enzymes and biochemical genetics. Journal of the American Medical Association 165: 835 -837.

Nagai K, Natori T, Nishino T, Kodaira F (2008) Epigenetic disregulation induces cell growth retardation in primary cultured glial cells. J. Biosci. Bioeng 105: 470-475.

Nakamura Y (2009) DNA variations in human and medical genetics: 25 years of my experience. J. Hum. Genet 54: 1-8.

Nebert DW, Vesell ES (2004) Advances in pharmacogenomics and individualized drug therapy: exciting challenges that lie ahead. Eur. J. Pharmacol 500: 267-280.

Nebert DW, Zhang G, Vesell ES (2008) From human genetics and genomics to pharmacogenetics and pharmacogenomics: past lessons, future directions. Drug Metab. Rev 40: 187-224.

Newbold RR, Padilla-Banks E, Jefferson WN (2006) Adverse effects of the model environmental estrogen diethylstilbestrol are transmitted to subsequent generations. Endocrinology 147: S11-17.

Okino ST, Pookot D, Li L-C, Zhao H, Urakami S, Shiina H, Igawa M, Dahiya R (2006) Epigenetic inactivation of the dioxin-responsive cytochrome P4501A1 gene in human prostate cancer. Cancer Res 66: 7420-7428.

Onica T, Nichols K, Larin M, Ng L, Maslen A, Dvorak Z, Pascussi J-M, Vilarem M-J, Maurel P, Kirby GM (2008) Dexamethasone-mediated up-regulation of human CYP2A6 involves the glucocorticoid receptor and increased binding of hepatic nuclear factor 4 alpha to the proximal promoter. Mol. Pharmacol 73: 451-460.

Paz MF, Yaya-Tur R, Rojas-Marcos I, Reynes G, Pollan M, Aguirre-Cruz L, García-Lopez JL, Piquer J, Safont M-J, Balaña C, Sanchez-Cespedes M, García-Villanueva M, Arribas L, Esteller M (2004) CpG island hypermethylation of the DNA repair enzyme methyltransferase predicts response to temozolomide in primary gliomas. Clin. Cancer Res 10: 4933-4938.

Peedicayil J (2008) Pharmacoepigenetics and pharmacoepigenomics. Pharmacogenomics 9: 1785-1786.

Phiel CJ, Zhang F, Huang EY, Guenther MG, Lazar MA, Klein PS (2001) Histone deacetylase is a direct target of valproic acid, a potent anticonvulsant, mood stabilizer, and teratogen. J. Biol. Chem 276: 36734-36741.

Plumb RS, Stumpf CL, Gorenstein MV, Castro-Perez JM, Dear GJ, Anthony M, Sweatman BC, Connor SC, Haselden JN (2002) Metabonomics: the use of electrospray mass spectrometry coupled to reversed-phase liquid chromatography shows potential for the screening of rat urine in drug development. Rapid Commun. Mass Spectrom 16: 1991-1996.

Plumb RS, Stumpf CL, Granger JH, Castro-Perez J, Haselden JN, Dear GJ (2003) Use of liquid chromatography/time-of-flight mass spectrometry and multivariate statistical analysis shows promise for the detection of drug metabolites in biological fluids. Rapid Commun. Mass Spectrom 17: 2632-2638.

Relling MV, Hancock ML, Rivera GK, Sandlund JT, Ribeiro RC, Krynetski EY, Pui CH, Evans WE (1999) Mercaptopurine therapy intolerance and heterozygosity at the thiopurine S-methyltransferase gene locus. J. Natl. Cancer Inst 91: 2001-2008.

Reo NV (2002) NMR-based metabolomics. Drug Chem Toxicol 25: 375-382.

Roden DM, George Jr AL (2002) The genetic basis of variability in drug responses. Nat. Rev. Drug Discov 1: 37-44.

Rønneberg JA, Tost J, Solvang HK, Alnaes GIG, Johansen FE, Brendeford EM, Yakhini Z, Gut IG, Lønning PE, Børresen-Dale A-L, Gabrielsen OS, Kristensen VN (2008) GSTP1 promoter haplotypes affect DNA methylation levels and promoter activity in breast carcinomas. Cancer Res 68: 5562-5571.

Rual J-F, Hirozane-Kishikawa T, Hao T, Bertin N, Li S, Dricot A, Li N, Rosenberg J, Lamesch P, Vidalain P-O, Clingingsmith TR, Hartley JL, Esposito D, Cheo D, Moore T, Simmons B, Sequerra R, Bosak S, Doucette-Stamm L, Le Peuch C, Vandenhaute J, Cusick ME, Albala JS, Hill DE, Vidal M (2004) Human ORFeome version 1.1: a platform for reverse proteomics. Genome Res 14: 2128-2135.

Sachidanandam R, Weissman D, Schmidt SC, Kakol JM, Stein LD, Marth G, Sherry S, Mullikin JC, Mortimore BJ, Willey DL, Hunt SE, Cole CG, Coggill PC, Rice CM, Ning Z, Rogers J, Bentley DR, Kwok PY, Mardis ER, Yeh RT, Schultz B, Cook L, Davenport R, Dante M, Fulton L, Hillier L, Waterston RH, McPherson JD, Gilman B, Schaffner S, Van Etten WJ, Reich D, Higgins J, Daly MJ, Blumenstiel B, Baldwin J, Stange-Thomann N, Zody MC, Linton L, Lander ES, Altshuler D; International SNP Map Working Group (2001) A map of human genome sequence variation containing 1.42 million single nucleotide polymorphisms. Nature 409: 928-933.

Sato N, Matsubayashi H, Fukushima N, Goggins M (2005) The chemokine receptor CXCR4 is regulated by DNA methylation in pancreatic cancer. Cancer Biol. Ther 4: 70-76.

Saunders MA, Liang H, Li W-H (2007) Human polymorphism at microRNAs and microRNA target sites. Proc. Natl. Acad. Sci. U.S.A 104: 3300-3305.

Schmidt CW (2004a) Metabolomics: what's happening downstream of DNA. Environ. Health Perspect 112: A410-415.

Schmidt C (2004b) Metabolomics takes its place as latest up-and-coming «omic» science. J. Natl. Cancer Inst 96: 732-734.

Selbach M, Schwanhäusser B, Thierfelder N, Fang Z, Khanin R, Rajewsky N (2008) Widespread changes in protein synthesis induced by microRNAs. Nature 455: 58-63.

Serpe L, Calvo PL, Muntoni E, D'Antico S, Giaccone M, Avagnina A, Baldi M, Barbera C, Curti F, Pera A, Eandi M, Zara GP, Canaparo R (2009) Thiopurine S-methyltransferase pharmacogenetics in a large-scale healthy Italian-Caucasian population: differences in enzyme activity. Pharmacogenomics 10: 1753-1765.

Shah MY, Pan X, Fix LN, Farwell MA, Zhang B (2011) 5-Fluorouracil drug alters the microRNA expression profiles in MCF-7 breast cancer cells. J. Cell Physiol 226: 1868-1878.

Shuldiner AR, O'Connell JR, Bliden KP, Gandhi A, Ryan K, Horenstein RB, Damcott CM, Pakyz R, Tantry US, Gibson Q, Pollin TI, Post W, Parsa A, Mitchell BD, Faraday N, Herzog W, Gurbel PA (2009) Association of cytochrome P450 2C19 genotype with the antiplatelet effect and clinical efficacy of clopidogrel therapy. JAMA 302: 849-857.

Sindrup SH, Brøsen K (1995) The pharmacogenetics of codeine hypoalgesia. Pharmacogenetics 5: 335-346.

Smirlis D, Muangmoonchai R, Edwards M, Phillips IR, Shephard EA (2001) Orphan receptor promiscuity in the induction of cytochromes p450 by xenobiotics. J. Biol. Chem 276: 12822-12826.

Srinivasan BS, Chen J, Cheng C, Conti D, Duan S, Fridley BL, Gu X, Haines JL, Jorgenson E, Kraja A, Lasky-Su J, Li L, Rodin A, Wang D, Province M, Ritchie MD (2009) Methods for analysis in pharmacogenomics: lessons from the Pharmacogenetics Research Network Analysis Group. Pharmacogenomics 10: 243-251.

Stearns V, Johnson MD, Rae JM, Morocho A, Novielli A, Bhargava P, Hayes DF, Desta Z, Flockhart DA (2003) Active tamoxifen metabolite plasma concentrations after coadministration of tamoxifen and the selective serotonin reuptake inhibitor paroxetine. J. Natl. Cancer Inst 95: 1758-1764.

Suzuki T, Tanaka R, Hamada S, Nakagawa H, Miyata N (2010) Design, synthesis, inhibitory activity, and binding mode study of novel DNA methyltransferase 1 inhibitors. Bioorg. Med. Chem. Lett 20: 1124-1127.

Synold TW, Dussault I, Forman BM (2001) The orphan nuclear receptor SXR coordinately regulates drug metabolism and efflux. Nat. Med 7: 584-590.

Takagi S, Nakajima M, Mohri T, Yokoi T (2008) Post-transcriptional regulation of human pregnane X receptor by micro-RNA affects the expression of cytochrome P450 3A4. J. Biol. Chem 283: 9674-9680.

Takagi S, Nakajima M, Kida K, Yamaura Y, Fukami T, Yokoi T (2010) MicroRNAs regulate human hepatocyte nuclear factor 4α, modulating the expression of metabolic enzymes and cell cycle. J. Biol. Chem 285: 4415-4422.

Takahashi H, Ishikawa S, Nomoto S, Nishigaki Y, Ando F, Kashima T, Kimura S, Kanamori M, Echizen H (2000) Developmental changes in pharmacokinetics and pharmacodynamics of warfarin enantiomers in Japanese children. Clin. Pharmacol. Ther 68: 541-555.

Takahashi H, Kashima T, Nomizo Y, Muramoto N, Shimizu T, Nasu K, Kubota T, Kimura S, Echizen H (1998a) Metabolism of warfarin enantiomers in Japanese patients with heart disease having different CYP2C9 and CYP2C19 genotypes. Clin. Pharmacol. Ther 63: 519-528.

Takahashi H, Kashima T, Nomoto S, Iwade K, Tainaka H, Shimizu T, Nomizo Y, Muramoto N, Kimura S, Echizen H (1998b) Comparisons between in-vitro and in-vivo metabolism of (S)-warfarin: catalytic activities of cDNA-expressed CYP2C9, its Leu359 variant and their mixture versus unbound clearance in patients with the corresponding CYP2C9 genotypes. Pharmacogenetics 8: 365-373.

Takeuchi F, McGinnis R, Bourgeois S, Barnes C, Eriksson N, Soranzo N, Whittaker P, Ranganath V, Kumanduri V, McLaren W, Holm L, Lindh J, Rane A, Wadelius M, Deloukas P (2009) A genome-wide association study confirms VKORC1, CYP2C9, and CYP4F2 as principal genetic determinants of warfarin dose. PLoS Genet 5: e1000433.

Tanaka Y, Nishida N, Sugiyama M, Kurosaki M, Matsuura K, Sakamoto N, Nakagawa M, Korenaga M, Hino K, Hige S, Ito Y, Mita E, Tanaka E, Mochida S, Murawaki Y, Honda M, Sakai A, Hiasa Y, Nishiguchi S, Koike A, Sakaida I, Imamura M, Ito K, Yano K, Masaki N, Sugauchi F, Izumi N, Tokunaga K, Mizokami M (2009) Genome-wide association of IL28B with response to pegylated interferon-alpha and ribavirin therapy for chronic hepatitis C. Nat. Genet 41: 1105-1109.

Teichert M, Eijgelsheim M, Rivadeneira F, Uitterlinden AG, van Schaik RHN, Hofman A, De Smet PAGM, van Gelder T, Visser LE, Stricker BHC (2009) A genome-wide association study of acenocoumarol maintenance dosage. Hum. Mol. Genet 18: 3758-3768.

Thai TH, Christiansen PA, Tsokos GC (2010) Is there a link betweendysregulated miRNA expression and disease? Discov Med 10:184-94.

The International HapMap Project (2003) . Nature 426: 789-796.

To KKW, Zhan Z, Litman T, Bates SE (2008) Regulation of ABCG2 expression at the 3' untranslated region of its mRNA through modulation of transcript stability and protein translation by a putative microRNA in the S1 colon cancer cell line. Mol. Cell. Biol 28: 5147-5161.

Tokizane T, Shiina H, Igawa M, Enokida H, Urakami S, Kawakami T, Ogishima T, Okino ST, Li L-C, Tanaka Y, Nonomura N, Okuyama A, Dahiya R (2005) Cytochrome P450 1B1 is overexpressed and regulated by hypomethylation in prostate cancer. Clin. Cancer Res 11: 5793-5801.

Tsuchiya Y, Nakajima M, Takagi S, Taniya T, Yokoi T (2006) MicroRNA regulates the expression of human cytochrome P450 1B1. Cancer Res 66: 9090-9098.

Tuma RS (2004) Proteomics: from signature to protein identification. J. Natl. Cancer Inst 96: 817.

Tung EWY, Winn LM (2010) Epigenetic modifications in valproic acid-induced teratogenesis. Toxicol. Appl. Pharmacol 248: 201-209.

Urnov FD, Wolffe AP (2001) Above and within the genome: epigenetics past and present. J Mammary Gland Biol Neoplasia 6: 153-167.

Valeri N, Gasparini P, Braconi C, Paone A, Lovat F, Fabbri M, Sumani KM, Alder H, Amadori D, Patel T, Nuovo GJ, Fishel R, Croce CM (2010) MicroRNA-21 induces resistance to 5-fluorouracil by down-regulating human DNA MutS homolog 2 (hMSH2). Proc. Natl. Acad. Sci. U S A 107: 21098-21103.

van Aken J, Schmedders M, Feuerstein G, Kollek R (2003) Prospects and limits of pharmacogenetics: the thiopurine methyl transferase (TPMT) experience. Am J Pharmacogenomics 3: 149-155.

van der Greef J, Martin S, Juhasz P, Adourian A, Plasterer T, Verheij ER, McBurney RN (2007) The art and practice of systems biology in medicine: mapping patterns of relationships. J. Proteome Res 6: 1540-1559.

Vreugdenhil E, Verissimo CS, Mariman R, Kamphorst JT, Barbosa JS, Zweers T, Champagne DL, Schouten T, Meijer OC, de Kloet ER, Fitzsimons CP (2009) MicroRNA 18 and 124a down-regulate the glucocorticoid receptor: implications for glucocorticoid responsiveness in the brain. Endocrinology 150: 2220-2228.

Wall JD, Pritchard JK (2003) Haplotype blocks and linkage disequilibrium in the human genome. Nat. Rev. Genet 4: 587-597.

Wang D, Lippard SJ (2004) Cisplatin-induced post-translational modification of histones H3 and H4. J. Biol. Chem 279: 20622-20625.

Watkins PB, Kaplowitz N, Slattery JT, Colonese CR, Colucci SV, Stewart PW, Harris SC (2006) Aminotransferase elevations in healthy adults receiving 4 grams of acetaminophen daily: a randomized controlled trial. JAMA 296: 87-93.

Wedlund PJ (2000) The CYP2C19 enzyme polymorphism. Pharmacology 61: 174-183.

Weinshilboum RM, Sladek SL (1980) Mercaptopurine pharmacogenetics: monogenic inheritance of erythrocyte thiopurine methyltransferase activity. Am. J. Hum. Genet 32: 651-662.

Westberry JM, Prewitt AK, Wilson ME (2008) Epigenetic regulation of the estrogen receptor alpha promoter in the cerebral cortex following ischemia in male and female rats. Neuroscience 152: 982-989.

Wilkinson GR (2005) Drug metabolism and variability among patients in drug response. N. Engl. J. Med 352: 2211-2221.

Woodson K, O'Reilly KJ, Hanson JC, Nelson D, Walk EL, Tangrea JA (2008) The usefulness of the detection of GSTP1 methylation in urine as a biomarker in the diagnosis of prostate cancer. J. Urol 179: 508-511; discussion 511-512.

Wuttke H, Rau T, Heide R, Bergmann K, Böhm M, Weil J, Werner D, Eschenhagen T (2002) Increased frequency of cytochrome P450 2D6 poor metabolizers among patients with metoprolol-associated adverse effects. Clin. Pharmacol. Ther 72: 429-437.

Xie W, Barwick JL, Downes M, Blumberg B, Simon CM, Nelson MC, Neuschwander-Tetri BA, Brunt EM, Guzelian PS, Evans RM (2000a) Humanized xenobiotic response in mice expressing nuclear receptor SXR. Nature 406: 435-439.

Xie W, Barwick JL, Simon CM, Pierce AM, Safe S, Blumberg B, Guzelian PS, Evans RM (2000b) Reciprocal activation of xenobiotic response genes by nuclear receptors SXR/PXR and CAR. Genes Dev 14: 3014-3023.

Yates CR, Krynetski EY, Loennechen T, Fessing MY, Tai HL, Pui CH, Relling MV, Evans WE (1997) Molecular diagnosis of thiopurine S-methyltransferase deficiency: genetic basis for azathioprine and mercaptopurine intolerance. Ann. Intern. Med 126: 608-614.

Yung R, Powers D, Johnson K, Amento E, Carr D, Laing T, Yang J, Chang S, Hemati N, Richardson B (1996) Mechanisms of drug-induced lupus. II. T cells overexpressing lymphocyte function-associated antigen 1 become autoreactive and cause a lupuslike disease in syngeneic mice. J. Clin. Invest 97: 2866-2871.

Zhou S-F, Wang B, Yang L-P, Liu J-P (2010) Structure, function, regulation and polymorphism and the clinical significance of human cytochrome P450 1A2. Drug Metab. Rev 42: 268-354.

Zhu H, Wu H, Liu X, Evans BR, Medina DJ, Liu C-G, Yang J-M (2008) Role of MicroRNA miR-27a and miR-451 in the regulation of MDR1/P-glycoprotein expression in human cancer cells. Biochem. Pharmacol 76: 582-588.

Permissions

The contributors of this book come from diverse backgrounds, making this book a truly international effort. This book will bring forth new frontiers with its revolutionizing research information and detailed analysis of the nascent developments around the world.

We would like to thank Despina Sanoudou, PhD FACMG Cibiol, for lending her expertise to make the book truly unique. She has played a crucial role in the development of this book. Without her invaluable contribution this book wouldn't have been possible. She has made vital efforts to compile up to date information on the varied aspects of this subject to make this book a valuable addition to the collection of many professionals and students.

This book was conceptualized with the vision of imparting up-to-date information and advanced data in this field. To ensure the same, a matchless editorial board was set up. Every individual on the board went through rigorous rounds of assessment to prove their worth. After which they invested a large part of their time researching and compiling the most relevant data for our readers. Conferences and sessions were held from time to time between the editorial board and the contributing authors to present the data in the most comprehensible form. The editorial team has worked tirelessly to provide valuable and valid information to help people across the globe.

Every chapter published in this book has been scrutinized by our experts. Their significance has been extensively debated. The topics covered herein carry significant findings which will fuel the growth of the discipline. They may even be implemented as practical applications or may be referred to as a beginning point for another development. Chapters in this book were first published by InTech; hereby published with permission under the Creative Commons Attribution License or equivalent.

The editorial board has been involved in producing this book since its inception. They have spent rigorous hours researching and exploring the diverse topics which have resulted in the successful publishing of this book. They have passed on their knowledge of decades through this book. To expedite this challenging task, the publisher supported the team at every step. A small team of assistant editors was also appointed to further simplify the editing procedure and attain best results for the readers.

Our editorial team has been hand-picked from every corner of the world. Their multi-ethnicity adds dynamic inputs to the discussions which result in innovative outcomes. These outcomes are then further discussed with the researchers and contributors who give their valuable feedback and opinion regarding the same. The feedback is then collaborated with the researches and they are edited in a comprehensive manner to aid the understanding of the subject.

Apart from the editorial board, the designing team has also invested a significant amount of their time in understanding the subject and creating the most relevant covers. They scrutinized every image to scout for the most suitable representation of the subject and create an appropriate cover for the book.

The publishing team has been involved in this book since its early stages. They were actively engaged in every process, be it collecting the data, connecting with the contributors or procuring relevant information. The team has been an ardent support to the editorial, designing and production team. Their endless efforts to recruit the best for this project, has resulted in the accomplishment of this book. They are a veteran in the field of academics and their pool of knowledge is as vast as their experience in printing. Their expertise and guidance has proved useful at every step. Their uncompromising quality standards have made this book an exceptional effort. Their encouragement from time to time has been an inspiration for everyone.

The publisher and the editorial board hope that this book will prove to be a valuable piece of knowledge for researchers, students, practitioners and scholars across the globe.

List of Contributors

Roxana-Georgiana Tauser
University of Medicine and Pharmacy "Gr. T. Popa." Iasi, Romania

Susan J. Hsiao
Department of Pathology, Columbia University Medical Center, New York, NY, USA

Alex J. Rai
Department of Pathology, Columbia University Medical Center, New York, NY, USA.
Special Chemistry Laboratory, New York Presbyterian Hospital, Columbia University
Medical Center, New York, NY, USA

Sonja Pavlovic, Branka Zukic and Gordana Nikcevic
Institute of Molecular Genetics and Genetic Engineering, University of Belgrade, Belgrade,
Serbia

Irena Mlinaric-Rascan, Miha Milek, Alenka Smid and Natasa Karas Kuzelicki
University of Ljubljana, Faculty of Pharmacy, Ljubljana, Slovenia

Suayib Yalcin
Hacettepe University Institute of Oncology, Turkey

Jorge Duconge and Odalys Escalera
University of Puerto Rico School of Pharmacy, Medical Sciences Campus, Pharmaceutical
Sciences Department, San Juan, Puerto Rico

Mohan Korchela and Gualberto Ruaño
Genetic Research Center, Hartford Hospital, Hartford, USA

Eva Gak and Rivka Inzelberg
Sagol Neuroscience Center (JSNC), Sheba Medical Center, Sackler Faculty of Medicine, Tel
Aviv University, Israel

Pothitos M. Pitychoutis, Despina Sanoudou, Christina Dalla and Zeta Papadopoulou-
Daifoti
Department of Pharmacology, Medical School, National and Kapodistrian University of
Athens, Greece

Maria Ana Redal
Molecular Medicine and Genomics Unit, Institute for Basic Sciences and Experimental
Medicine and Department of Cellular and Molecular Biology, Hospital Italiano de Buenos
Aires School of Medicine, Buenos Aires, Argentina

Santiago Isolabella
Clinical Pharmacology Section, Internal Medicine Service and Department of Pharmacology and Toxicology, Hospital Italiano de Buenos Aires School of Medicine, Argentina Central Pharmacy Service, Hospital Italiano de Buenos Aires, Argentina

Waldo Horacio Belloso, Paula Scibona and Leonardo Garfi
Clinical Pharmacology Section, Internal Medicine Service and Department of Pharmacology and Toxicology, Hospital Italiano de Buenos Aires School of Medicine, Argentina

José Pedro Gil
Department of Physiology and Pharmacology, Drug Resistance Unit, Division of Pharmacogenetics, Karolinska Institutet, Stockholm, Sweden. Department of Biomedical Sciences, University of Algarve, IBB-Institute for Biotechnology and Bioengineering, The Centre for Molecular and Structural Biomedicine, Gambelas, Portugal. Department of Biological Sciences, The Harpur College of Arts and Sciences, Binghamton University, Binghamton, the New York State University, NY, USA

C. Ortner, C. Ciliberto and R. Landau
University of Washington, Seattle, WA, USA

Andrzej Mariusz Fal and Marta Rosiek-Biegus
Wroclaw Medical University, Wroclaw, Poland

Roberto Canaparo
University of Torino, Italy

www.ingramcontent.com/pod-product-compliance
Lightning Source LLC
Chambersburg PA
CBHW070737190326
41458CB00004B/1201